The Micro-Organisms of the Human Mouth

The Micro-Organisms of the Human Mouth

The Local and General Diseases Which are Caused by Them

Unaltered reprint of the original work by
WILLOUGHBY D. MILLER (1853–1907)
published in 1890 in Philadelphia

With an introductory essay by KLAUS G. KÖNIG (Nijmegen)

128 figures and 3 plates

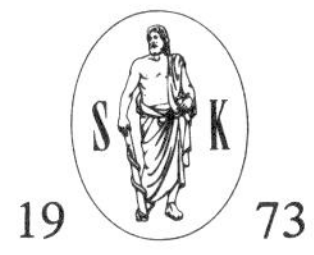

19 73

S. Karger · Basel · München · Paris · London · New York · Sydney

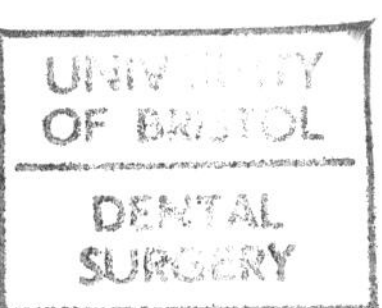

S. Karger · Basel · München · Paris · London · New York · Sydney
Arnold-Böcklin-Strasse 25, CH–4011 Basel (Switzerland)

Printed in Switzerland by Graphische Anstalt Schüler AG, Biel
ISBN 3–8055–1614–2

W. D. Miller and his Contributions to Dental Science

by Klaus G. König, Nijmegen

Willoughby Dayton Miller (1853–1907) was the first dentist in history with a thorough training in the natural sciences. He had studied mathematics and physics at the University of Ann Arbor, Michigan from 1871 to 1875 and intended to follow additional courses in Europe.

While he studied in Edinburgh, his bank went bankrupt and he lost nearly all his money. Miller then travelled to Berlin where he continued his studies, but in his difficult financial situation he had to earn money. It was not easy for Miller to find a job, but he was lucky to make the acquaintance of an American dentist, Frank Abbot, living and practicing in Berlin, and Miller asked him for help. Dr. Abbot found him a job as a translator, and in addition asked Miller to give lessons to his wife and daughter. How much the ladies learned from Miller in the natural sciences is not known. However, an important side effect of the lessons was that Miller soon became engaged, and determined to marry, Miss Caroline Abbot. Moreover, Miller began to like his future father-in-law's profession and, supported by this generous man, returned to the United States to study dentistry.

In Spring 1879 Miller graduated as Doctor of Dental Surgery from the Philadelphia Dental College. Returning to Berlin he assisted in the office of his father-in-law and continued his studies of natural and medical sciences, especially microbiology. The latter had achieved enormous progress under the stimulating influence of Robert Koch whose methods appealed to the research-minded dentist. He worked hard and the dental problems he tackled were solved with a critical sense of logic, a thoroughness and a versatility of methods which is amazing even to the sophisticated research worker of the late 20th century.

Between 1881 and 1907 Miller published 164 scientific articles in

German, American and English journals. Of the few books he wrote, the most famous one was first published in German in 1889, under the title 'Die Mikroorganismen der Mundhöhle'. Better known internationally and more often cited is the English version of this book which has been reprinted in the present edition. 'The Micro-Organisms of the Human Mouth' was published in Philadelphia a year after the German original. The American edition of 1890 is not only better known nowadays than the German edition, but its text had been partly revised besides being translated, and a whole new chapter (III) was added by the author. Several reasons seem to justify a new edition of this book. First of all, it is so extremely rare that it is nearly inaccessible, although no part of it is obsolete. To say the least, it is a unique document of the first major attempt to solve a number of unsolved dental problems in a scientific way. The etiology of dental caries for which the book is most famous, is only one of them. Miller was an outstanding histopathologist, and the results of his investigations of carious dentine and of infections of the pulp, for their time, were a step from the Stone Age to Modern Science. The vicinity of Miller's small laboratory to the institute of Robert Koch obviously explains the keen interest of the Professor of Dentistry not only in oral but also in general microbiology. Miller's methods of determination and differentiation of strains were as versatile as his very limited facilities would permit (his research laboratory measured about 30 square feet). Miller's limitations were compensated for by his awareness of the pitfalls, and he knew that an oral microbiologist must not rely on morphology: '. . . the form of a fungus alone by no means always entitles us to draw conclusions as to its specific character'. Miller's self-critical attitude also becomes apparent when he refers to his great many attempts 'to cultivate the supposed bacterium of greenstain, but so far without success', or when he questions the validity of an earlier success in isolating from the mouth 'the bacterium of brick-colored deposit': 'My present opinion however, is that the one I obtained is not the one I have been seeking' (p. 91 and 92). Few scientists will know that Miller did not claim the 'chemico-parasitical' explanation of the caries process to be his own invention, although in retrospect he deserves full credit for the caries theory bearing his name: '. . . in the decay of the hard tooth-structures 'two factors have always been in operation: (1) the action of acids, and (2) the action of germs'. 'This theory – which for the sake of distinction may be called the septic – is rather an amplification of the chemical theory than a contradiction of it. Most probably the work of decalcification is entirely performed by the action of acids, but these acids are, we think, secreted by the germs themselves . . .' (p. 134). This is not a citation from Miller, but Miller's citation of Milles and Underwood (Transact. Int. Med. Congr. 1881) to whom Miller gives ample credit.

Miller's comprehension for the possibilities of caries prevention, derived from his ideas of the etiology of caries, was remarkably clear and would have credibility had it been written yesterday: '. . . it must be apparent that there are four ways by which we may counteract or limit the ravages of this disease. We may endeavour (1) by hygienic measures to secure the best possible development of the teeth; (2) by repeated, thorough, systematic cleansing of the oral cavity and the teeth, to so far reduce the amount of fermentable substances as to materially diminish the production of acid, as well as to rob the bacteria of the organic matter necessary to their rapid development; (3) by prohibiting or limiting the consumption of such foods or luxuries, which readily undergo acid fermentation, to remove the chief source of the ferment products injurious to the teeth; (4) by the proper and intelligent use of antiseptics to destroy the bacteria, or at least to limit their number and activity' (p. 223).

What Miller wanted to say by mentioning as a possibility the 'proper and intelligent use of antiseptics' is elaborated in his book in great detail and is worth serious consideration by all those working on this problem today: 'If a very thorough mechanical cleansing has not preceded the antiseptic, its action upon the centers of decay will be equal to little more than zero' (p. 225 and 226). This remark is only one of the many warnings Miller gave as limitations to his general idea. Needless to say, Miller knew from his own investigations that even under optimum conditions not more than a temporary reduction of microbial counts was to be expected after the application of antiseptics.

One of the most interesting facettes of the book is Miller's misconception about the etiologic role of plaque. This is the more surprising since Miller nearly always was right with the interpretation of what he observed, if he was able to observe it. His failure to recognize the importance of plaque, and his persistance in denying it is perhaps explained by his clinical experience being inferior to that of his famous colleagues and opponents G.V. Black and J.L. Williams.

There is no doubt that Miller payed some attention to aggregates on the surface of teeth, because he states that he isolated 'more than one hundred different kinds of bacteria from the *juices and deposits* in the mouth' (p. 68; emphasis supplied by the editor). Nevertheless, Miller remained reluctant, and from his many experiments, when using bacteria-containing saliva for acid production in vitro, he seemed to believe in the cariogenic effect of free acid in the oral cavity.

Under the impression of the evidence accumulated by Black and Williams, Miller in 1902 published an article on 'The Presence of Bacterial Plaques on the Surface of the Teeth, and Their Significance', in Dental Cosmos 44, 425–446; May (No. 5) 1902. He begins by defending himself and citing quotations from his earlier writings in which he had pointed at the presence of 'masses of bacteria' in a 'matrix' on the tooth surface – but the matrix he refers to is the enamel cuticle which is 'thickened and invaded by masses of bacteria'. Miller then enlarges on Williams' opinion that all softening of enamel in the caries process 'is due to the action of acids, and chiefly or wholly to the acids excreted by bacteria in situ'. Miller continues: 'Others, in commenting upon his communication, have, it seems to me, gone rather farther than Williams himself, and the view seems now to be rather prevalent that the bacteria coating the surface of the enamel cover or invest themselves with a gelatinous substance, underneath which they produce their acids directly in contact with the enamel, and that only acids produced beneath those films and protected from dissipation in the saliva by the films are responsible for the beginning of caries. Acids distributed in the saliva have no influence in causing caries'. Miller then goes on citing Black: 'Caries of the teeth has its beginning when the conditions of the mouth are such that micro-organisms causing caries form gelatinous plaques, by which they are glued to the surface of the teeth'. Miller's lack of appreciation of these views culminates in the comment 'I am not convinced that the nature of this film has been determined with sufficient clearness, or whether its significance and importance may not have been somewhat overrated'.

From this statement it is obvious that Miller did not think of extracellular formation of polysaccharide as a specific factor in the cariogenic environment of the teeth. As a matter of fact Miller, in his book (pages 19, 22 and 23), did mention dextran formation as one of the metabolic activiteis bacteria may exert on carbohydrates, and he described the example of *Leuconostoc mesenteroides* in the molasses of sugar factories; this was mentioned, however, solely for the purpose of giving – as introduction – a complete systematic survey of what Miller called the 'vital manifestations of microorganisms'.

Miller's lack of recognition of the importance of plaque, and his experimenting in vitro with incubation mixtures of oral fluid and different carbohydrates explains why he considered starch to be more cariogenic than sucrose. In a mixture of saliva and bacteria where there is no diffusion barrier, and where incubation for hours blurs the details of the degradation, addition of starch as substrate may result in formation of more acid than addition of sucrose. Miller thought that 'sugar, being readily soluble, is soon carried away or so diluted with the saliva as to be rendered harmless, whereas amylaceous matter (i.e. starch; edit.) adheres to the teeth for a greater length of time and consequently manifests a more continued action than sugar' (p. 207). Miller, however, adds a – presumably personal – communication saying that 'Busch, on the contrary, is of the opinion that 'baker caries' is due rather to the inhalation of sugar-dust than to that of flour-dust' (p. 207).

In spite of all limitations, Miller's 'Micro-Organisms of the Human Mouth' is highly rewarding reading matter; every page of it reflects stimulating ideas of a sparkling, creative mind – one of the greatest in dental science we ever had.

THE

MICRO-ORGANISMS OF THE HUMAN MOUTH.

THE LOCAL AND GENERAL DISEASES WHICH ARE CAUSED BY THEM.

BY

WILLOUGHBY D. MILLER, D.D.S., M.D.,

PROFESSOR AT THE UNIVERSITY OF BERLIN.

WITH ONE HUNDRED AND TWENTY EIGHT ILLUSTRATIONS, ONE CHROMO-LITHOGRAPHIC AND TWO PHOTO-MICROGRAPHIC PLATES.

PHILADELPHIA:

THE S. S. WHITE DENTAL MFG. CO.

1890.

PREFACE.

THE impetus given to the study of bacteriology by the introduction of the exact methods of bacteriological investigation now in vogue, has led to discoveries in the domain of dental and oral pathology which are of the greatest importance not to the dental surgeon alone but equally to the practitioner of general medicine.

It has been established beyond all question that myriads of micro-organisms are constantly present in the human mouth, and that these, under favorable circumstances, are capable of manifesting an action of the utmost significance upon the local as well as the general health of the patient. Not alone are they responsible for the vast majority of those diseases of the teeth and contiguous parts which the dental surgeon is called upon to treat, but they also give rise to other local and general disorders of the most serious nature.

These various disturbances are produced partly by the direct action of micro-organisms and their products upon the teeth and the mucous membrane of the mouth, partly by constant swallowing of large masses of bacteria, partly by carrying them into the lungs, particularly in cases of violent inspiration, and, finally, by their obtaining an entrance into the blood or lymph-vessels in the various ways described in Chapter XI.

The existence of a most excellent nursery for bacteria at the very portal of the human body is a fact which has only recently begun to receive the attention which its importance demands.

It has been my endeavor in the following pages to bring about a better understanding of the nature and extent of bacteritic growths in the human mouth, of the disastrous effects which they are capable of producing, and, accordingly, a more proper appreciation of the importance of dental surgery and dental hygiene as a branch of general medicine.

The contents of the book consist chiefly of original investigations which, in part, have appeared in different American, English, and German journals, and in part appear here for the first time.

The first three chapters are designed more particularly for those of my readers who may not have occupied themselves with bacteriological studies, it being, in my opinion, utterly impossible for anyone to obtain a proper understanding of the action of micro-organisms in the mouth without a knowledge of at least the elementary principles lying at the foundation of the science of bacteriology.

Of those works to which I am indebted for aid in my labor, I wish to mention in particular the Lehrbuch der Mikroorganismen, by Flügge, and Die Fortschritte in der Lehre von den pathogenen Mikroorganismen, by Baumgarten.

I take pleasure in acknowledging the very valuable assistance rendered me by my friend Mr. Frank Thilly, of Cincinnati, Ohio, in the preparation of the manuscript.

THE AUTHOR.

BERLIN, May, 1890.

CONTENTS.

PART I.

GENERAL BACTERIOLOGICAL STUDIES, WITH SPECIAL REFERENCE TO THE BACTERIA OF THE HUMAN MOUTH.

CHAPTER I.

CHAPTER II.

CHAPTER III.

CHAPTER IV.

CHAPTER V.

CHAPTER VI.

CHAPTER VII.

CHAPTER VIII.

CHAPTER IX.

PART II.

THE PATHOGENIC MOUTH-BACTERIA, AND THE DISEASES WHICH THEY PRODUCE.

CHAPTER X.

CHAPTER XI.

CHAPTER XII.

LITERATURE.

[1] DE BARY. Vergl. Morphologie und Biologie der Pilze. S. 490.

[2] FLÜGGE. Die Mikroorganismen. Leipzig, 1886. S. 76.

[3] FRANK. Leunis' Synopsis der drei Naturreiche. Bd. III. Specielle Botanik, Kryptogamen. § 842.

[4] ZOPF. Die Spaltpilze. S. 1.

[5] CORNIL et BABES. Les Bactéries. P. 173.

[6] EHRENBERG. Organisation, Systematik und geographisches Verhältniss der Infusionsthierchen. Berlin, 1830. Die Infusionsthierchen als vollkommene Organismen. Leipzig, 1838.

[7] LEEUWENHOEK. Opera omnia sive arcana naturæ ope microscopiorum exactissimorum detecta. 1722.

[8] NENCKI. Beiträge zur Biologie der Spaltpilze. 1880.

[9] COHN und MENDELSOHN. *Cohn's Beiträge.* Bd. III, Heft 1.

[10] R. KOCH. Aetiologie der Wundinfectionskrankheiten. Leipzig, 1878. S. 46.

[11] G. KLEMPERER. Ueber die Beziehung der Mikroorganismen zur Eiterung. (Aus dem Laboratorium der 2. medicinischen Klinik zu Berlin. *Zeitschr. f. klin. Med.* 1885. Bd. X, S. 158.)

[12] D. BIONDI. Contribuzione all' etiologia della suppurazione. (*La Riforma medica*, 1886. No. 34-36.)

[13] A. ZUCKERMANN. Ueber die Ursache der Eiterung. (*Centralbl. f. Bacteriologie und Parasitenkunde.* 1887. Bd. I, No. 17.)

[14] KREIBOHM und ROSENBACH. Experimentelle Beiträge zur Frage: Kann Eiterung ohne Mitbetheiligung, etc. (*Archiv f. klin. Chirur.* 1888. Bd. XXXVII, S. 737.)

[15] GRAWITZ und W. DE BARY. Ueber die Ursachen der subcutanen Entzündung und Eiterung. (*Virchow's Archiv.* Bd. CVIII, S. 67.)

[16] SCHEURLEN. Weitere Untersuchungen über die Entstehung der Eiterung, ihr Verhältniss zu den Ptomaïnen und zur Blutgerinnung. (*Fortschritte d. Medicin.* 1887. No. 23, S. 762.)

[17] NATHAN. *Archiv f. klin. Chirurgie.* Bd. XXXVII, Heft 4.

[18] GRAWITZ. Beitrag zur Theorie der Eiterung. (*Virchow's Archiv.* Bd. CXVI, Heft 1, S. 116.)

[19] HOPPE-SEYLER. Physiologische Chemie.

[20] MILLER. Ueber Gährungsvorgänge im Verdauungstractus und die dabei betheiligten Spaltpilze. (*Deutsche med. Wochenschr.* 1885. No. 49.)

[21] FLÜGGE. Die Mikroorganismen. Leipzig, 1886.

[22] PASTEUR. Annales de Chimie et Physiologie. 1857.

[23] HUEPPE. Ueber die Zersetzung der Milch. (*Mitth. a. d. Reichsgesundheitsamt.* Bd. II, S. 307.)

[24] BLACK. Gelatine-forming Micro-organisms. (*Independent Practitioner.* 1886. P. 546.)

[25] PRAZMOWSKI. Untersuchungen über die Entwickelung ùnd Fermentwirkung einiger Bacterienarten. Leipzig, 1880.

[26] BRIEGER. Ueber Spaltungsproducte der Bacterien. (*Zeitschr. f. physiol. Chemie.* Bd. VIII, Heft 4 und Bd. IX, Heft 1.)

[27] FITZ. *Berichte der Chem. Gesell.* 1873, Bd. VI, S. 48; 1876, Bd. IX, 2, S. 1348; 1878, Bd. XI, S. 42; 1879, Bd. XII, 1, S. 474; 1880, Bd. XIII, 1, S. 1309; 1882, Bd. XV, 1, S. 867; 1883, Bd. XVI, S. 844; 1884, Bd. XVII, S. 1189.

[28] BOUTROUX. Sur la fermentation lactique. (*Comptes rendus.* Bd. LXXXVI, P. 605. 1878.)

[29] FLÜGGE. Die Mikroorganismen. S. 486.

[30] NENCKI. Ueber die Zersetzung der Gelatine und des Eiweisses bei der Fäulniss u. s. w. Bern, 1876.

[31] BRIEGER. Ueber Ptomaïne. Weitere Untersuchungen über dieselben, 1885, und Untersuchungen über Ptomaïne. 3. Theil. 1886.

[32] VAUGHAN. Ueber die Anwesenheit von Tyrotoxikon in giftigem Speiseeise und in giftiger Milch, seine wahrscheinliche Beziehung zur Cholera infantum. (*Archiv f. Hygiene.* Bd. VII, S. 420.)

[33] HANSEN. Contributions à la connaissance des organismes qui peuvent se trouver dans la bière et la moût de bière et y vivre. (*Meddelser fra Carlsberg-laboratoriet.* 1879. Heft 2.)

[34] W. LEUBE und E. GRESER. Ueber die harnstoffzersetzenden Pilze im Urin. (*Virchow's Archiv.* Bd. C, S. 555.)

[35] SCHLÖSING und MÜNTZ. *Comptes rendus.* Bd. LXXXIX, Pp. 891 et 1074; Bd. LXXXIV, P. 301; Bd. LXXVII, Pp. 203, 353.

[36] GAYON et DUPETIT. *Comptes rendus.* 1882. Bd. XCV, Pp. 664, 1365.

[37] DEHÉRAIN et MAQUENNE. Sur la réduction des nitrates, etc. (*Comptes rendus.* 1882. II. Bd. XCV, Pp. 691, 732, 854.)

[38] HERAEUS. Ueber das Verhalten der Bacterien im Brunnenwasser. (*Zeitschr. f. Hygiene.* Bd. I.)

[39] WARRINGTON. *Journal of the Chem. Society.* August, 1888. P. 727.

[40] BINZ. Arzneimittellehre. S. 197, 198.

[41] LIBORIUS, FLÜGGE. Die Mikroorganismen. S. 455.

[42] HOPPE-SEYLER. Physiologische Chemie. S. 188.

[43] ELLENBERGER und HOFMEISTER. Der Speichel der Wiederkäuer. (*Bericht über das Veterinärwesen im Königreich Sachsen.* 1885. S. 119.)

[44] THE SAME. Die Function der Speicheldrüsen der Haussäugethiere. (*Archiv f. wissensch. u. prakt. Thierheilk.* 11. 1885.)

[45] ROUX. Gazz. med. veterin. di Milano. 1871. (See Hoppe-Seyler[19].)

[46] HERMANN. Physiologie. S. 94.

[47] KIRK. A Contribution to the Etiology of Erosion. (*Dental Cosmos.* 1887. P. 50.)

[48] LEEUWENHOEK. Opera omnia, etc. Bd. II, S. 40, 1722.

[49] MANDL. Comptes rendus hebd. des Séances de l'Académie des Sciences. Bd. XVII, P. 213.

[50] BÜHLMANN. Müller's Archiv f. Anatomie. 1840.

[51] HENLE. Pathologische Untersuchungen. 1840.

[52] ERDL. *Allgemeine Zeitung f. Chirurgie von Rohatzsch.* 1843. No. 19. S. 159.

[53] FICINUS. Ueber das Ausfallen der Zähne. (*Walter's und Ammon's Journal für Chirurgie*, etc. 1847. Bd. VI, Heft 1.)

[54] ROBIN. Histoire naturelle des végétaux parasites. 1853.

[55] ROBIN. Des végétaux qui croissent sur les animaux vivants. Paris, 1847. P. 42.

[56] KLENCKE. Die Verderbniss der Zähne. Leipzig, 1850.

[57] HALLIER. Die pflanzlichen Parasiten, etc. Leipzig, 1866.

[58] LEBER und ROTTENSTEIN. Ueber d. Caries der Zähne. Berlin, 1867.

[59] VIGNAL. Recherches sur les Microorganismes de la bouche. (*Archives de physiol. norm. et pathol.* 1886. No. 8.)

[60] MILLER. Zur Kenntniss der Bakterien der Mundhöhle. (*Deutsche med. Wochenschr.* 1884. No. 47.)

[61] LEWIS. *Lancet.* September, 1884.

[62] MILLER. Ueber einen Zahn-Spaltpilz, Leptothrix gigantea. (*Berichte der Botanischen Gesellschaft.* 1883. S. 224.)

[63] MILLER. Biological Studies on the Fungi of the Human Mouth. (*Indep. Practitioner.* 1885. Pp. 227, 283.)

[64] BLACK. Trans. of Ill. State Dental Society. 1886.

[65] WATT. Chemical Essays.

[66] VIGNAL. *La France médicale.* Août 25, 1887.

[67] HUEPPE. *Deutsche med. Wochenschr.* 1884. Nos. 48, 49.

[68] ESCHERICH. Die Darmbacterien des Säuglings. 1886.

[69] BAGINSKY. *Deutsche med. Wochenschr.* 1888. No. 20.

[70] KRÄUTERMANN. Sicherer Augen- und Zahnarzt. 1732. (See Schlenker [72].)

[71] BOURDET. Recherches et observations sur toutes les parties de l'art du dentiste. 1757. P. 95.

[72] SCHLENKER Die Verderbniss der Zähne

[73] v. CARABELLI. Handbuch der Zahnheilkunde.

[74] EUSTACHIUS. Opuscula anatomica et de dentibus. 1574.

[75] JOHN HUNTER. Diseases of the Teeth, etc. 1778.

[76] JOSEPH FOX. The History and Treatment of the Diseases of the Teeth and Gums. 1806.

[77] THOMAS BELL. Anatomy, Physiology, and Diseases of the Teeth. 1831.

[78] E. NEUMANN. Ueber das Wesen der Zahnverderbniss. (*Archiv f. klin. Chirurgie.* Bd. VI, Heft 1, S. 117.)

[79] HERTZ. *Virchow's Archiv.* Bd. XLI, S. 441.

[80] KÖCKER. Principles of Dental Surgery. P. 111.

[81] HEITZMANN and BOEDECKER. Inflammation of Dentine (Eburnitis). (*Indep. Pract.* 1886. P. 120.)

[82] THE SAME. Contributions to the History of the Development of the Teeth. (*Indep. Pract.* May, 1887, to July, 1888.)

[83] FRANK ABBOTT. Caries of the Human Teeth. (*Dental Cosmos.* 1879. February, March, April.)
[84] HEITZMANN. *New England Journal of Dentistry.* Vol. I, P. 193.
[85] FAUCHARD. Le chirurgien-dentiste. Paris, 1728, 1746, 1786.
[86] PFAFF. Abhandlung von den Zähnen. 1756.
[87] LINDERER. Handbuch der Zahnheilkunde. 1837 and 1842.
[88] W. ROBERTSON. A Practical Treatise on the Human Teeth, etc. 1835.
[89] ROGNARD. *Gaz. des hôpit.* 1838.
[90] MAGITOT. La salive. Paris, 1867.
[91] WEDL. Pathologie der Zähne. 1870.
[92] J. TOMES. Dental Surgery. 1873. P. 734.
[93] J. TAFT. Operative Dentistry.
[94] MAGITOT. Etudes et expériences sur la salive. Paris, 1867.
[95] MILLES and UNDERWOOD. Transact. Internat. Med. Congr. 1881.
[96] AD. WEIL. Vorträge, gehalten zu München in der Sitzung des ärztlichen Vereins. 1880. S. 187.
[97] ARKÖVY. Diagnostik der Zahnkrankheiten.
[98] BASTYR. *Oesterreichisch-Ung. Vierteljahrsschr. f. Zahnheilk.* 1885-86. S. 355.
[99] A. GYSI. *Dental Cosmos.* 1887. No. 4.
[100] W. X. SUDDUTH. *Indep. Pract.* 1888. P. 579.
[101] PEIRCE. *Ibid.* 1888. P. 583.
[102] G. ALLAN. *Internat. Dent. Journal.* 1889. No. 3.
[103] BLACK. Dental Caries. (American System of Dentistry. Vol. I. 1886.)
[104] BRIDGMAN. *Trans. Odont. Soc. of Great Britain.* 1861-63. Vol. III, P. 369.
[105] CHASE. *Correspondenzbl. f. Zahnärzte.* 1880. S. 190.
[106] MILLER. *Dental Cosmos.* 1881 P. 91.
[107] J. TOMES. A System of Dental Surgery. 2d Edition. P. 720.
[108] MAGITOT. Recherches sur la carie des dents. 1871.
[109] J. and C. S. TOMES. Dental Surgery. 2d Edition. 1873. P. 722.
[110] WEDL. Pathologie der Zähne. S. 334.
[111] O. WALKHOFF. Mikroskopische Untersuchungen über pathologische Veränderungen des Dentins. (*Monatsschr. f. Zahnheilk.* 1885. S. 12.)
[112] BLACK. American System of Dentistry. Vol. I, P. 741.
[113] F. J. CLARK. *Indep. Pract.* 1883. P. 134.
[114] ALFRED GYSI. Dental Caries under the Microscope. (*Dental Cosmos.* April, 1887.)
[115] A. WEIL. Zur Histologie der Zahnpulpa. (*Habilitationsschrift.* München, 1887.)
[116] MILLER. Einfluss der Mikroorganismen auf die Caries der menschlichen Zähne. (*Archiv für experimentelle Pathologie.* Bd. XVI. 1882.)
[117] J. and C. S. TOMES. Dental Surgery. 1887. 3d Edition. P. 246.
[118] THE SAME. *Ibid.* 2d Edition. P. 301.
[119] MILLES and UNDERWOOD. *Trans. of the Odont. Soc. of Great Britain.* 1884 P. 222.
[120] ATKINSON. *Indep. Pract.* 1888. Pp. 580, 581.
[121] ELLENBERGER und HOFMEISTER. *Archiv f. wissensch. u. prakt. Thierheilk.* Bd. XI, S. 162.

[122] HESSE. *Deutsche med. Wochenschr.* 1885. No. 24.

[123] COLEMAN. *Trans. of the Odont. Soc. of Great Britain.* 1861 to 1863. P. 82.

[124] BRIDGMAN. *Ibid.* P. 369.

[125] MM. GALIPPE et VIGNAL. Note sur les microorganismes de la carie dentaire. (*L'Odontologie.* Mars, 1889.)

[126] MAGITOT. Traité de la carie dentaire. 1867. P. 60.

[127] MUMMERY. *Trans. of the Odont. Soc. of Great Britain.* New Series. 1870. Vol. II, P. 7.

[128] W. C. BARRETT. An Examination of the Condition of the Teeth of Certain Prehistoric Races. (*Indep. Pract.* October, 1883.)

[129] MILLER. Prehistoric Teeth. (*Ibid.* 1884. P. 40.)

[130] BLACK. American System of Dentistry. P. 730.

[131] KOCH. Ueber Desinfection. (*Mittheilungen aus dem Kaiserl. Gesundheitsamt.* Bd. I, S. 234.)

[132] BLACK. Antiseptics. (*Dental Review.* 1889. Nos. 2 and 3.)

[133] v. KACZOROWSKI. Der aetiologische Zusammenhang zwischen Entzündung des Zahnfleisches und anderweitigen Erkrankungen. (*Deutsche med. Wochenschr.* 1885. Nos. 33, 34, 35.)

[134] WITZEL. Deutsche Zahnheilkunde in Vorträgen. Heft 4, S. 99 u. f.

[135] BUSCH. Verhandlungen der deutschen odontologischen Gesellschaft. Bd. I.

[136] MILLER. *Indep. Pract.* June, 1884.

[137] TASSINARI. *Centralblatt für Bacteriologie und Parasitenkunde.* 1888. Bd. IV, S. 449.

[138] HUNTER. A Treatise on the Venereal Disease. 1786. P. 391.

[139] LETTSOM. Transactions of the Medical Society of London. Aug. 2, 1786.

[140] STRICKER. Die Bedeutung des Mundspeichels. 1889. S. 138.

[141] EBERLE. Die Verdauung. 1834. S. 34.

[142] SENATOR. Untersuchungen über d. fieberhaften Process. 1873. S. 6.

[143] RAYNAUD et LANNELONGUE. *Bulletin de l'Académie de méd.* 18 Janvier, 1881.

[144] PASTEUR. *Ibid.*, 18 et 25 Janvier, 1881.

[145] VULPIAN. *Ibid.*, 29 Mars, 1881.

[146] STERNBERG. Bulletin of the National Board of Health. April 30, 1881.

[147] GRIFFIN. *Archivio per le scienze mediche.* Vol. V, Fasc. 3.

[148] GAGLIO et DI MATTEI. Sulla non essistenza di una proprietà tossica della saliva umana. (*Arch. per le scienze med.* 1882. Vol. VI, Fasc. 1. Referat im *Centralbl. f. klin. Med.* 1883. S. 261.)

[149] A. FRÄNKEL. Verhandl. d. 3. Congr. f. innere Med. 1884.

[150] MILLER. *Deutsche med. Wochenschr.* 1884. No. 25.

[151] KLEIN. Ein Beitrag zur Kenntniss der Pneumokokken. (*Centralbl. f. med. Wissensch.* 1884. No. 30. S. 529.)

[152] KREIBOHM. Flügge, Mikroorganismen. S. 257.

[153] A. FRÄNKEL. *Zeitschr. f. klin. Med.* 1886. Bd. X, S. 401.

[154] BAUMGARTEN. Lehrbuch d. pathol. Mykologie. 1888. S. 245.

[155] KREIBOHM. Lit. 152. S. 260.

[156] BLACK. *Indep. Pract.* August, 1887.

[157] KOCH. *Mitth. a. d. Kais. Gesundheitsamt.* Bd. II, S. 42.

[158] GAFFKY. *v. Langenbeck's Archiv.* Bd. XXVIII, Heft 3, S. 500.

[159] BIONDI. Breslauer ärztliche Zeitschr. September, 1887. No. 18.

[160] ZAKHAREVITSCH. Vrach No. 34. S. 523.

[161] BAUME. Lehrbuch der Zahnheilkunde. S. 644.

[162] v. MOSETIG-MOORHOF. *Oesterr.-Ung. Vierteljahrsschr. f. Zahnheilkunde.* 1885. Heft 2.

[163] ZAWADZKI. *Gaz. lekarska.* 1886. No. 8. (From the *Deutsche med. Wochenschr.*)

[164] v. METNITZ. Ein Fall von acuter Osteomyelitis des Unterkiefers mit tödtlichem Ausgange. (*Osterr.-Ung. Vierteljahrsschr. f. Zahnheilk.* 1887. Heft 1.)

[165] CONRAD. *Archives of Dentistry.* November, 1886.

[166] RITTER. *Deutsche Monatsschrift f. Zahnheilkunde.* December, 1886.

[167] PARREIDT. Zur Antiseptik beim Zahnausziehen. (*Deutsche Monatsschr. f. Zahnheilk.* 1888. Heft 7, S. 254.)

[168] BUSCH. *Deutsche med. Wochenschr.* 1885. No. 24.

[169] PORRE. *Dental Record.* October, 1887.

[170] BAKER. *Ibid.* July, 1888.

[171] PONCET. *Gaz. des Hôpit.* No. 19.

[172] FRIPP. *Dental Record.* August, 1887.

[173] RITTER. *Monatsschr. f. Zahnheilk.* 1886. No. 8.

[174] COOPMAN. *Correspondenzbl. f. Zahnärzte.* Januar, 1888. S. 56.

[175] MARSHALL. *Dental Cosmos.* December, 1888. P. 891.

[176] PIETRZIKOWSKI. *Oesterr.-Ung. Vierteljahrsschr. für Zahnheilk.* 1886. S. 363.

[177] HARRISON ALLEN. *Dental Cosmos.* 1874. P. 569.

[178] SCHMID. *Oesterr.-Ung. Vierteljahrsschr. f. Zahnheilk.* 1885. Heft 1.

[179] RITTER. *Correspondenzbl. f. Zahnärzte.* October, 1888.

[180] GALIPPE. Die infectiöse arthro-dentäre Gingivitis. 1888. (Uebersetzung von Manassewitsch.)

[181] ODENTHAL. Cariöse Zähne als Eingangspforte infectiösen Materials und Ursache chronischer Lymphdrüsenschwellungen am Halse. (Inaugural dissertation. Bonn, 1887.)

[182] UNGAR. Sitzung der Niederrhein. Gesellschaft für Natur und Heilkunde zu Bonn, 1884. Mai 17.

[183] v. BERGMANN. Erkrankungen der Lymphdrüsen. (Gerhardt's Handbuch der Kinderkrankheiten. Bd. VI, Abth. 1, S. 253, 254.)

[184] ARKÖVY. Diagnostik der Zahnkrankheiten.

[185] ROTHMANN. Patho-Histologie der Zahnpulpa, etc. 1888.

[186] JAFFÉ. Lungengangrän, durch einen verschluckten Kirschkern erzeugt. (*Allgem. med. Zeitung.* 1886. S. 233.)

[187] LEYDEN und JAFFÉ. Ueber putride (fœtide) Sputa. (*Deutsches Archiv f. klin. Med.* 1867. Bd. II, S. 488.)

[188] JAMES ISRAEL. Ein Beitrag zur Pathogenese der Lungenaktinomykose. (*Archiv f. klin. Chir.* 1886. Bd. XXXIV, Heft 1, S. 160.)

[189] BAUMGARTEN. Jahresbericht. 1 Jahrgang. S. 142.

[190] BAGINSKY. *Deutsche med. Wochenschr.* 1888. No. 20.

[191] BEDNAR. Krankheiten der Neugeborenen und Säuglinge. 1854. S. 54.

[192] HENOCH. Klinik der Unterleibskrankheiten, S. 589 und Beiträge zur Kinderheilkunde. Bd. I, S. 111, und Bd. II, S. 309.

[193] NAUNYN. Ueber das Verhältniss der Magengährungen zur mechanischen Magen-Insufficienz. (*Archiv f. klin. Med.* Bd. XXXI, S. 225.)

[194] LEUBE. *Archiv f. klin. Med.* Bd. XXXIII, S. 4.

[195] DE BARY. Zur Kenntniss der niederen Organismen im Mageninhalte. (*Archiv f. exper. Pathol. u. Pharmakol.* 1886. Bd. XX, S. 243.)

[196] FRERICHS. Wagner's Handwörterbuch der Physiol. Bd. III. 1 Abth. S. 869.

[197] EWALD. Die Lehre von der Verdauung. 1886. S. 104.

[198] ESCHERICH. Beiträge zur antiseptischen Behandlungsmethode der Magen-Darmerkrankungen des Säuglings. (*Therap. Monatshefte.* 1887. S. 390) und Die desinficirende Behandlungsmethode der Magen-Darmkrankheiten des Säuglingsalters. (*Centralbl. f. Bacteriol. u. Parasitenkunde.* 1887. Bd. II, No. 21.)

[199] MINKOWSKI. Ueber die Gährungen im Magen. 1888.

[200] MILLER. *Deutsche med. Wochenschrift.* 1885. No. 49.

[201] MACFADYAN. Flügge. Mikroorganismen. 1885. S. 590.

[202] SUCKSDORF. Das quantitative Vorkommen von Spaltpilzen im menschlichen Darmcanal. (*Archiv f. Hygiene.* 1886. Bd. IV.)

[203] BAUMGARTEN. *Centralbl. f. klin. Med.* 1884, No. 2.

[204] MILLER. *Deutsche med. Wochenschr.* 1885, No. 49. 1886, No. 6.

[205] KOCH. Zweite Serie zur Erörterung der Cholerafrage. (*Deutsche med. Wochenschr.* 1885. No. 19, etc.)

[206] PEDLEY. On the Pathology of Riggs's Disease. (*Dental Record.* May, 1887.)

[207] BLAND SUTTON. *Ibid.* May, 1887.

[208] REEVE. *Indep. Pract.* Vol. VI, P. 367.

[209] PATTERSON. *Dental Cosmos.* 1885. P. 669.

[210] BENNETT. *Dental Record.* May, 1887. Pp. 229, 233.

[211] ARKÖVY. Diagnostik der Zahnkrankheiten. 1885. S. 232.

[212] SCHECH. Krankheiten der Mundhöhle, des Rachens und der Nase.

[213] LÖFFLER. *Mitth. a. d. Kais. Gesundheitsamt.* Bd. II, S. 480.

[214] BULKLEY. On the Dangers arising from Syphilis in the Practice of Dentistry

[215] DULLES *Medical and Surgical Reporter.* January, 1878.

[216] OTIS. Lectures on Syphilis. New York, 1887. P. 102.

[217] LANCERAUX. Proceedings Académie de Médicine de Paris. (*L'Union Médicale.* 1889. P. 655.)

[218] GIOVANNI. Lo Sperimentale. 1889. P. 262.

[219] LELOIR. Leçons sur la Syphilis. 1886. P. 62.

[220] LYDSTON. *Journal of the American Medical Association.* 1886. P. 654.

[221] RODDICK. *Montreal Medical Journal.* August, 1888. P. 93.

[222] PARKER. *Western Dental Journal.* February, 1890.

[223] BOLLINGER. *Centralbl. f. d. med. Wissensch.* 1877. No. 27.

[224] BOSTRÖM. Verh. d. Congr. f. innere Med. Wiesbaden, 1885. S. 94.

[225] JAMES ISRAEL. Neue Beobachtungen aus dem Gebiet der Mykose des Menschen. (*Virchow's Archiv.* 1878. Bd. LXXIV, S. 15.)

[226] PONFICK. Ueber eine wahrscheinlich mykotische Form von Wirbelcaries. (*Berliner klin. Wochenschr.* 1879. S. 345.)

[227] JAMES ISRAEL. Klinische Beiträge zur Aktinomykose des Menschen 1885.

[228] HOCHENEGG. Zur Casuistik der Aktinomykose des Menschen. (*Wiener med. Presse.* 1887. No. 16–18.)

[229] ROTTER. Demonstration von Impfaktinomykose. (*Tagebl. der Naturforscher-Versammlung.* Wiesbaden, 1887. S. 272)

[230] PARTSCH. Einige neue Fälle von Aktinomykose des Menschen. (*Deutsche Zietschr. f. Chirurgie.* 1886. Bd. XXIII, S. 498.)

[231] MOOSBRUGGER. Ueber die Aktinomykose des Menschen. (See *Baumgarten's Jahresbericht,* 1886. S. 317.)

[232] ROSER. *Deutsche med. Wochenschr.* 1886. No. 22. S. 369.

[233] BRAUN. Ueber Aktinomykose des Menschen.

[234] LAURENT. Handbuch der ges. Medicin. S. 263.

[235] PLAUT. Neue Beiträge zur systematischen Stellung des Soorpilzes in der Botanik. Leipzig, 1887.

[236] KLEMPERER. Ueber die Natur des Soorpilzes. (*Centralblatt für klin. Med.* 1885. No. 50. S. 849.)

[237] BAGINSKY. Ueber Soorculturen. (*Deutsche med. Wochenschr.* 1885. No. 50. S. 866.)

[238] GRAWITZ. Ueber die Parasiten des Soors, etc. (*Virchow's Archiv.* 1886. Bd. CIII, S. 393.)

[239] FRÄNKEL. Grundriss der Bacterienkunde.

[240] ZOPF. Pilzthiere oder Schleimpilze. 1885.

[241] DE BARY. Morphologie und Biologie der Pilze. 1884. S. 453.

[242] WORONIN. Pringsheim's Jahrbücher für Wissensch. Botanik. 1878. Bd. XI.

[243] KOCH. Mitth. aus d. Kais. Gesundheitsamt. 1881. Bd I.

[244] EIDAM. *Allg. landwirthschaft. Zeitung.* 1880. No. 97.

[245] FLÜGGE. Die Mikroorganismen. S. 110.

[246] BAUMGARTEN. Lehrb. d. path. Mykologie. 1888. S. 72.

PART I.

General Bacteriological Studies,

WITH

SPECIAL REFERENCE TO THE BACTERIA OF THE HUMAN MOUTH.

The Micro-Organisms of the Human Mouth.

CHAPTER I.

INTRODUCTORY.

Fungi belong to that class of Cryptogamia which are designated as Thallophyta (Thallophytes).

Their position in the vegetable kingdom may be indicated by the following classification:

- Plants.
  - Cryptogams, flowerless plants reproducing chiefly by spores.
    - Thallophytes,
      - *Fungi*,
      - Algæ,
      - Lichens.
    - Leafy Cryptogams.
  - Phanerogams, flowering plants reproducing by seeds.

The Cryptogams differ from the Phanerogams in the absence of flowers, and in that they do not propagate themselves by means of seeds, in which the future plant is already present in embryo, but by means of spores, *i.e.* by simple bodies or cells, which show no differentiation corresponding to the parts of the future plant.

As leaf-bearing Cryptogams, we designate those spore-forming plants which have leaves, stems, and often also roots. These represent a higher stage of development than the Thallophytes, inasmuch as the latter do not have the parts mentioned.

Thallophytes are very commonly divided into Fungi, Algæ, and Lichens: Fungi being characterized as cells *without* chlorophyl, which subsist on preformed organic substances; Algæ as cells *with* chlorophyl, living on inorganic substances; Lichens as a combination of cells with and without chlorophyl, also living on inorganic substances.

This classification has, however, recently been justly pronounced untenable, since it is not possible to make the presence or absence of chlorophyl a criterion for determining the fungal or non-fungal character of any growth. The fungi comprise not only Thallophytes without, but also such with chlorophyl, and indeed some of the most characteristic members of this group of Thallophytes contain chlorophyl (de Bary[1]). Secondly, fungi and algæ show so marked a similarity in regard to their morphology and conditions of reproduction, that a separation on the chlorophyl basis alone scarcely seems desirable. In the third place, recent investigations have demonstrated with considerable certainty that lichens are not entitled to recognition as a separate group of organisms, being nothing more than a mixture of fungi and algæ, in which the former live as parasites upon the latter (Flügge[2]). Again, the view has been steadily gaining ground that bacteria have very little in common with the pure fungi, and accordingly should not be classed with them.

For the present I have, however, retained the old division, particularly as the question of arranging and classifying the Thallophytes has not yet been definitely settled. (See Lit. 1, 2, 3, 4.)

From a hygienic point of view we recognize four chief groups of fungi:

1. Fission-fungi (Bacteria) . . . Schizomycetes.
2. Mould- or Thread-fungi (Fungi proper, Moulds) . . . . . Hyphomycetes.
3. Bud-fungi (Yeast-fungi, Yeast) . . Blastomycetes.
4. Animal-fungi (Pilzthiere) . . Mycetozoa.

Of these four groups, bacteria command by far the greatest interest. They are the chief agents in the production of those intense decompositions designated as fermentation, putrefaction, etc. By this means they not only prevent the accumulation of dead animal and vegetable matter upon the earth's surface, but, at the same time, produce from the complicated organic substances of the latter the simple compounds, carbonic acid (CO_2) and ammonia (NH_3), which are absolutely necessary to the continuance of a chlorophyl-bearing vegetation.

Without these processes all higher vegetation, and consequently all animal life, would in the course of time become extinct. Unfortunately, however, the activity of the bacteria is by no means restricted to the performance of this important rôle in the household of nature. They are also capable of exerting a most deleterious influence on the living animal body, and have been recognized as the exciting cause of the majority of all diseases to which mankind is subject.

Mould-fungi (Moulds), although very widely distributed in nature, do not by far play so important a part as the fission-fungi. They do not produce as intense decompositions of organic substances, nor, with the exception of certain cutaneous diseases, are they capable of bringing about such disturbances in the human body as result from the invasion of fission-fungi. Many diseases of plants and of lower animals (insects) have, however, been traced to the agency of mould-fungi.

Bud-fungi (yeast-fungi) exert even less disturbing influence on human life than moulds; with the single exception of thrush, no disease is at present known to be due to their action.

Our knowledge of the physiological and hygienic significance of the "animal-fungi" is, as yet, very inaccurate.

The lower Mycetozoa (Monadina) occur as parasites on algæ and fungi, as well as on higher plants. They have also been found in enormous quantities in the human intestines, in diseased as well as in healthy conditions, without it being possible to assign to them an indubitably pathogenic action.

SHORT OUTLINE OF THE MORPHOLOGY AND BIOLOGY OF BACTERIA.

Bacteria are microscopic, spherical or elongated, unicellular organisms, which live upon preformed organic substances, and increase by fissation, or through the medium of spores.

Each cell possesses a cell-membrane and protoplasmic contents; the latter is usually homogeneous, seldom containing vacuoles or granules (Beggiatoa). The deposits of lime-salts, so common with other Thallophytes, have been but very rarely observed in growths of bacteria.

Many kinds of bacteria possess the power of locomotion, and consequently were formerly often classed among the infusoria.

The size of the cells of the different kinds of bacteria varies very considerably, nor are the cells of one and the same kind always of the same size. The micrococcus of progressive suppuration in rabbits has a diameter of only 0.15μ*; several millions of this micro-organism could easily dance, if not upon the point, at least upon the head of a pin. On the other hand, Beggiatoa mirabilis is 35μ thick, and Spirochæte plicatilis attains a length of 225μ or $\frac{1}{4}$ millimeter.

1. Forms of Bacteria.

According to de Bary, the chief forms of bacteria are:

1. Cocci: isodiametric, or at least but very slightly uniaxially elongated single cells.

2. Rod-forms: uniaxially elongated, cylindrical, less frequently spindle-shaped cells, or short chains of the same.

3. Screw-forms: rods which are twisted after the pattern of a corkscrew, partly with shallow, partly with steep spirals.

To the *first* group (coccus-forms) belong:

a. Micrococci: cells spherical, or nearly so (Fig. 1, *a*, *c*, *d*).

b. Macrococci, Megacocci: remarkably large cocci.

c. Diplococci: biscuit-shaped cells, which arise during the fissation of cocci (Fig. 1, *b*).

It would probably be more correct to consider diplococci simply as transition-forms.

---

*μ = mikro-millimeter = $\frac{1}{1000}$ millimeter.

To the *second* group (rod-forms) belong:

d. Bacilli: rods, *i.e.* cells, whose longitudinal axis visibly exceeds the transverse (Fig. 1, *p*).

FIG. 1.

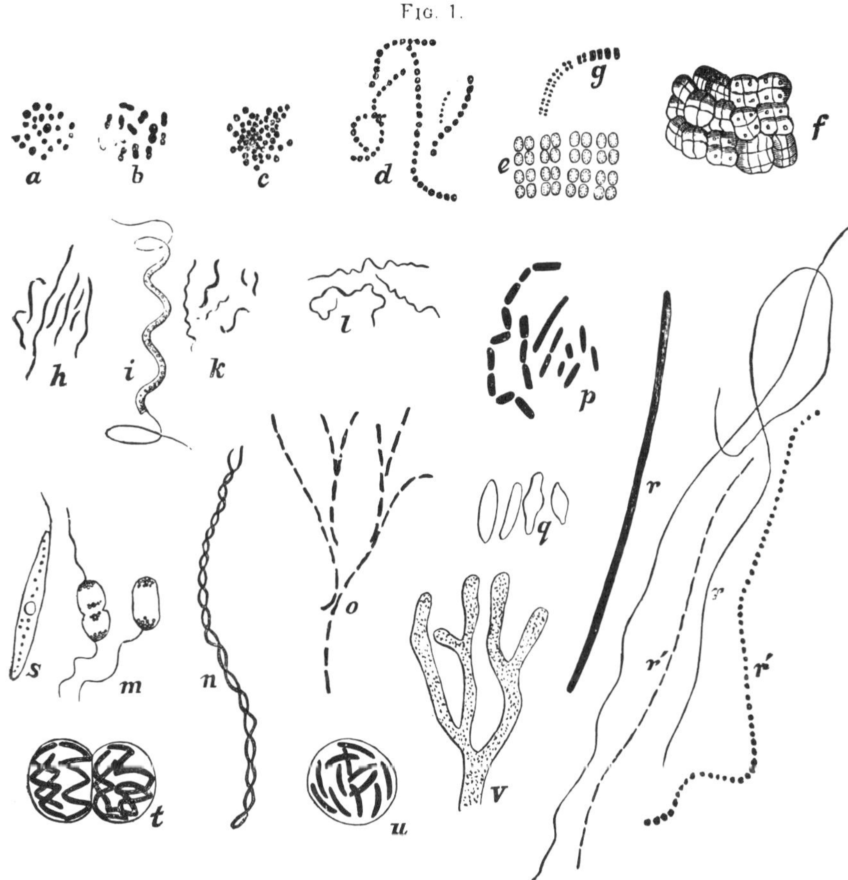

FORMS OF BACTERIA.

a, Cocci. *b*, Diplococci. *c*, Cluster-cocci (Staphylococci). *d*, Coccus chains (Streptococci, Torula). *e*, Surface-shaped colonies (Merismopedia). *f*, Packet-shaped colonies (Sarcina). *g*, A double coccus chain produced by a single fissation of each member in a direction at right angles to the long axis of the chain. *h*, Vibriones. *i*, *k*, Spirilla. *l*, Spirochætes. *m*, Spiromonades. *n*, Spirulina. *o*, Cladothrix. *p*, Rods (bacilli). *q*, Clostridium. *r*, Leptothrix (threads). *r'*, Articulated threads. *s*, Rhabdomonas. *t*, *u*, *v*, Zooglœa. (In part after Flügge & Zopf.)

e. Clostridium: spindle-shaped cells (Fig. 1, *q*).

f. Leptothrix: thread-shaped cells, or chains of cells (Fig. 1, *r*, *r'*).

g. Beggiatoa: long, thick, rigid threads, which deposit grains of sulphur in their protoplasm.

h. Crenothrix: thread-forming water-fungi, whose threads (which may be either unicellular or composed of chains of cocci and rods) are inclosed by a sheath, and increase in diameter from base to apex.

i. Cladothrix: thread-forming bacteria with false branchings (pseudo-branchings), (Fig. 1, *o*).

Some writers question the correctness of classing Beggiatoa, Crenothrix, and Cladothrix under bacteria.

To the *third* group (screw-forms) belong:

j. Vibriones: rods or threads with a slight undulating curve or twist (Fig. 1, *h*).

k. Spirilla: rigid rods and threads with pronounced screw-like windings (Fig. 1, *i*, *k*).

l. Spirochætes: flexible threads with narrow, unequal windings, sometimes as many as sixty in one thread (Fig. 1, *l*). The genera Vibrio, Spirillum, Spirochæte, are not separated from each other by any sharp line of division; an organism which one would describe as a vibrio might by another be designated as a spirillum; what one terms spirillum another calls spirochæte, etc. Furthermore, micro-organisms belonging to the second group not unfrequently show a slight curve or twist in some of their cells, without thereby being entitled to be placed among the screw-forms.

Threads, whose ends are wound about each other like a braid of hair, have been termed Spirulina (Fig. 1, *u*).

Each of the three fundamental forms (spheres, rods, and screws) is subject to extensive modifications, according to the circumstances under which it is cultivated, and it is not always easy to determine whether the particular organism under examination should be classed as a coccus or a bacillus, as a bacillus or a vibrio, etc. Whether these modifications can be carried so far by any condition or conditions of cultivation that a micro-organism normally occurring in any one of the three fundamental forms is transformed into another (for example a coccus into a bacillus), or that a monomorphous organism becomes pleomorph, is a question upon which much has been said pro and con, but which we cannot discuss here. Suffice it to say, that at present the great mass of evidence points to the conclusion that such transformations cannot be brought about in the manner indicated. On the other hand, there are many kinds of bacteria that manifest two or all of the fundamental forms at the same time. These have been designated as pleomorphous, in contradistinction to those which produce only one form (monomorphous). (See Zopf.)

The following forms are classed by Zopf[4] and others among the bacteria; Flügge speaks of them as being of doubtful relation to the bacteria, while Cornil and Babes[5] make of some of them a sort of connecting link between the bacteria and infusoria:

1. Monades: large, spherical, oval, or short cylindrical cells, provided with cilia, often in pairs (Fig. 1, *m*).
2. Rhabdomonas: large spindle-shaped ciliated cells (Fig. 1, *s*).
3. Spiromonas: leaf-like, flat cells, "twisted around an imaginary axis in the direction of their length."

2. Cumulative Forms of Bacteria.

Besides these forms of the single cells, we recognize various configurations which result from the accumulation or combination of *several* cells. These are:

1. Thread-forms or Chain-forms: *i.e.* forms produced by a succession of single cells. To these belong:
   - *a.* Streptococci (Chain cocci): cocci which appear chiefly in chains, sometimes improperly called Torula (Fig. 1, *d*).
   - *b.* Leptothrix: long, articulated threads, composed of single cells (cocci or rods), (Fig. 1, *r′*).
2. Cluster-forms, *i.e.* groups, produced by the aggregation of cells without definite arrangement, particularly Staphylococci,* which are mostly found in clusters (Fig. 1, *c*).
3. Surface- or Mass-forms, which are produced by fissation in two or three directions, such as merismopedia: plate-shaped colonies, produced by fissation in two directions (Fig. 1, *e*), and

* σταφυλή, A cluster of grapes

sarcina: packet-shaped groups, produced by fissation in three directions (Fig. 1, *f*).

4. Zooglœa-forms, produced by the gelatinization of the membranes of the accumulated cells, in such a way that the latter become imbedded in a mass of jelly (Palmella- or Zooglœa-condition, Fig. 1, *t*, *u*, *v*). Where the jelly is very thick and cartilaginous, the term Ascococcus is applied; where only the outer layers of a Zooglœa are gelatinized, the term Clathrocystis. Threads, or pieces of threads, imbedded in round masses of jelly, have been named Myconostoc (Fig. 1, *t*, *u*).

Pseudo-branching (Cladothrix) may also be regarded as a cumulative form (Fig. 1, *o*).

3. Reproduction of Bacteria.

The reproduction of bacteria takes place in three different ways: by fissation, in the same manner as seen in the infusoria

Fig 2.

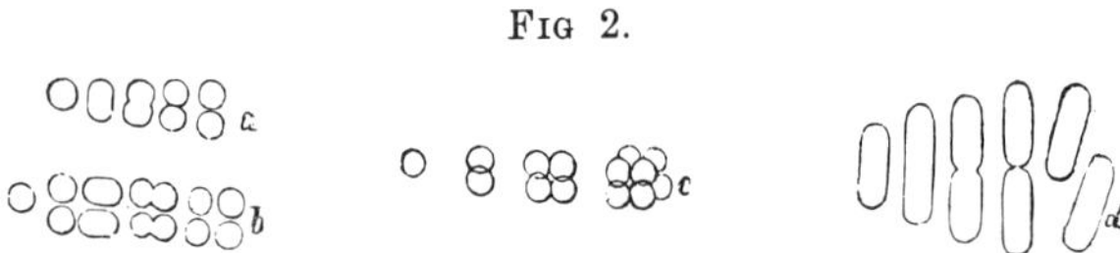

Proliferation of Bacteria by Fissation.

a and *d*, Fissation in one direction; *b*, in two; *c*, in three directions.

Fig. 3.

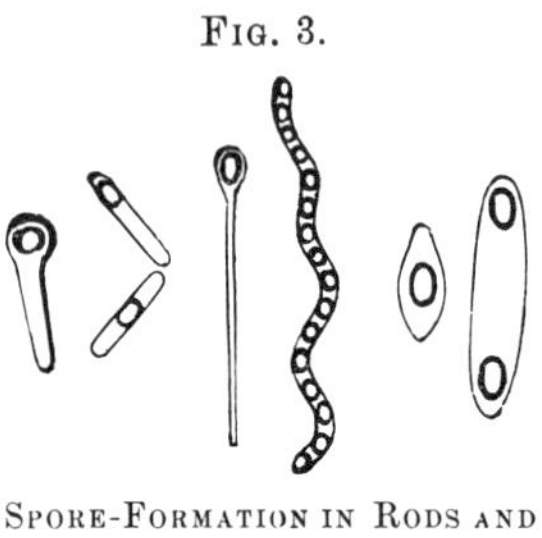

Spore-Formation in Rods and Threads.

(After Zopf.)

Fig. 4.

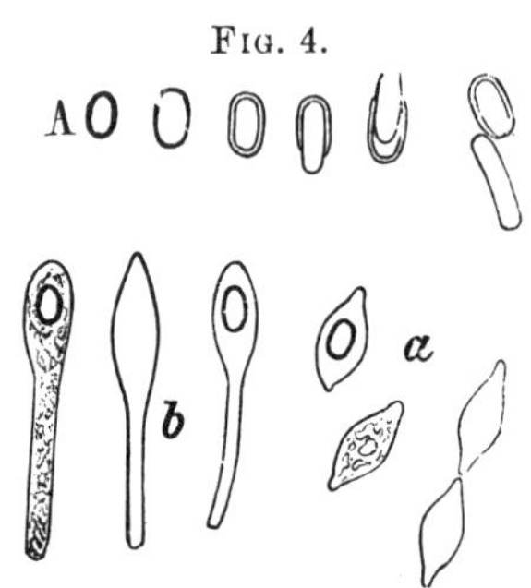

Formation of Spores in Bacillus butyricus.

A, Germination of a spore.

(After Prazmowski.)

(Fig. 2), by spores (Figs. 3 and 4), or by the separation of certain cells from their original cyclus, and their development into new combinations, morphologically identical with those from which they sprang. By some these cells are called cocci, by others spores (arthrospores).

The spores (Fig. 3) are spherical or ovoidal bodies, with sharp contours and strongly refractive contents. They are formed chiefly in media of which the available nourishment for bacteria has been already, for the most part, consumed. Considered from a hygienic stand-point they are of great interest, since they offer more resistance to influences of every nature (chemical, thermal, etc.) than the vegetative cells (as the active growing cells may be designated in contradistinction to the inactive, resting, spores). Formation of spores has been observed in various rod- and some screw-forms, and recently also in the case of a micrococcus. Bacteria with endogenous spore-formation are called endospore; those without endogenous spore-formation are called arthrospore.

4. The Origin of Bacteria.

It has long been known that various kinds of bacteria are found in the atmosphere, water, soil, etc. This fact was first established by Ehrenberg[6] (1828), although Leeuwenhoek[7] had observed microscopic organisms in the human mouth as early as 1675. Regarding their origin, a long and violent dispute was carried on for many years between those who claimed that they were produced spontaneously in solutions of organic matter (*generatio spontanea, sive æquivoca, abiogenesis*), and those who believed that they could originate only from pre-existing germs. The exact methods of sterilization practiced in the last ten years have alone made it possible to establish the fact beyond all question, that the proposition "*omnis cellula e cellula*" is quite as applicable to these low forms of life as to the higher animal organism. The appearance of bacteria in solutions supposed to have been sterilized, simply proves that the latter were either *not* thoroughly sterilized in the beginning, or that they were afterwards infected from without.

The question whether the number of species of bacteria remains constant, or whether, in the course of centuries, through the propagation of varieties in the Darwinian sense, new species arise, has not been finally decided. The tendency seems to be to accept the latter view, although positive evidence for the origin of new species has not yet been adduced.

5. Life-Conditions of Bacteria.

I designate as life-conditions of bacteria those circumstances relative to food, air, temperature, etc., which are indispensable to their development.

Nencki's[8] analysis gives for bacteria the following chemical composition: water 84.81 per cent., albumen 13.03 per cent., fat 1.20 per cent., ashes 0.64 per cent., undetermined residue 0.32 per cent.

According to this analysis a nutrient solution for bacteria should be composed of albumen, carbohydrates, and small quantities of salts; a conclusion which has been completely confirmed by experience, which has taught that such solutions invariably form the best culture media.

The juices and accumulations in the human mouth at all times present such a medium. Artificially it may be prepared in different ways, perhaps most easily by means of the following mixture: water 100.0, peptone 2.0, sugar 1.0, beef extract 1.5.

The solid culture media introduced by Koch, which are prepared by the addition of gelatine or agar-agar, are similarly composed.

The composition and concentration of the culture medium are of the greatest importance. The organic substances, albumen, peptone, sugar, etc., are without question the most suitable culture media, although formerly mineral solutions were extensively used. One of these, recommended by Nägeli, has the following composition: water 100 c.cm., tartrate of ammonia 1.0, phosphate of potassium 0.1, sulphate of magnesium 0.02, chloride of calcium 0.01. Such mineral solutions are, however, as a rule, by no means so well adapted to culture experiments as the media now in use.

For each species of bacteria there seems to be a certain concentration of the culture medium best suited to its growth, although it has not as yet been possible to establish definite laws governing this principle, or to say just what degree of concentration is best adapted to each. So much, however, is certain, that whereas no degree of dilution protects culture media against bacteria, a too large proportion of solid matter or a too small proportion of water impedes, or entirely prevents, their development.

The chief condition for the formation of spores appears to be an at least partial exhaustion of the available nourishment in the solution, while a certain influence is also exerted by its temperature and composition. The first condition is presented in most perfect form by the necrotic tooth-pulp, a fact which, on account of its great importance, will be referred to at more length in a later chapter.

6. Influence of Various Conditions on the Growth of Bacteria.

a. Action of Temperature.

Temperature naturally exerts an unlimited influence upon the vegetation of bacteria. That temperature which permits the most rapid increase (designated as the optimum) varies considerably for the different kinds, for the most, however, ranging between 25° and 40° C. Above 40° the development rapidly diminishes, and ceases almost or entirely at 41°; below 5°, on the other hand, proliferation takes place very slowly, if at all. Many bacteria will not grow at a temperature below 20°; some even not under 30° C.

The temperature most favorable for the majority of bacteria, particularly for the pathogenic varieties, is 37° or 38° C. In this respect, again, the oral cavity presents an excellent culture medium.

b. Action of Oxygen.

The access of atmospheric air exerts special influence upon the vegetation of bacteria. In accordance with this fact, we distinguish three groups of bacteria. For the development of the first, oxygen is absolutely necessary; they are called aërobic. Bacteria of the second group thrive better without oxygen, or even absolutely demand the exclusion of air for their development; they are called anaërobic. The third group of bacteria flourish either with or without oxygen, at least for a certain length of time; Hueppe characterizes them as facultatively anaërobic. Most bacteria appear to belong to the first group, but comparatively few purely anaërobic bacteria being at present known.

The capability of certain bacteria to proliferate and to manifest their specific action without access of air, may explain the progress of tooth caries under air-tight fillings, in cases where the softened dentine was not thoroughly removed before inserting the filling.

c. Action of Acids and Alkalies.

Acids and alkalies, especially the former, even in very dilute solutions, retard the development of bacteria. Some species, however, show important deviations from this rule; thus, for example, the acetic acid bacterium grows best in an excess of one to two per cent. of acetic acid, while Micrococcus ureæ will bear a high degree of alkalinity. A bacterium which I have examined produces in solutions of carbohydrates 0.75 per cent. of lactic acid, but perishes in this solution in a few days, through the action of its own product. With comparatively few exceptions, a neutral medium is best adapted to the development of bacteria.

d. Action of Light, Electricity, and Pressure.

Light, electricity, and pressure have very little or no influence upon the development of bacteria, nor upon their specific vital manifestations. (See Cohn and Mendelsohn.[9]) The assertion that combined fillings of tin and gold, or of amalgam and gold, etc., prevent the development of bacteria by means of the electricity which they produce, is utterly without scientific foundation.

That even weak electric currents sometimes appear to have a slight retarding action upon the development of bacteria, may be easily demonstrated by the following simple experiment:

A tube of culture gelatine is richly infected with a bacterium which grows rapidly at room temperature without liquefying the gelatine; it is then poured upon a glass plate in the customary manner. While the gelatine is still liquid, place upon the plate a metallic strip, one end of which is composed of tin, the other of gold.

On the border of the tin, a retardation in the development of the bacteria will be observed; the gelatine remains clear (Fig. 5). In a few days the tin (electro-positive pole) will appear surrounded by a white zone 10 to 30 mm. in diameter; the reaction

FIG. 5

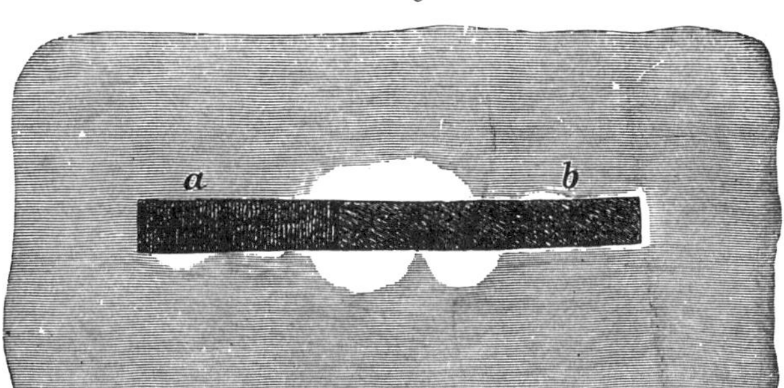

APPARENT PREVENTION OF THE GROWTH OF BACTERIA BY ELECTRIC ACTION.

a, Gold; *b*, Tin, on a plate of culture gelatine. In the parts indicated by the white color no development of bacteria occurs. Reaction around the tin strongly acid; around the gold alkaline.

in this zone will be found to be strongly acid. The retardation in the development is to be ascribed not to the electricity, but to the acid.

On the border of the gold the reaction will be found to be alkaline. The development of the bacteria is here also retarded, but much less than on the margin of the tin (the electro-positive pole).

7. ANTAGONISM AMONG THE BACTERIA.

The principle of the struggle for existence and of natural selection plays an important, though not fully understood, part in the life of bacteria. If we bring a number of different kinds of bacteria into a common culture medium, it will be found that they do not all develop with equal rapidity; *one* kind will always attain the supremacy. If we infect a second nutrient medium with this culture and continue the operation through a series of generations, we may find that at last only one kind remains, the others having been crowded out. It depends upon the composition of the solution, the temperature, and various other conditions, as to which species will gain the victory. It may also happen that at first one kind prevails, and that later, through a change in the character of the medium, another kind gains the upper hand; or again, in one part of the medium—for example, on the surface—one kind may prevail, in another part another. In the human mouth this struggle for existence seems to play an important part; otherwise we should invariably expect to find a much larger number of different kinds of bacteria than are actually present. The attempt to make use of this principle in therapeutics, by bringing large numbers of harmless bacteria into the human body in order to drive out others of a pathogenic nature (Cantani), has hitherto not been accompanied by the results which we had been led to hope for.

8. Self-Destruction of Bacteria.

The growth and ferment activity of bacteria are always more or less influenced by their own waste products. Lactic acid fermentation not only ceases when the acidity of the solution has reached 0.75 to 0.80 per cent., but the bacteria themselves are often destroyed by the action of the acid which they have produced. The vital action of yeast cells is also hemmed by the alcohol which accumulates in the solution, and for the same reason the ammoniac fermentation of urine ceases when the amount of ammonium carbonate produced amounts to 13 per cent. (Flügge).

Some products of putrefaction appear to exert a similar action upon the life of bacteria. Up to the present, however, it has not been possible to determine with certainty to which of the many products of putrefaction this action is to be ascribed.

VITAL MANIFESTATIONS OF BACTERIA.

As vital manifestations of bacteria, are to be considered all those phenomena which are excited by their presence in the substrata which they inhabit. It is immaterial whether the latter consist of dead substances, or of living animal or vegetable organisms.

I. Action of Bacteria upon the Living Vegetable or Animal Body.

It is a belief of very old date, which found expression in the writings of Varro as early as the first century B.C., that diseases of an epidemic character are produced by some invisible living element, a *contagium vivum, contagium animatum;* not, however, until the first quarter of the present century, was this belief placed on a scientific basis by the celebrated physician and naturalist, Hufeland. In the year 1835 it received a strong actual support by the discovery of Bassi that a fatal disease of the silkworm (muscardine), was produced by a mould-fungus (Botrytis Bassiana). A few years later de Bary, Kühn and others, established the parasitic nature of a number of diseases in grain, and in the years 1851 to 1857, Rayer, Brauell, and Pollender followed with the discovery of the anthrax bacillus. From this time on, the attention of physicians and naturalists has been constantly directed more and more to these low forms of life as the exciting causes of disease. Micro-organisms were found to be present in various disorders, and finally, within the last few years, since the introduction of Koch's well-known culture methods, the parasitic nature of a large number of diseases has been indubitably established.

I will here name only anthrax, relapsing fever, abdominal typhus, lepra, gonorrhœa, tuberculosis, lupus, cholera, pneumonia, syphilis, malaria, glanders, erysipelas, diphtheria, puerperal fever, and suppurative processes.

We distinguish bacteria according to their action upon living bodies, as (1) pathogenic and (2) non-pathogenic. Pathogenic are all micro-organisms which, when brought into contact with any part of a living organism under favorable conditions, multiply and give rise to either local or general disturbances.

No sharp line of distinction can, however, be drawn between pathogenic and non-pathogenic bacteria, for every bacterium brought into the animal organism *in sufficiently large masses* will be able to maintain itself for a certain length of time and to excite more or less inflammatory reaction.

Pathogenic in a high degree are those bacteria which, like the anthrax bacillus, produce dangerous disturbances, even though singly inoculated into the organism; very slightly pathogenic are those which can cause disturbances only when introduced in large quantities. *Non*-pathogenic are those, which, brought into the organism in large numbers, soon disappear without having produced any apparent disturbance.

Pathogenic bacteria exert very different and diverse influences upon different species of animals. An animal of one species may manifest symptoms of disorder soon after inoculation, while members of another species may remain altogether unaffected by it. Even different varieties of one and the same species do not always manifest the same degree of susceptibility when inoculated with the same bacterium; *e.g.* house mice inoculated with the bacillus of mouse septicæmia in a skin pocket succumb within forty to sixty hours, whereas field mice suffer no inconvenience from the inoculation. Koch[10] explains this phenomenon by the difference of the blood of these two nearly related varieties.

A species or variety is consequently said to be either susceptible (disposed) or unsusceptible (immune, refractory). With every animal the degree of susceptibility varies at different times, according to the condition of the body at the time being (temporary susceptibility). Furthermore, since in all epidemics the disease does not rage everywhere with equal severity, but attains its greatest intensity at certain circumscribed points or localities, it is customary to speak also of a local disposition or susceptibility.

Bacteria are further divided into *parasitic:* such as live in or upon living organisms, and *saprophytic:* such as are confined to dead substances. Most parasitic bacteria, however, are also able to live upon dead matter, and may consequently be cultivated in artificial media, while on the other hand pure saprophytes occasionally take on the habitus of parasites.

Such parasites as thrive *only* in or upon living organisms are classed by de Bary as strictly obligatory parasites. To this class several species occurring in the oral cavity *seem* to belong. Saprophytes which find their conditions of existence fulfilled only in dead substances, are called obligatory saprophytes. Parasites which occur in the interior of an organism are called endophytic; those which vegetate only on the surface, epiphytic. Bacteria which on being introduced into the human or animal organism lead to formation of pus, are designated as pyogenic.

Very careful investigations made by Klemperer,[11] Biondi,[12] Zuckermann,[13] and many others, have led to the conclusion that "chemical irritants, when free from micro-organisms, cannot produce suppuration." Kreibohm and Rosenbach,[14] Grawitz and de Bary[15] obtained other results. According to them, certain chemical substances, as oil of turpentine, ammonia, nitrate of silver, etc., may under favorable conditions call forth suppuration. Scheuerlen[16] was also able to cause suppuration by the action of an alkaloid of putrefaction (cadaverine), without the agency of micro-organisms. Nathan[17] repeated the experiments of Grawitz and de Bary, and also found that suppuration took place after injections of oil of turpentine, ammonia, and nitrate of silver; in all cases, however, he was able by means of the culture method to establish the presence of micro-organisms. Nevertheless Grawitz,[18] in a subsequent communication, maintains the correctness of his previous conclusions.

It has been suggested that these conflicting results may be explained by the fact that different investigators have made use of different animals in their experiments. While the advocates of the theory: no suppuration without micro-organisms, have used chiefly rabbits, guinea-pigs and rats, Kreibohm and others employed dogs.

As the matter stands at present, the burden of proof seems to be in favor of the view that, in case of dogs at least, certain substances may, under specified conditions, produce suppuration without the agency of micro-organisms.

II. Action upon Lifeless Matter.

Bacteria are furthermore designated, with reference to their action upon the substratum, as:

1. Zymogenic, or fermentation bacteria.
2. Chromogenic, or color-forming bacteria.
3. Aërogenic, or gas-forming bacteria.
4. Saprogenic, or putrefaction bacteria.

1. *Fermentation Bacteria.*

Ferment bacteria are such as bring about those changes in the substratum which have been designated as fermentation. According to Hoppe-Seyler,[19] these changes are intense decompositions of complicated organic compounds, through which substances arise "which have together less heat of combustion than those bodies out of which they were formed." By others, fermentation is described as a process of decomposition, which is inaugurated and continued by a substance called a ferment, without the ferment itself suffering any change; this kind of action is frequently designated as catalysis, *καταλυσις* (*καταλύω*) dissolution. During the process of fermentation the medium gradually loses its nutritive power; it becomes used up. The substances which are thereby produced are very numerous, and of very different character. Many of them, the ptomaïnes, have exceedingly poisonous properties. It is highly probable that all bacteria, pathogenic as well as non-pathogenic, when brought into a suitable substratum, possess the property of producing changes which must be designated as fermentation. The fermentation of nitrogenous, and more particularly of albuminous substances, which is accompanied by the development of large quantities of gaseous and stinking products, is called putrefactive fermentation, or simply putrefaction, and the bacteria causing this kind of fermentation are putrefactive or saprogenic bacteria.

Many years ago I[20] called attention to the fact that the course of the fermentation frequently depends more upon the substratum than upon the micro-organism. Bacteria which grow upon white of egg, producing an intensely offensive smell and a strong alkaline reaction, when brought into carbohydrates exhibit entirely different phenomena, viz. acid reaction and total absence of bad smell.

We cannot therefore draw a sharp line between putrefactive and fermentative bacteria. According to my observation there are but a limited number of bacteria which will, under all circumstances, produce putrefaction. These might be called obligatory saprogenic bacteria, in contradistinction to those which produce putrefaction only under certain specified conditions; these latter might be called facultatively saprogenic.

Bacteria produce a series of well-characterized fermentations, whose nature has, however, in many points not yet been fully explained. These fermentations are, according to Flügge's classification:[21]

A. Fermentation of carbohydrates.

B. Fermentation of the polyvalent alcohols.

C. Fermentation of fatty acids.

D. Putrefaction.

E. Oxidation of alcohol to acetic acid. To these we add:

F. Ammoniacal fermentation.

G. Diverse processes of oxidation and reduction first observed in the soil, but probably going on under various other conditions.

A. *Fermentation of Carbohydrates.*

Carbohydrates, when acted upon by different bacteria, undergo a series of fermentations which may be considered under the following heads:

a. Lactic acid fermentation.

b. Mannite, or mucous fermentation.

c. Dextrane fermentation.

d. Butyric acid fermentation.

e. Diverse fermentations which cannot be classed under the above heads.

Among the carbohydrates, the sugars in particular are fermentable in a high degree; other carbohydrates, however, as dextrine, starch, cellulose, etc., may also undergo fermentation under the action of certain micro-organisms. Tappeiner (Flügge[21]) observed a fermentative decomposition of cellulose in the alimentary canal of ruminants; also two kinds of cellulose fermentation in artificial mixtures. The former took place in neutral 1 per cent. beef extract solutions, in which purified cotton or paper pulp was suspended, carbonic acid, marsh gas, and small quantities of sulphuretted hydrogen, aldehyde, isobutyric acid, and acetic acid being formed; the latter in alkaline beef-extract solutions, carbonic acid and hydrogen being formed, with the same by-products as before. Nothing at all is known concerning the occurrence of such fermentations in the human mouth. They might possibly come into consideration in the decomposition of cotton used in the treatment of teeth.

a. Lactic Acid Fermentation.

Lactic acid fermentation of carbohydrates takes place spontaneously in milk, in the juice of the sugar-beet, in the accumulations in the oral cavity, etc., and may be artificially induced by a large number of different bacteria in saccharine solutions. It proceeds most rapidly at a temperature of from 30°–38° C. The course of the fermentation varies greatly, according to the bacterium by which it is produced. Sometimes there seems to be a perfectly even decomposition of the molecules of sugar into two molecules of lactic acid, according to the equation $C_6H_{12}O_6$ (grape sugar)$=2C_3H_6O_3$ (lactic acid), no appreciable quantity of carbonic acid or hydrogen being formed. At other times the fermentation is of a more violent nature, large quantities of carbonic acid and hydrogen being formed, with other by-products, as acetic, formic, succinic, and possibly butyric acid.

It is usually assumed that lactic acid fermentation must always be accompanied by a development of carbonic acid. I was, however, struck by the fact that in certain cultures an evolution of gas always failed to take place. In order to arrive at a positive conclusion in regard to this point, I undertook an experiment in a large glass vessel containing a liter of beef-extract-sugar-solution, which I inoculated with a small piece of carious dentine. Then a rubber cork, carrying a bent glass rod, was coated with sealing-wax and pressed into the heated opening of the glass vessel, thus hermetically sealing it. The vessel, being placed in the incubator, exhibited after a few hours a rapid development of bacteria and an acid reaction. No bubbles of gas were seen to be ascending through the solution, or to have accumulated upon its surface, as is frequently the case in such cultures. Hereupon the end of the escape-tube was made to dip into lime-water, in which the smallest quantity of CO_2 escaping from the flask would be readily detected by the cloudiness occasioned by the formation of the carbonate of lime, but after twelve hours no cloudiness had appeared. I then heated the flask, in order to drive out any carbonic acid possibly formed; the lime-water, however, still remained clear. I repeated this experiment with an apparatus for collecting the gas over mercury. In a culture in which 1.75 grams of lactic acid were produced, only one little bubble of gas was collected, which might as well have been caused by an imperceptible rise in the temperature of the incubator as by actual gas formation.

From these experiments I can draw no other conclusion than that the fermentation produced by the micro-organisms in question is not accompanied by development of carbonic acid. This process, writes Flügge (Lit. 2, p. 483), which wholly fails to evolve gases, does not meet the requirements of the ordinary definition of fermentation, and can consequently not be considered as such.

The fermentation ceased in all cases which I have thus far examined, when the substratum showed 0.75 per cent. of acid. In the mouth, however, the fermentation can proceed without interruption, since the acid formed is either washed away or combines with the lime of the teeth and tartar.

As early as 1857, Pasteur[22] showed that the transformation of sugar into lactic acid depended upon the presence of a species of micro-organism.

The name of Bacillus acidi lactici (lactic acid bacterium) has been given to a bacillus, first cultivated by Hueppe,[23] from sour milk. Although very many different bacteria are known which possess the power of converting carbohydrates into lactic acid, it is thought that Hueppe's bacterium should be designated as *the* lactic acid bacterium, since it is "by far the most frequent cause of spontaneous lactic acid fermentation."

This bacillus forms short, plump rods, from 1–1.7μ long and 0.3–0.4μ thick; it is immotile, forms spores. Below 10° C.

and above 45.5° C. all development ceases, the optimum lying between 35° and 42° C. It possesses inverting action, and transforms not only dextrose, but also cane-sugar, milk-sugar, and mannite into lactic acid. Its ferment-action is regularly accompanied by the development of carbonic acid.

It is not improbable that this bacillus plays an essential part in fermentations of the human mouth. The frequency of its occurrence in the oral cavity has, however, not yet been determined, although I have several times cultivated a micro-organism from the mouth which, in point of morphology and physiology, seems to be identical with Hueppe's bacterium.

b. Mannite Fermentation.

Mannite fermentation (mucous or gum fermentation) is caused by an exceedingly small coccus (Micrococcus viscosus) which grows in chains in various saccharine beverages, in wine, beer, etc., and in saccharine juices. In consequence of the fermentation these liquids become slimy, viscous (stringy).

The products of fermentation are a kind of gum (viscose), closely resembling dextrine, also mannite and carbonic acid. The optimum of temperature is 30° C. Black[24] observed a similar fermentation, caused by the action of various mouth-bacteria (micrococci) in saccharine solutions. One coccus, occurring in chains, cultivated in peptone bouillon with 2 per cent. of sugar, "gelatinized" the fluid so entirely in twenty-four hours that it did not run out when the tube was inverted. The optimum of temperature was above 100° F. The products of fermentation were not examined. This fermentation, which is most probably a kind of gum fermentation, explains, according to Black, the mucous coating on the teeth and tongue in case of sordes in fever.

c. Dextrane Fermentation.

Dextrane fermentation occurs spontaneously under the action of a micrococcus, Leuconostoc mesenterioïdes, in the juice of the beet and in the molasses of sugar factories, and can also be induced artificially in saccharine solutions. The masses of bacteria (zooglœa) form a jelly of cartilaginous consistency, which completely fills the vessels containing the molasses. The products of fermentation are a jelly-like substance, dextrane and carbonic acid. The optimum of temperature lies between 25°–35° C. As cane-sugar is easily inverted, it serves the purpose of fermentation as well as grape-sugar.

d. Butyric Acid Fermentation.

Few trustworthy observations have been made in regard to the butyric acid fermentation of carbohydrates. The experiments of Fitz, and more recently those of Flügge, have made it appear probable that several species of bacteria are able to cause a fermentation of carbohydrates, in which butyric acid results as

FIG. 6.

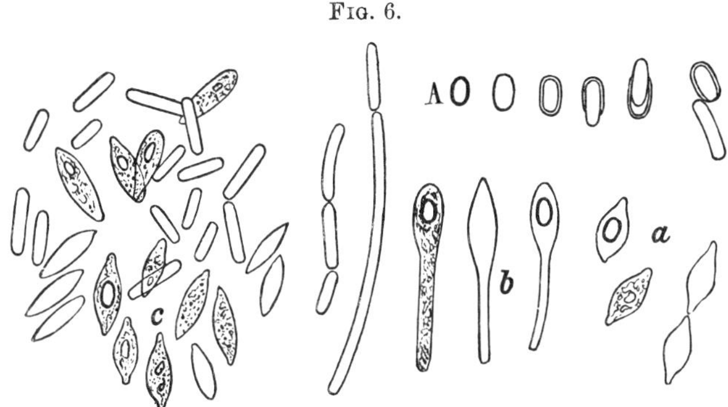

BACILLUS BUTYRICUS.
a, *b*, Tadpole- and Spindle-shapes, partly with spores; *c*, Zooglœa condition. A, Germination of a spore. (After Prazmowski.)

the principal product. These seem to be, for the most part, anaërobic, which makes it difficult to obtain them in pure culture. Butyric acid, as well as lactic acid fermentation, was formerly supposed to be due to the action of a single organism. This bacterium of butyric acid fermentation (Bacillus butyricus, Clostridium butyricum, Vibrion butyrique, etc.), whose morphology, development, etc., have been thoroughly investigated by Prazmowski,[25] appears in form of rods from 2–12μ long and about 1.0μ broad, either single or in long chains, or in zooglœa (Fig. 6); frequently the rods grow out into long threads. During spore-formation the cells exhibit peculiar changes of form; spindle, ellipsoidal, or tadpole shapes appear, which in certain parts attain to a diameter of 2.6μ. (Fig. 6, *a*, *b*.) The plasma of the cells is thereby condensed and becomes highly refractive; the membrane also appears considerably thickened. This change of form is soon followed by the formation of the spores. The Bacillus butyricus is typically anaërobic; access of air impedes or entirely prevents its development and fermentative action.

In solutions of carbohydrates (starch, sugar, dextrine), and of lactates, this micro-organism produces butyric acid under evolution of carbonic acid and hydrogen. The fermentation is most intense when air is excluded; optimum temperature, 35° to 40° C.

The butyric acid fungus shows a peculiar reaction in regard to iodine, which is also incidental to several other bacteria. "Under certain conditions it gives rise to a compound which is colored blue to dark violet by iodine, and which consequently is to be regarded as an analogon of starch." This reaction occurs when the micro-organism is cultivated in solutions of starch, cellulose, glycerine, and lactate of lime, rarely when solutions containing dextrine and sugar are made use of. The young rods are colored blue, the older ones dark violet; some only in scattered transverse zones, others in continuo. The reaction depends also upon the intensity of the fermentation.

The conditions obtaining in some parts of the human mouth are not adverse to the development of the butyric acid bacterium; hitherto, however, no proof has been adduced for the statement, regularly found in hand-books of dentistry, that butyric acid is formed in the oral cavity. In the first place, no micro-organism has as yet been discovered in the mouth which gives rise to this fermentation, nor has any trace of butyric acid ever been detected in it. In regard to this point, however, experiments of a sufficiently exhaustive nature are still wanting.

That butyric acid may be formed in the oral cavity *as a by-product* in lactic acid fermentation, is at least highly probable. The fermentation of a large quantity of saliva and starch yielded about 2.0 c.cm. of lactic acid, and a few drops of a liquid faintly smelling of butyric acid, but the quantity was too small to allow of a more accurate determination.

e. Diverse Fermentations.

Brieger[26] examined a number of bacteria, especially pathogenic, in regard to their products of decomposition. A coccus which occurs in the human fæces always splits 3 per cent. cane- or grape-sugar solutions in the same manner, producing ethyl-alcohol within the short space of twenty-four hours. Traces of acetic acid are also appreciable. A pathogenic bacillus, also found in the fæces, forms in grape-sugar solutions propionic acid, accompanied by minute quantities of acetic acid. The coccus of pneumonia decomposes cane- and grape-sugar solutions into acetic acid, and very minute quantities of formic acid, under evolution of large quantities of carbonic acid. (The solutions had been saturated with freshly precipitated carbonate of lime.)

Typhus bacilli split grape-sugar solutions, or starch, into acetic and lactic acids, and ethyl alcohol. Staphylococcus pyogenes aureus, when cultivated in bouillon containing glycogen (3 : 100) and a quantity of freshly precipitated carbonate of lime, forms very small quantities of organic acids (principally oxalic acid).

Fitz[27] has also observed several carbohydrate fermentations; among others, one in which ethyl alcohol appeared as chief product. As products of milk-sugar fermentation, he found ethyl alcohol and other substances not further determined. Cane-sugar yielded butyl alcohol, butyric acid, and traces of lactic and succinic acids. Starch yielded butyric and acetic acid; inuline, which fermented as easily as starch, gave alcohol and volatile acids.

Boutroux[28] found gluconic acid as a product of the fermentation of milk-sugar.

B. *Fermentation of Polyvalent Alcohols.*

In his communications concerning "schizomycetes fermentations," Fitz has described a number of different fermentations of polyvalent alcohols: glycerine, erythrite, mannite, dulcite, and quercite. Glycerine yielded normal butyl alcohol, with profuse generation of carbonic acid and hydrogen, normal butyric acid, and traces of a higher fatty acid (probably capronic).

A second experiment showed as chief product capronic acid, and as by-products butyric and lactic acids. In other cases of glycerine fermentation Fitz discovered traces of acetic acid, with butyl alcohol as principal product. The Bacillus butyricus fermented glycerine, so that butyric acid, as well as acetic, capronic, and lactic acids, were formed. Different experiments with erythrite yielded alcohol, butyric, acetic, also traces of formic and succinic acids. Mannite yielded butyl and ethyl alcohol, butyric and succinic acids, with a variable quantity of capronic, acetic, lactic, and formic acids. Dulcite gave many volatile and some non-volatile acids; quercite gave normal butyric acid, etc.

Fitz probably employed impure cultures in all his experiments, which would explain the large number of products of fermentation. It is not to be supposed that these fermentations play an important part in the mouth, as the necessary nutrients are not present in sufficient quantities, or in part are altogether wanting.

C. *Fermentation of Fats, Fatty Acids, and Oxyacids.*

Fats exposed to the air soon become rancid, as is well known, and give off a more or less strongly marked odor of fatty acids. This change is due to a decomposition of the fats into glycerine and fatty acid, under the action of micro-organisms.

The following fatty and oxyacids and their salts are also fermentable: formic and acetic acids, lactic acid (oxypropionic acid), glycerinic acid, malic (oxysuccinic) acid, tartaric (dioxysuccinic acid, citric (oxytricarballylic) acid.

Formate of lime yields $CaCO_3$, CO_2, and H;

Acetate of lime yields $CaCO_3$, CO_2, and CH_4.

According to Fitz, lactate of lime undergoes four different fermentations. In the first are formed propionic acid, and as by-products, acetic and succinic acids and alcohol; in the second, propionic and valeric acids; in the third, butyric and propionic acids; in the fourth, butyric acid, with ethyl and butylic alcohol as by-products.

Glycerate of lime produces tartrate of lime, with succinic acid and ethyl alcohol as by-products; according to Fitz, also acetic acid and traces of formic and succinic acids.

Malate of lime also undergoes several kinds of fermentation, forming propionic, butyric, acetic, and lactic acids.

Tartrate of lime yields propionic or butyric acid, and, according to Fitz, alcohol, acetic, and traces of succinic acids.

Finally, citrate of lime yields acetic acid, with ethyl alcohol and succinic acid as by-products. (See Flügge, Micro-organisms, p. 489.)

In accordance with the various fermentative processes specified in the foregoing pages, a particle of starch introduced into the oral cavity would undergo about the following successive changes: In the first place it is, in part at least, transformed into grape-sugar by the diastase of the saliva (ptyaline). This, in turn, is split into lactic acid through the action of various bacteria in the mouth. The lactic acid unites with the lime of the teeth, or tartar, forming lactate of lime. The latter, according to the investigations of Fitz and others just referred to, may then undergo various fermentations, giving rise to new acid products and to the formation of the corresponding lime-salts, from which, by still other processes of fermentation, acids are again derived. The process, however, most probably ceases after the formation of lactate of lime.

D. *Putrefaction.*

When the decomposition of a culture medium is accompanied by the development of stinking, for the most part gaseous products, ammonia, sulphuretted hydrogen (NH_3, SH_2), etc., the process is commonly designated as putrefaction. Albuminous substances are especially liable to putrefaction; also the albuminoids (glue-giving substances), peptones, and lastly, some substances related to the albuminous bodies,—leucine, tyrosine, indol, etc.

It is evident, however, that this definition by no means involves a precise chemical or bacterio-chemical process, and that the presence or absence of stinking gases cannot be made an absolute criterion by which to judge of the real nature of the changes going on in a medium containing bacteria.

The appearance of putrefactive products in any fermentation does not depend alone upon the kind of fermentation and the kind of bacterium, but more especially upon simultaneously occurring processes which have little or nothing whatever to do with the decomposition of the decaying substance. If, for instance, a tooth-pulp decomposes in a closed root-canal, an incredible amount of bad-smelling gas may be formed, so that on opening the pulp-chamber the whole room will be impregnated with the odor. But if a tooth-pulp is allowed to decompose in the open air, hardly any disagreeable smell will be noticed, although the decomposition of the nutrient medium caused by the fungi may be identical in both cases. In the latter case, under free access of air, those products of putrefaction which are accountable for the offensive odor are further decomposed (oxidized) by the oxygen of the air, which is activated by the hydrogen liberated during the process of decomposition; they consequently do not manifest their presence at all. Where, however, the access of air is limited, or the air altogether excluded, the oxidation of these products cannot take place and they escape unchanged from the solution. The products of fermentation remain the same in both cases, but their subsequent fate is different.

A solution of white of egg, infected with saliva and kept at blood temperature, soon gives rise to a stinking smell and an alkaline reaction (NH_3 and SH_2). But upon addition of about 2 per cent. of cane-sugar to a similarly infected solution, no bad smell will be detected; free NH_3 and SH_2 are not evolved; the reaction is acid. Nevertheless, we have no reason to doubt that the white of egg undergoes the same decomposition in both cases.

The products arising from the decomposition of these albuminous substances are very numerous. According to Flügge,[29] they are: carbonic acid, hydrogen, free nitrogen, sulphuretted hydrogen, phosphuretted hydrogen, marsh gas, formic, acetic, butyric, valeric, palmitic, acrylic, crotonic, glycolic, lactic, and valerolactanic acids; oxalic and succinic acids, leucine, glycocoll, glutaminic, asparaginic, and amidostearinic acids; ammonia, carbonate of ammonia, sulphide of ammonia; numerous amine bases, propylamine, trimethylamine, etc.; indol, scatol, scatol-carbonic acid; tyrosine and its derivatives of the aromatic series, and lastly the ptomaïnes.

The large number of acids included in this list does not by

any means justify the assumption that a putrefying mixture must have an acid reaction; this is not the case, for the simultaneously formed basic products are more than sufficient to neutralize the acids, so that the resulting reaction is alkaline. We must further consider that by no means are all of the substances named generated in every process of putrefaction. The number of ascertained putrefactive products of the individual bacteria seldom exceeds six, they being generally stinking gases (H_2S, etc.), ammonia, peptone, trimethylamine, and fatty acids; reaction alkaline.

Ptomaïnes.

This name has been given to certain nitrogenous waste products of bacteria, closely resembling vegetable alkaloids, which are formed in putrefying mixtures. As they were found repeatedly, and at first chiefly in decaying corpses, Selmi called them ptomaïnes (πτῶμα, corpse). According to Brieger, the principal authority on this subject, and upon whose exposition my remarks are based, Panum was the first to isolate a chemical putrid poison, a ptomaïne. The alkaloid of Panum had an action upon the animal body similar to that of snake-poison and curare. Then Schmiedeberg and Bergmann obtained from putrefying yeast a very minute quantity of a substance acting toxically on frogs and dogs, which they called "sepsine." Zuelzer and Sonnenschein isolated a substance from macerated corpses which acted like atropine, and Rörsch and Fasbender one showing properties similar to digitaline.

Furthermore, there were gained from corpses an oil having the odor of propylamine, a substance resembling coniin, "septicine," an amorphous base similar to nicotine, and aqueous extracts with action like that of curare. Selmi obtained non-crystalline products, which, in regard to their reaction and toxic properties, might have been mistaken for morphine, coniine, atropine, or delphinine. A strychnine-like base was also found in putrid maize, and von Nencki[30] obtained in chemically pure condition a ptomaïne isomeric with collidine.

In 1883, Brieger[31] began his experiments with the basic products of putrefaction, which soon proved very successful. From

putrefied meat, fish, glue, and yeast, from old cheese and digesting fibrine, and from pure cultures of pathogenic bacteria, he isolated a large number of ptomaïnes, some of which were found to be non-poisonous, others poisonous in the highest degree. Of the poisonous ptomaïnes, the following are deserving of particular mention:

1. Peptotoxine, gained from fibrin, casein, brain-matter, liver, and muscular tissue.
2. Neurine, from putrefied meat.
3. A base similar to ethylenediamine, from putrefied fish.
4. Muscarine, from the same source.
5. Mydaleïne, and another not distinctly defined ptomaïne, from putrefying parts of corpses.
6. A ptomaïne having toxical effects on guinea-pigs, found in cultures of typhus bacilli on meat-pap, which did not present any of the characteristic symptoms of putrefaction; also another poison called typhotoxicon.
7. Tetanin, from cultures containing principally tetanus bacilli. This base, which is formed along with profuse quantities of ammonia, produced the same symptoms in mice, frogs, and guinea-pigs, which accompany tetanus in man.

The following ptomaïnes were designated as non-poisonous:

1. Neuridine, in putrefying cheese, meat, and glue.
2. Gadinine, in putrefying fish.

3–6. Cadaverine, putrescine, saprine, choline, in putrefying parts of corpses.

Brieger furthermore isolated a non-poisonous base from cultures of Staphylococcus pyogenes aureus on meat-pap. Pure cultures of Streptococcus pyogenes yielded, besides the normal components of meat (xanthine, etc.), especially large quantities of trimethylamine.

Vaughan[32] isolated a poisonous alkaloid, which he called tyrotoxicon, from a cheese which had occasioned extensive poisoning, as well as from the milk and cream used in the preparation of vanilla ice-cream, which had also proved poisonous.

The question now arises whether the products which may possibly be formed in an unclean mouth can exert any deleterious influence on the mucous membrane of the oral cavity, or upon the general state of health, and whether the alkaloids which doubtless form in putrid pulps have any irritating action upon the peridental tissues. The fact, established by Odenthal, that glandular swellings in the region of the lower jaw occur especially as concomitants of dental caries, seems to justify the assumption that the resorption of the putrefactive products attending the decomposition of a tooth-pulp is an important agent in the above-named disturbance.

E. *Oxidation of Alcohol to Acetic Acid.*

The exciting cause of acetic acid fermentation, the vinegar fungus (Mycoderma aceti), usually appears in the form of cocci, or diplococci, either singly or in chains (Fig. 7). According to Hansen,[33] Zopf, and others, it also grows in rod and leptothrix forms. The formation of very long chains and so-called involuted forms is specially characteristic of the vinegar fungus (Fig. 7, *a*). It grows best at 30° to 35° C., and forms a covering or pellicle on the surface of fermenting liquids, which attains a thickness of 50 to 100 mm. The cells of this fungus transfer the oxygen of the air to the medium, and thus possess the specific faculty of oxidizing the alcohol in fermented liquors to acetic acid; $C_2H_5, OH + O_2 = CH_3, COOH + H_2O$. The fermentation takes place most rapidly when a minute quantity of acetic acid (1 to 2 per cent.) is already present. More than 10 per cent. prevents the continuance of the fermentation; under 10° C. and over 35° C. the formation of acetic acid ceases. The deficiency of alcohol and the high temperature render the occurrence of the specific acetous fermentation in the mouth highly improbable.

Fig. 7

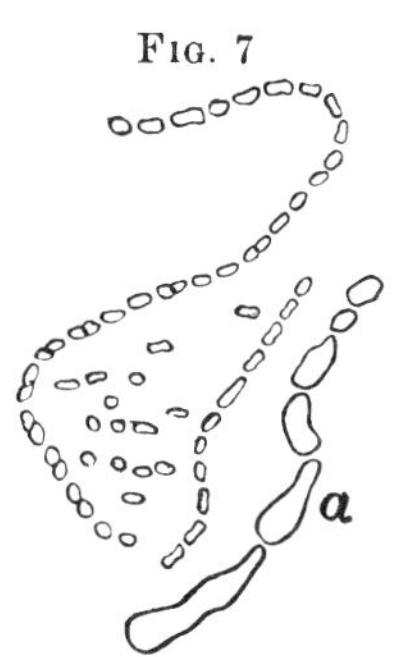

Bacterium of Acetic Acid Fermentation (Mycoderma aceti). *a*, Involution forms.

An oxidation of alcohol to acetic acid also occurs in a certain degree when alcohol is exposed to the air on large surfaces (wood shavings); also when the oxygen is transferred to the alcohol by means of sponge platinum. For obvious reasons this process does not occur in the mouth.

F. *Ammoniacal Fermentation.*

Various bacteria, Ascococcus Billrothii, Micrococcus ureæ, Bacillus ureæ, etc., occasion a fermentation of urea leading to the formation of carbonate of ammonia, and imparting an intensely alkaline reaction to the solution. W. Leube and E. Greser[34] obtained pure cultures of four different bacteria which have the power to decompose urea. Two of them, a small bacillus (Bacterium ureæ) and a coccus (Micrococcus ureæ), showed intense urea-decomposing properties. The other two possessed this property in a less marked degree. Lungsarcina also effected an intense decomposition of urea.

G. *Nitrification and Denitrification.*

Finally, certain processes of oxidation and reduction which take place in the soil have been found to be due to the presence of micro-organisms, and must consequently be classed under fermentations. Schlösing and Müntz[35] established this fact for the case of natural nitrification, which, according to their experiments, must be regarded as a process of fermentation, resulting from the action of a specific micro-organism. In their experiments they used filtered and sterilized drainage-water (l'eau d'égout), or weak alkaline solutions containing mineral substances, a salt of ammonia, and organic matter. When these solutions were sterilized, infected with soil and exposed to the air, a nitrate-forming fermentation ensued, which was occasioned by very small oblong microbes (ferment nitrique). Continuous exclusion of air destroyed the ferment nitrique; it occurs very extensively, but was not found in the atmosphere.

The conditions for the consummation of this process are (1) access of oxygen, (2) a certain degree of humidity, (3) weak alkalinity, and (4) the presence of organic matter. Below 5° C. nitrification proceeds very slowly; at a higher temperature the intensity of the fermentation increases, until 37° C. is reached, which represents the maximum. At a still higher temperature it decreases rapidly, and at 50° C. (!) yields but minute quantities of nitrates.

On the other hand, Gayon and Dupetit[36] found four different microbes which reduced nitrates, sometimes to nitrites, sometimes to ammonia, nitrogen, and nitrous oxide (denitrification.)

Drainage-water, to which saltpetre was added (0.02 to 1 litre), infected with spoiled urine, showed a gradual decrease of the nitrate under development of numerous microbes.

When the culture was sterilized, or chloroform, or any other antiseptic added to it, no process of reduction took place. The presence of organic matter and a limited access of air were the conditions of fermentation. The optimum of temperature was found to lie between 35° and 40° C.

Salicylic acid, in antiseptic doses, did not impede the process of reduction, but soon disappeared itself. Nitrates of sodium, ammonium, and calcium were reduced in the same way as nitrates of potassium. Dehérain and Maquenne[37] obtained similar results. Their first experiment yielded the following figures for one hundred parts of the gas formed:

CO_2	80.5
N_2O	8.2
N	11.3

The second experiment yielded—

CO_2	67.3
H	31.5
N	1.2

These processes of oxidation and reduction have also recently been observed in pure cultures.

It appears from Heraeus's[38] investigations that they may be occasioned by a large number of different species of bacteria. He made experiments with several known kinds, and also with twelve unknown kinds, which he cultivated from water, soil, etc. Of the latter, two reduced nitric acid to nitrous acid and ammonia, and converted urea into carbonate of ammonia. Two consumed nitric acid without reduction; one of them transforming urea into salts of ammonia, the other not. None of these twelve varieties manifested any oxidizing influence. Heraeus succeeded, however, in isolating, from garden soil, two species which led to the formation of nitrous acid in saccharine solutions, in urine, etc.

The following well-known species also showed the power of oxidation: Micrococcus (Bacillus) prodigiosus, typhus and anthrax bacilli, Finkler-Prior's and Denecke's spirilla, Staphylococcus citreus. Brieger's and Miller's bacteria yielded inconstant results. Contrary to Schlösing and Müntz, Heraeus found these organisms in the atmosphere also. The latter declares Pasteur's "anaërobium" to be untenable; there are, on the contrary, bacteria which call forth reductions under all circumstances, as well as those which occasion oxidations.

Wherever bacteria find a favorable nutrient medium, in concentrated urine, saccharine solutions, meat-juices,—that is, wherever there are large quantities of organic matter,—the reducing bacteria will preponderate; but wherever the condition of the nutrient medium prevents rapid proliferation, the oxidizing bacteria will gain the ascendency.

Warrington[39] was able to note only a reduction of nitrates to nitrites; gaseous products did not appear. His experiments with artificial mixtures showed but minute traces of nitrification.

Fresh corpses, imbedded in powdered charcoal, are said not to putrefy, but to decay in such a way that after several months only bones and fat remain, while the charcoal contains a quantity of nitric acid.[40] We probably have here to do with a process similar to or identical with nitrification, the oxygen condensed in the charcoal taking the place of the atmospheric air. The question whether these processes occur in the human mouth will be discussed in Chapter V. It appears to me not at all improbable that the appearance of nitrous acid in the oral cavity is due to the reduction of nitrates.

2. *Chromogenic Bacteria.*

Many kinds of bacteria occasion so-called pigment fermentations in which coloring-matter is produced; green, red, and yellow colors predominate, brown, blue, and violet being of less frequent occurrence. The colors sometimes appear in the membrane or protoplasm of the cells, which is usually the case with bacteria that form yellow coloring-matter. More frequently, only the culture medium becomes colored, the cells remaining colorless. This is the case with all bacteria that form green coloring matter, with the exception, perhaps, of Bacterium chlorinum (Engelmann) and Bacillus virens (van Tieghem). Access of atmospheric air is essential to the production of pigment fermentation.

H. Kronecker first called attention to a liquefying bacillus whose cultures in bouillon showed no color when the access of air was limited, but when shaken with air an intensely green color instantly appeared. I have noted a similar result in the case of other bacteria. Liborius[41] proved for a large number of pigment bacteria "that all these coloring-matters are formed only where there is free access of air."

Chromogenic bacteria are widely distributed in nature. When a plate of nutritive agar-agar is exposed to the air for some time, and then kept in a moist chamber, colonies of various kinds of chromogenic bacteria generally develop upon it. They have their representatives among the pathogenic, as well as the non-pathogenic organisms.

Fig. 8.

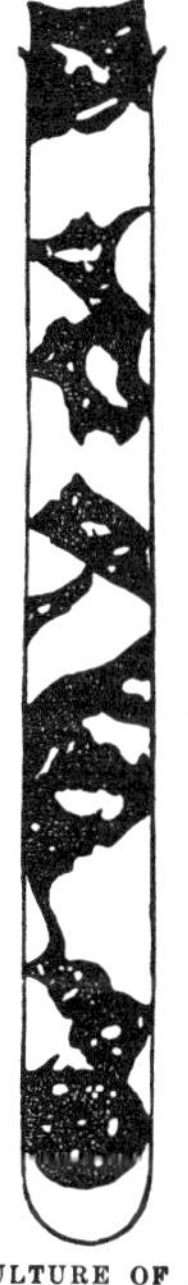

Culture of a Gas-forming Bacterium from the Stomach, in Bread-Sugar Gelatine. One day old. ½ : 1.

3. *Aërogenic Bacteria.*

Various kinds of gases, CO_2, H, N, SH_2, CH_4, NH_3, etc., are often formed as waste products of bacteria, as well as of fungi in general. According to Flügge, the functional activity of the lower fungi must always be accompanied by the development of CO_2. Nevertheless the quantity of CO_2 evolved from many cultures is excessively small, and is to be considered as a product of intermolecular respiration only (see also page 20).

In fermentations of carbohydrates, lactic and butyric acid, mannite and cellulose fermentations, and various others, CO_2, H, and CH_4 are principally or exclusively formed, the former often in such quantities that the course of the fermentation is exceedingly violent (Fig. 8).

The fermentation of albuminous substances (putrefaction) is

accompanied by the development of CO_2, H, N, SH_2, PH_3, CH_4, NH_3. In cellulose fermentations CO_2, H, and CH_4, in alcohol fermentations CO_2 and H are produced.

The formation of gas occasions manifold disorders in the human stomach and intestinal tract. In putrefying pulps it is the frequent cause of periostitis and abscess formation, since the gases generated force their way through the apical foramen or even carry particles of the putrid pulp along with them, thereby causing a severe irritation of the pericementum.

4. *Saprogenic Bacteria* (*Bacteria of Putrefaction*).

This term has been applied to such bacteria as are endowed with intense putrefactive properties. They occur among the saprophytes, as well as among the parasites. Many pathogenic bacteria possess saprogenic properties; thus, for example, Bacillus saprogenes (I, II, III), Bacillus pyogenes fœtidus, Brieger bacillus, etc. The cause of putrefaction lies in the faculty possessed by many, if not by most, bacteria, of decomposing albuminous substances in such a manner as to give rise to characteristic products of decomposition. (See Putrefaction, page 27.)

CHAPTER II.

NUTRIENT MEDIA FOR BACTERIA IN THE ORAL CAVITY.

THE organic and inorganic substances found in the mouth, which may serve as nutriment for micro-organisms, are the following:

1. Normal saliva.
2. Buccal mucus.
3. Dead epithelium.
4. Dental tissue softened by acids.
5. Exposed pulps.
6. Exudations of the gums, conditioned by the irritation of tartar, etc.
7. Accumulation of particles of food.

1. SALIVA.

Normal, human, mixed saliva is a colorless liquid, usually slightly clouded by epithelium; it is more or less slimy, slippery, and viscous, differing with different individuals. Normally the submaxillary and sublingual glands furnish a viscous secretion, whereas that of the parotid is more dilute. In healthy persons it has a weak alkaline or neutral reaction; its specific gravity is 1.002 to 1.006. Under the conditions mentioned in Chapter VIII, the reaction frequently becomes acid. If kept standing, especially at blood temperature, it will putrefy sooner or later, according to the amount of organic matter it contains; in the presence of starch or sugar no real putrefaction takes place, but a process of fermentation ensues, giving rise to an acid reaction and sour smell, accompanied by the formation of carbonic acid.

The analysis of C. Schmidt and Jacubowitsch[42] gives the following chemical ingredients of human saliva:

Water	995.16
Soluble organic substances	1.34
Epithelium	1.62
Sulphocyanide of potassium	0.06
Chloride of calcium (KCl) and chloride of sodium (NaCl)	0.84
Other inorganic salts	0.98
	1000.00

The composition of the saliva of such animals as have been particularly studied with reference to this point, differs essentially from that of human beings. According to Ellenberger and Hofmeister, the parotid saliva contains in 1000 parts:

a. in horses:	
Water	991.613
Dry substance	8.387
Organic substance	2.429
Mineral salts	5.958
Salts soluble in water	4.580
ClNa	2.364
CO_3 alkali	1.775
Phosphates of the alkalies and sulphates	0.441
$CaCO_3$ insoluble in water	1.378

b. in cows:	
Water	990.000
Dry substance	10.000
Organic substance	0.400
Mineral salts	9.600
Salts soluble in water	9.550
ClNa	0.440
CO_3 alkali	7.460
Sulphates and phosphates of alkalies	1.650
$CaCO_3$ insoluble in water	0.050

The great amount of carbonate of the alkalies is specially noteworthy; it imparts a strong alkaline reaction to animal saliva, and is well calculated to neutralize such acids as may be formed in the animal mouth, thus tending to prevent the appearance of caries.

Ellenberger and Hofmeister[43, 44] have carefully examined the saliva of various animals (domestic mammals). According to their researches, all the glands of the oral cavity of horses, cattle, sheep, pigs, and dogs contain a ferment which converts starch-paste into sugar and dextrine, while soluble modifications of starch appear as intermediate stages. The saliva of cattle, sheep, dogs, rabbits, etc., as well as that of horses and cows, differs essentially from human saliva, in the strong alkaline reaction.

The inorganic ingredients (salts) contained in human saliva are, besides chloride of potassium and chloride of sodium, combinations of carbonic and phosphoric acids with calcium, potassium, natrium, and magnesium, calcium and natrium carbonate preponderating (Hoppe-Seyler). Clear saliva exposed to the air becomes cloudy through the precipitation of carbonate of lime (Hoppe-Seyler), a fact which should be borne in mind in any attempt to account for the formation of *tartar*. Human saliva also contains slight traces of a nitrous compound, as is shown by the appearance of a blue color upon adding saliva slightly acidified with very dilute sulphuric acid to a dilute solution of iodide of potassium containing starch. The presence of nitrites in the human saliva is probably to be accounted for by a reduction of the nitrates introduced into the mouth with food and drink.

If human saliva from an unclean mouth be acidified with muriatic acid, and a small quantity of chloride of iron added, a beautiful red color almost always appears, which indicates a compound of sulphocyanogen. The manner in which this compound is formed in the human mouth is unknown. It has been supposed to have some connection with carious teeth, or, according to others, with smoking; the latter view is unquestionably erroneous, for I have repeatedly found the above-mentioned combination in the mouths of non-smokers.

The human saliva, as may be readily seen from the analysis, is very poor in organic ingredients. It contains traces of an albuminous substance which is coagulated by heat, also invariably a small quantity of mucine; in the saliva of dogs 0.662–2.604 grams were found in 1000 (Hoppe-Seyler). Consequently, the saliva turns slightly yellow when boiled with nitric acid, changing to orange upon the addition of an alkali. The addition of sulphate of copper ($CuSO_4$) and caustic potash (KHO) produces a violet color. Alcohol, acetic acid, etc., cause a white flaky or fibrous precipitate.

Lastly, human saliva invariably contains a diastatic ferment, called ptyaline, which is identical with that found in the secretion of the pancreatic glands, in the juices of the stomach and intestines, in blood-corpuscles, in the liver, in the secretion of the tonsils, etc. This ferment also occurs in the saliva of guinea-pigs and rabbits, rarely in that of dogs (Hoppe-Seyler); Roux[45] failed to detect it in the saliva of horses. Ellenberger and Hofmeister, on the other hand, invariably found ptyaline in the saliva of dogs and horses.

Through the action of ptyaline, starch is converted into dextrine and a kind of sugar (called ptyalose by Nasse), which is directly fermentable and has the property of reducing the oxide of copper. The process of saccharification begins instantly, so that it is immaterial for the ensuing fermentation whether the saliva be mixed with starch or with sugar. Theoretically, the acid reaction would set in at the same time and with equal intensity in both cases. Indeed, it seems as if saliva mixed with starch ferments not only sooner, but also forms a larger quantity of acid than sugar. (See Chapter VIII.)

Ptyaline is able to convert comparatively large, though not unlimited, quantities of amylum into sugar. In an experiment made by Krüger, 4.672 grams of amylum were converted into ptyalose by 1 gram of pancreatic juice, within the space of thirty minutes. Now, since 1 gram of pancreatic juice contains only 0.014 of organic matter, of which, again, the ferment represents but a small fraction, it is evident that 1 gram of the ferment can transform a multiple of 314 grams of amylum into sugar in half an hour. Ptyaline differs from the vegetable diastase, (1) in the dissimilarity in the sugars formed; in the latter case, not ptyalose, but maltose, is produced; (2) in respect to the very different temperatures at which the ferments are most active, ptyaline acting most rapidly at 35° to 40° C., vegetable diastase at 70° C.

A sufficient quantity of pure saliva for the purpose of experimentation may be obtained, after very thoroughly cleansing the teeth and entire oral cavity, by placing a crystal of muriate of cocaine upon the back of the tongue or by painting the surface of the tongue and cheeks with sulphuric ether. If the mouth is then held wide open over a glass or porcelain vessel, the saliva will flow out in clear thin drops from the parotid or in long, viscous streams from the sublingual and submaxillary glands. Saliva thus obtained is but slightly clouded, but forms a white precipitate when left standing. If a small quantity of this precipitate be placed upon an object-glass in a drop of water, covered with a cover-glass and a small drop of dilute sulphuric acid allowed to flow underneath, a formation of gas-bubbles will be observed (CO_2), while under 20 to 40 diameters the needles characteristic of sulphate of lime will appear. By means of molybdate of ammonia, phosphoric acid may also be easily detected in this precipitate. The latter, therefore, consists partly of carbonates and partly of phosphates (lime-salts), and sufficiently explains the formation of tartar. There is, consequently, no need of having recourse to the theory, which for various reasons is untenable, that tartar consists of the calcareous remains of bacteria.

Pure saliva exposed to the air undergoes putrefaction, not as rapidly, however, as is generally asserted in text-books of physiology; on the contrary, sometimes very slowly, so that no bad smell may be detected before several days have elapsed. Only when the saliva is mixed with organic matter from the mouth does it soon show marked signs of putrefaction.

This may be easily understood when we take into consideration the fact that human saliva contains only about 0.15 per cent. of organic matter, and is, therefore, but a very indifferent culture medium for bacteria, since experience has taught that a good culture medium must contain a much greater quantity of organic matter. As before mentioned, if sugar is added to the saliva no sign of putrefaction will appear, but a fermentation takes place which engenders an acid reaction and a sour smell.

The view, entertained by many dentists, that saliva possesses antiseptic properties, seems to me to be unfounded. Those constituents of human saliva which have antiseptic properties are present in too small quantities to be able in any way to impede the development of bacteria. The fact that the human mouth is so favorable a place of habitation for so many kinds of bacteria, is of itself sufficient to prove the absolute incongruity of such an idea. What would we think of a man who would put a piece of meat in saliva, in the hope of keeping it from decay? The comparative rarity of diseases of the gums, in spite of the large number of bacteria in the mouth, is due, not to the antiseptic action of the saliva, but to the great power of resistance of the gums, and to their comparative unsusceptibility to infectious agents. It is well known that in removing tartar from badly kept teeth we often wound the gums with impunity, in a manner which on other parts of the body would be very likely to lead to a serious infection.

2. The Buccal Mucus.

The secretion of the mucus-glands of the mouth is identical with the mucus secreted by the submaxillary and sublingual glands, which gives the saliva of these glands its viscous and slippery character.

Hermann[46] calls the mucus "a clear, slimy, viscous *alkaline* fluid"; according to others, it has an *acid* reaction; most probably the reaction of mucus, as well as of saliva, is subject to variations dependent upon the general state of health. (See also Chapter VIII.)

It is so difficult to obtain a pure secretion of the mucus-glands, that the method proposed by Kirk[47] seems to be the only means of determining the reaction with any degree of certainty, for a large number of cases. Mucus mixes with water without being dissolved, is equally insoluble in alcohol, ether, chloroform, and dilute mineral acids; soluble, on the other hand, in dilute alkalies and excess of mineral acids. It does not coagulate when boiled, belongs to the albuminoids, and serves as a nutrient for bacteria.

3. Dead Epithelial Cells.

These cells, for the most part from the surface of the mucous membrane, form a flaky precipitate in saliva left standing, or are deposited, mixed with mucus and particles of food, upon the teeth, particularly in places which are not exposed to the friction of mastication. Under the microscope they appear as flat, irregular, many-sided cells, which are frequently covered with bacteria, especially in vitiated or spoiled saliva (Fig. 9). The fact that these cells are often found in a state of partial destruction by bacteria would seem to indicate that they form a not unfavorable nutrient for certain kinds at least, a view which is also supported by the chemical analysis.

Fig 9.

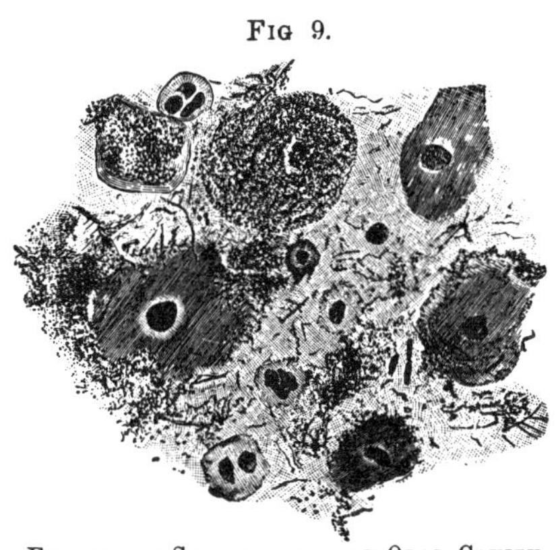

Epithelial Scales from the Oral Cavity.
Partly destroyed by cocci. Ca. 500 : 1.

4. Tooth-Cartilage.

The organic matrix of dentine belongs to the glue-giving substances. When decalcified dentine is boiled for any length of time, a gelatinous material is obtained, which solidifies on cooling.

Dry gelatine from dentine forms an odorless and colorless, or faintly yellowish mass, like bone-glue, which swells up in cold water, dissolves easily in hot, but is insoluble in alcohol and ether. At blood temperature dentine gelatine, like other gluey substances, is easily decomposed by bacteria, and my personal experience has shown it to be a good medium for culture experiments.

5. The Dental Pulp.

On account of its delicate structure and the abundance of blood, the dental pulp presents an exceedingly favorable nutrient medium, and therefore very easily putrefies. By means of a dead pulp spontaneous inoculations (auto-infections) readily occur, from which very dangerous local or general poisonings may result.

6. Exudations of the Gums.

The gums, when irritated by accumulations of tartar or food, or by sharp edges, protruding fillings, roots, etc., furnish particularly favorable conditions of nutrition for certain species of bacteria. The apparently strictly obligatory parasitic bacteria of the mouth, Spirochæte dentium and Spirillum sputigenum, find here the peculiar conditions essential to their development. It is a very interesting fact, and one showing what a powerful influence the nature of the culture medium may have upon the growth of bacteria, that though numberless attempts have been made to construct a culture medium adapted to the wants of these bacteria, they have all signally failed, so exactly must the natural conditions be imitated before they can be induced to grow.

7. Accumulation of Particles of Food.

The chief source of nutrition for the oral bacteria is, however, furnished by the particles of food collecting between the teeth, or in fissures, depressions, cavities of decay, etc., or adhering even to their free surfaces. These, consisting chiefly of albuminous substances and carbohydrates, mixed with the other nutrient matter mentioned under 1 to 6, present an almost perfect culture medium for bacteria.

After these introductory remarks, we shall now proceed to the study of the bacteria of the human mouth, a subject which has justly attracted a vast deal of attention in dental, as well as in medical circles, within the last few years.

CHAPTER III.

THE DEVELOPMENT OF THE STUDY OF MICRO-ORGANISMS IN THE ORAL CAVITY.

THE celebrated Dutch scientist, Leeuwenhoek,[48] was the first to observe that microscopically small organisms exist in the human mouth in great numbers. In a treatise bearing the date 1683, he gives descriptions and diagrams of several kinds of bacteria from the mouth, which show that the inferiority of his instruments compared with those now in use did not prevent his obtaining a very fair view, particularly of Spirillum sputigenum. In spite of the utmost care which Leeuwenhoek bestowed upon the teeth and oral cavity, "*quo fit, ut dentes mei adeo puri maneant et candidi, ut paucos mihi coætaneos hoc pacto raro videas, nec gingivæ meæ . . . unquam sanguinem emittant,*" he was nevertheless able to detect five different kinds of animalcula in a certain white matter between the teeth. "*Ac fere semper magna cum admiratione vidi dictæ illi materiæ inesse multa exigua admodum animalcula jucundissimo modo se moventia.*"

FIG. 10.

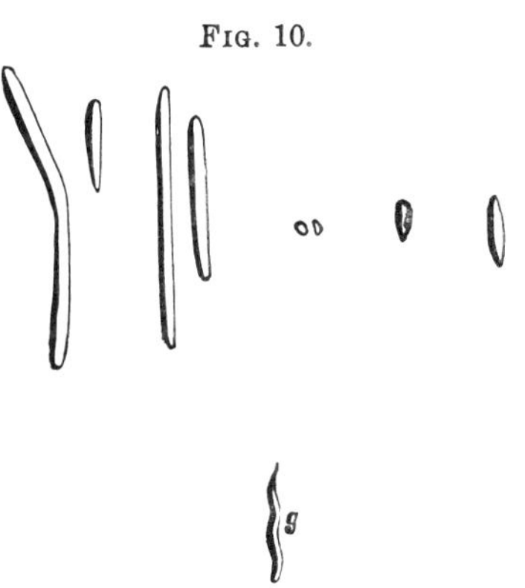

"ANIMALCULA" FROM THE MOUTH.
g, Spirillum sputigenum.
(After Leeuwenhoek.)

Leeuwenhoek's diagrams are reproduced in Fig. 10. The micro-organism marked *g* will immediately be recognized as the Spirillum sputigenum, now so well known. While conversing with an old man, Leeuwenhoek noticed the rather deplorable condition of his teeth and asked him when he had last brushed them, to which the latter replied that he was not in the habit of brushing his teeth at all. Leeuwenhoek, who never allowed any opportunity to pass by unheeded, immediately made the request to be allowed to make an examination of the old man's saliva and of the greasy deposit ("materia alba") upon his teeth. In this deposit he found so many animalcula, "*ut tota aqua vivere videatur.*" This observation agrees perfectly with our present knowledge as to the occurrence of mobile bacteria (Spirillum sputigenum, etc.) in the oral cavity.

Lebeaume compared tartar, as the breeding-place and habitation of these animalcula, to coral formations. Mandl[49] supposes tartar to form through the accumulations of the calcareous remains of vibrios, which he describes as rod-vibrios. Heat, spirituous liquors, and muriatic acid were found to destroy them.

Bühlmann[50] observed the thread-forming bacteria of the mouth and called them simply fibers, without expressing any definite opinion concerning their animal or vegetable nature.

Henle[51] was the first to give expression to the view that these buccal organisms were of a vegetable nature.

Erdl[52] (1843) treated carious teeth with muriatic acid, thereby loosening from the crown of the tooth a delicate, colorless membrane, composed of cells, which, in his opinion, is of a parasitic nature (*vide* Chapter VI).

A considerable advance in the study of the micro-organisms of the human mouth, as well as of the mouths of various domestic animals, was made by Ficinus,[53] a physician of Dresden, from whose dissertation on this subject the following passage is taken: "If a small quantity of the yellowish-white slimy substance found upon every tooth is brought under the microscope, fibers of a peculiar nature will be found, which have already been mentioned by Leeuwenhoek and drawn by Bühlmann. Between these lie dense masses of very small granules, epithelial cells, and mucus corpuscles. Occasionally a few infusoria, which have accidentally entered the mouth with food and drink, move across the field of vision. The interstices remaining between the masses of granular substance, when examined under high power and by good light (particularly on addition of a little water or saliva), afford the surprising revelation of a large number of small roundish, or oblong bodies, which wander about with lively, rotatory movements. Only when their motion abates, particularly when they arrive at objects which afford them nutriment, can their shape be more accurately distinguished.

"In the contraction in the middle of the body a lip-like protuberance may sometimes be observed, which I suppose to be the mouth, since it guides the organism in its approach to objects. It is, therefore, a hairless, probably also mailed, infusorium with an abdominal aperture, whose exterior is not unlike that of the paramæcium and the kolpoda."

FIG. 11.

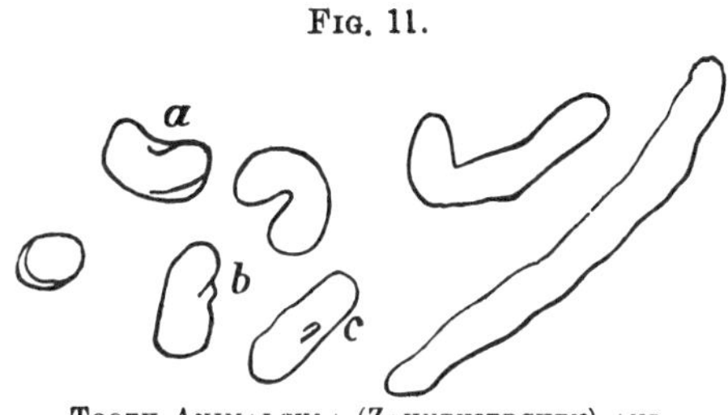

TOOTH-ANIMALCULA (ZAHNTHIERCHEN) AND BÜHLMANN'S FIBERS.
a, b, c, Zahnthierchen with abdominal aperture.
(After Klencke.)

Ficinus proposed for these animalcula the generic name Denticola.

Robin[54, 55] (1847) called them Leptothrix buccalis, and classed them among the algæ.

Klencke[56] continued the researches of Bühlmann and Ficinus, and furnished us with drawings of these tooth-animalcula (Zahnthierchen), as well as of the denticolæ or fibers of Bühlmann, supposed to be produced by the coalition of the animalcula. They are reproduced in Fig. 11. These diagrams are also interesting, because they exemplify the great influence which a preconceived notion may exert upon what is seen under the microscope. Klencke had learned from Ficinus that the tooth-animalcula presumably possessed an abdominal aperture (Fig. 11, *a*, *b*, *c*), and he consequently, not doubting the correctness of Ficinus's observation, saw it very distinctly.

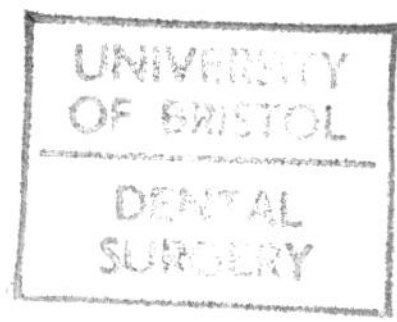

METHODS OF BACTERIOLOGICAL INVESTIGATION.

It was not my design, when I began the preparation of this book, to present even a summary of the various methods employed in bacteriological investigations. These have become so numerous within the last few years that an exhaustive treatment of the subject is a work of itself, and must be sought in treatises devoted to that alone. For these reasons I passed over this important matter in the German edition, with a bare mention. Since, however, some have expressed disappointment at this omission, I have concluded to present in this edition a brief summary of the most important methods now in use. This task I now undertake all the more willingly, because I am convinced that some of my readers in the dental and medical professions may in this way obtain a certain knowledge of the methods of bacteriological experimentation, which they would not do if they were obliged to consult a separate work for that purpose, and furthermore, because for every one, a knowledge of at least the fundamental principles of research very much facilitates the ready understanding of the results obtained by them. I must repeat, however, that it is only the most important and most commonly used methods that I propose briefly to consider here. In the first place, let me say that there is at present no science which opens up so broad and fruitful fields of study, and is so accessible to every one, as the science of bacteriology. Of course, we often find ourselves confronted by an apparently insoluble problem; but on the whole the study of bacteriology compared with that of chemistry is, we may almost say, child's play. This is testified to by the fact that a course of six weeks usually suffices to put one in possession of nearly all the important methods of bacteriological research. The application of the methods, however, sometimes involves an immense amount of time, and hard, patient labor.

Definitions of a Few Terms used in the Following Pages.

Agar-agar: the name given to various algæ growing on the coast of the East Indian archipelago, particularly Gracilaria lichenoïdes, Euchema spinosum, Gigartina speciosa, etc., which on boiling with water yield a jelly that solidifies at temperatures above that of the human body.

Platinum needle: a piece of platinum wire, about two and one-half inches long, with one end melted into the end of a glass rod (Fig. 12).

Fig. 12.

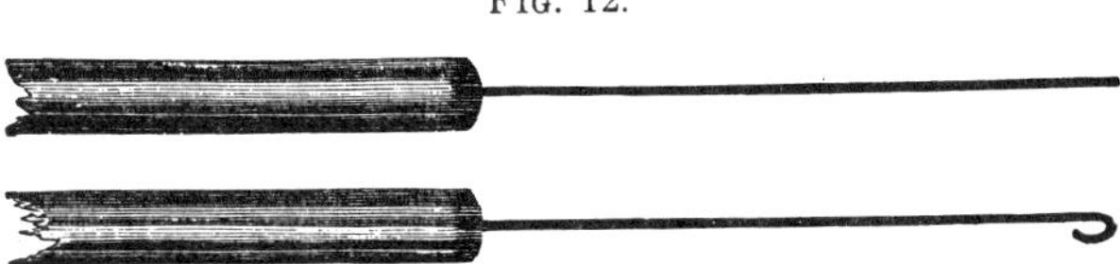

Platinum Needles.

Damp chamber: a shallow glass vessel whose bottom is covered by a piece of wet bibulous paper, and over which a second somewhat larger vessel is inverted (Fig. 13, *b*); or the arrangement illustrated in Fig. 13, *a*, may be used. Damp chambers may, however, be constructed of almost any two vessels,—for example, of two soup-plates.

Colony: a cryptogamous growth on the surface of, or within a layer of solid nutritive material, proceeding from one cell and

Fig. 13 *a*. Fig. 13 *b*.

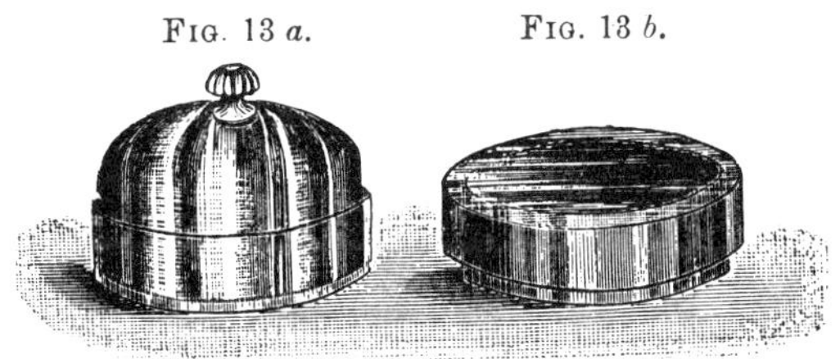

Damp Chambers.

consisting of a number of cells, varying from a few to myriads. The larger colonies are plainly visible to the naked eye, and their color, form, structure, density, etc., furnish a ready means for distinguishing between different kinds of micro-organisms without the aid of the microscope, or often when even the microscope fails to furnish the necessary information.

Apparatus.

The accessories absolutely necessary for beginning work in bacteriology are very few and inexpensive. I began work with an outfit which cost about twenty dollars (of course not including microscope), and gradually added one instrument after another.

For one hundred and twenty-five dollars a laboratory may be furnished with about all the apparatus necessary for carrying on extensive general work, including the incubator and microtome, but not the microscope.

Following is a list of the most essential apparatus:

1. A microscope. I would recommend those who are anxious to obtain a microscope at the least possible momentary expense by all means to procure a good stand, with two objectives of low power, and the necessary oculars to give a magnification of 200 to 300 diameters. With these one may carry on a very extensive series of bacteriological investigations; in fact, with help of the methods of pure culture, one can accomplish very much without a microscope at all.

When, however, the question of the morphology and mode of development of bacteria, or their distribution in tissues, etc., is to be considered, an oil-immersion lens will be necessary (price $25 to $150). It is poor policy to buy a cheap stand, because it will soon be out of order, and when subsequently one wishes to complete the apparatus by adding new lenses, etc., it will be found inadequate, and will have to be thrown away.

2. An incubator: zinc, $12.50; copper, $35 to $100.
3. A hot-air sterilizer for glass plates, etc., $6.
4. A steam sterilizer (Koch's Dampfcylinder), $6.
5. A spiral burner (automatic), $5.
6. A thermo regulator, $5 to $10.
7. A microtome with freezing arrangement (complete), $30.
8. Two gas-burners, $2.
9. Two dozen glass plates and benches, $1.50.
10. Six damp chambers, $3.
11. Leveling apparatus, for pouring cultures (complete), $4.

This apparatus consists of a tripod supported by three screws, two shallow glass vessels, one slightly smaller, resting upon three corks placed upon the bottom of the larger, a perfectly plane glass cover, and a spirit-level. In use, the glass cover is first adjusted and made perfectly horizontal by the help of the spirit-level and tripod; it is then removed, and the inner vessel filled with cold (iced) water and the cover replaced. The outer vessel acts simply as a receiver for the excess of water in the inner. A small glass plate placed upon the cover is not only horizontal, but is also cooled, so that in pouring the gelatine upon it there is no

FIG. 14.

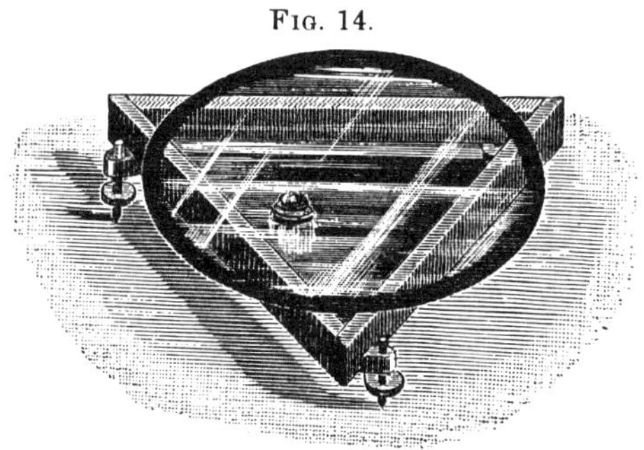

LEVELING APPARATUS.
For pouring culture-materials.

danger of its running off at one side. For pouring agar-agar the simpler form of the apparatus represented in Fig. 14 should be used.

12. A pair of scales (0.1–20.0 grams), a water-bath, one dozen small glass dishes and watch-glasses, one dozen Petri'sche Schalen (miniature damp chambers), measuring-glass, pipette, test tubes, bottles of various size for holding preparations, also some with ground stoppers for staining materials, a wash-bottle, object- and cover-glasses, a few hollow object-glasses for drop-cultures, various-sized porcelain evaporating-dishes, two platinum needles, brushes, spatula, filters, filter-paper, cotton, wire baskets for culture-tubes, scissors, pincers; further, for inoculation experiments, a sterilizable syringe, two vaccination-needles, mice-cages, etc.

The principal reagents made use of in staining bacteria are absolute alcohol, aniline water,* cedar oil, oil of cloves, Gram's solution (iodine 1, iodide of potassium 2, distilled water 300), various staining materials, of which the most important are

* A saturated solution of aniline oil in water, made by thoroughly shaking four parts aniline in one hundred parts water, then filtering.

fuchsine, methylene blue, methyl violet, gentian violet, vesuvine (in concentrated alcoholic solutions, to be diluted on using), bismarck brown (aqueous solution).

In preparing tissues for examination, naturally the various hardening, fixing, decalcifying, imbedding, and mounting solutions may be required which are used in general histological work, although most tissues may be cut and stained with excellent results in the simple manner described in connection with the preparation of decayed dentine. For staining tissues, picro-carmine and picro-lithio-carmine receive the preference.

Pure Culture.

By a pure culture we understand a cryptogamous growth in which only one kind of micro-organism is represented. For example, a culture containing only cells which belong in the developmental cyclus of the tubercle bacillus, is a pure culture of that bacillus. As soon, however, as a single cell of another species finds its way into the culture, it becomes an impure culture. Passing over the various methods which were formerly employed for obtaining pure cultures in liquids (fractional and dilution cultures of Klebs, Nägeli, etc.), we will describe in brief only the methods of cultivating micro-organisms on solid media, introduced by Vittadini and Brefeld, and perfected by Koch.

I will confine myself to the two methods most commonly employed for cultivating on gelatine or agar-agar. These are: 1, line cultures; 2, dilution cultures.

Line Cultures.

The principle of line cultures may be made clear by the following illustration: Suppose we were to dip a wet glass rod into a bag containing a mixture of timothy and clover seeds, so that a vast number of seeds of both kinds adhere to the rod, and then draw it over prepared ground; at first, great numbers of seeds will be left in the wake of the rod; gradually, however, they will become less and less, until at last only single seeds may be deposited. When these seeds grow, we will have in the first part of the track a mixture of timothy and clover, but in the last part separate stocks of timothy and clover, growing singly, or in pure cultures. To apply this method to the cultivation of bacteria, let us suppose that we wish to obtain a pure culture of the bacteria from the white deposit about the necks of the teeth. We proceed in the following manner: Having melted a tube of nutritive agar-agar, we carefully remove the cotton stopper, hold the mouth of the tube for a moment in the flame of a Bunsen burner, to destroy all germs sticking to it, then pour the material upon a sterilized glass plate, using the apparatus No. 11. As soon as this has stiffened, which takes place in about one or two minutes, we take up some of the deposit upon the point of a sterilized platinum needle, draw it lightly over the surface of the culture medium ten or fifteen times, and place the plate in a damp chamber at the temperature of the human body. In the course of a day or two we will invariably find that an abundant growth has taken place along the lines. On the first line it will be very thick, and on each succeeding line it will gradually become thinner, till on the last line the growth will appear only as a few isolated points (Fig. 15). These points usually represent pure cultures. If they are not pure, they can be made so by vaccinating from them a second plate in the manner just indicated. A portion of a culture made in this manner is represented in Fig. 15. In making line cultures on nutritive gelatine we pro-

FIG. 15.

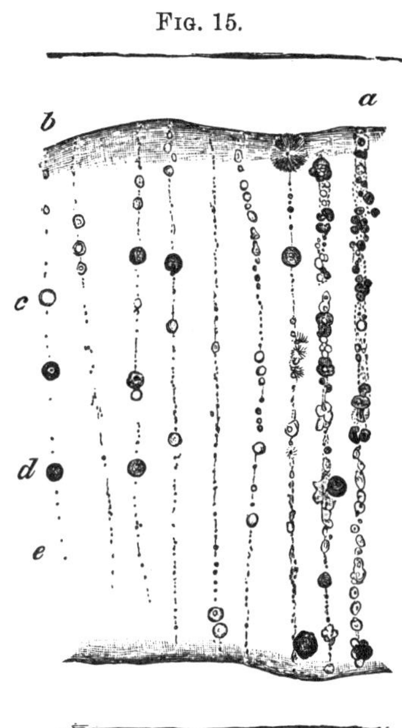

LINE CULTURE ON NUTRITIVE AGAR-AGAR.

The number of colonies in each line gradually decreases from a to b, until in the last line we have only twelve to fifteen colonies in which at least three different micro-organisms are represented, the colonies c, d, and e plainly differing from each other to the naked eye. The first colony in the third line from a is a mould. Natural size.

ceed in exactly the same manner, except that the cultures must be kept at a temperature just below that at which the gelatine used liquefies. Instead of the ordinary glass plates, Petri'sche Schalen may often be used to great advantage.

Dilution Cultures.

We may illustrate the principle of dilution cultures in the following manner: Suppose we have a handful of seeds of various kinds which are invisible to the naked eye, and we are given the task to separate the seeds, or at least to obtain pure cultures of

FIG. 16.

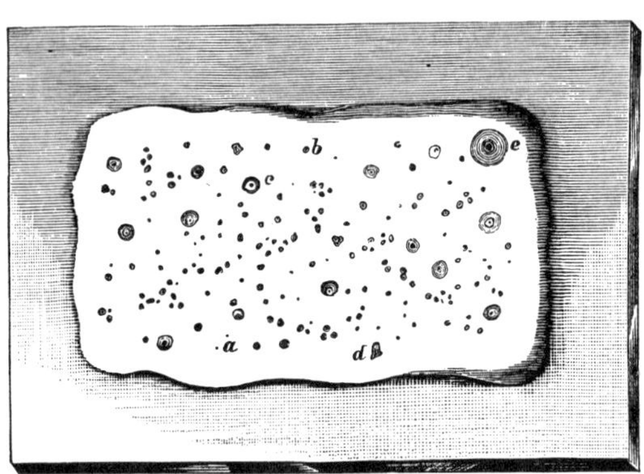

SECOND DILUTION OF A GELATINE-CULTURE FROM THE WHITE DEPOSIT ON THE TEETH.

a, very small; *b*, medium-sized; *c*, very large, round colonies; *d*, irregular colony. The different sizes represent different rapidities of growth. Culture three days old.

them. We may accomplish the task in the following manner: We go out to the field and cast the seed broadcast upon the ground which has been prepared for the sowing, wait till they spring up and ripen, then gather the different plants which are produced into separate heaps. In this way we obtain pure cultures of all the different plants represented in the original handful of invisible seeds.

In applying this principle to the pure cultivation of micro-organisms we proceed as follows: Having melted three tubes of nutrient gelatine by gently warming them over a gas flame, we transfer to one of them, on the point of a platinum needle, a small quantity of the material which we wish to examine, and shake the gelatine gently to distribute the micro-organisms throughout the mass. The quantity of soil in one tube is, however, so small, and the organisms would lie so closely together that we would not be able, as a rule, to distinguish between the separate colonies. We consequently transfer, on a loop of platinum wire, three or four small drops or beads from the first tube (first dilution) to a second tube (second

FIG. 17.

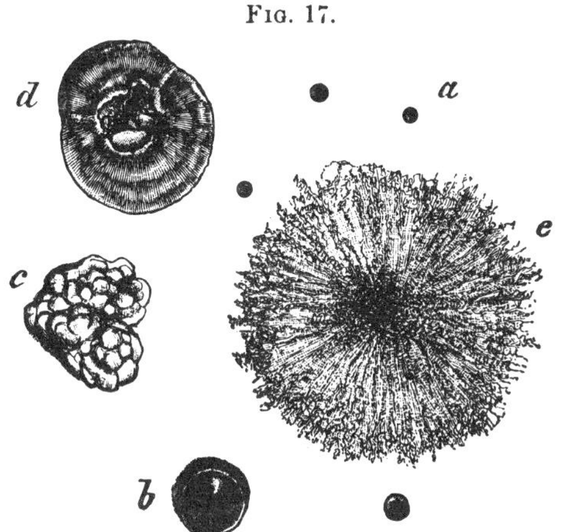

COLONIES FROM THE PLATE ILLUSTRATED IN FIG. 15, UNDER A POWER OF FIFTY DIAMETERS.
a, *b*, *c*, *d*, Colonies of four kinds of bacteria; *e*, Mould colony.

dilution), and if thought necessary six to eight beads from the second to a third tube (third dilution). We now pour the contents of the three tubes upon three separate plates, which are put into a damp chamber as soon as the gelatine has solidified.

If the plates are examined after about forty-eight hours, we will find, as a rule, that the first dilution has become completely opaque, through the development of innumerable colonies; the second plate will appear thickly studded (Fig. 16) with mostly whitish points (colonies), while the third plate will show but very few colonies, or possibly none at all. The number of colonies on the different plates will of course depend upon the number in the original material. In these colonies we have pure cultures or growths of all the different organisms present in the material used, as far as they are cultivable in gelatine. At this time, but much better a day or two later, it may be seen by the unaided eye (better, naturally, under a low power of the microscope) that the colonies do not all present the same appearance. In color they may be white, yellowish, dirty white, gray, brownish gray, brown, orange, red, etc., or they may impart color to the gelatine; they may be perfectly round or irregular, thick or thin, transparent or opaque, moist or dry, homogeneous or knotty, soft or cartilaginous, etc. Some liquefy the gelatine, others do not. Under the microscope, other differences of structure not discernible to the naked eye may be made out. (See Fig. 17.) By transferring one or more colonies of each kind to tubes of gelatine or agar-agar, as described below, we obtain larger, pure growths, in a form in which they may be kept a greater length of time without becoming impure.

TEST-TUBE CULTURES.

When it is desired to obtain pure growths in larger masses, and in a form in which they may be kept for a longer time, we make use of the so-called tube cultures. These are obtained by inoculating tubes of nutrient gelatine or agar-agar with separate colonies, either from line or dilution cultures. Placing the plate under a low power of the microscope (50 diameters), we adjust an isolated colony, which we pick up with the bent point of a platinum needle directly under the microscope (an operation which requires some practice), and transfer at once to the tube, puncturing the gelatine with the needle to a depth of about one and a half inches, the tube being held in the left hand, with the mouth downward, to prevent the falling in of germs from the air. Larger colonies may be picked up without the aid of the microscope, provided only we have satisfied ourselves beforehand by the microscopic examination that the colony is really isolated, and that no small colony of some other species, invisible to the naked eye, is lying near it. These test-tube growths also generally furnish a ready means of distinguishing between different species (Fig. 18, and plate, Figs. 1–4), although sometimes two different organisms grow so nearly alike that they cannot be distinguished by this means alone.

FIG. 18.

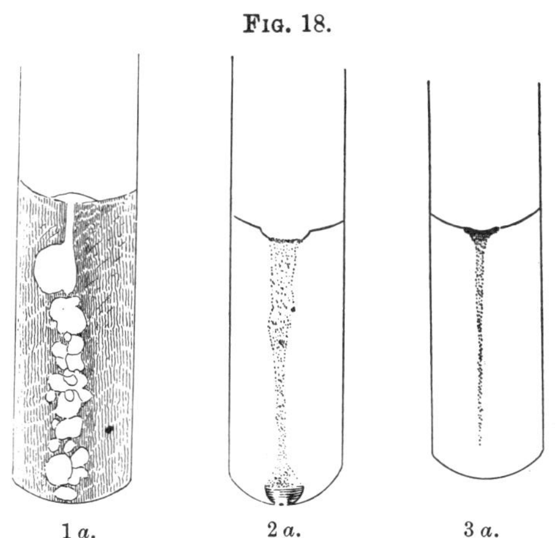

TEST-TUBE CULTURES OF THREE DIFFERENT BACTERIA.
All of same age.

Pure cultures in bouillon are obtained in the same manner, though in this case we naturally cannot invert the tube, and particular caution is requisite to prevent impurification during the process of inoculation.

OTHER SOLID CULTURE MEDIA.

It sometimes happens that two different micro-organisms, cultivated on gelatine or agar-agar, present characteristics of growth so similar to each other that it is not possible to distinguish between them, or that they do not grow at all on these media. In such cases we have recourse to other media, such as coagulated blood-serum, boiled potato, boiled egg, starch-paste, etc. I cannot enter into a description of the method of preparing blood-serum. Any one wishing to undertake this by no means very easy task, must refer to the works on this subject. I would certainly advise any one, unless he needs a very large quantity of the material, to buy it, if possible, already prepared. It is congealed, after sterilization, in shallow glass vessels, or in test tubes placed obliquely, so as to obtain the greatest possible surface. Only line or puncture cultures can be made with this material; it is particularly adapted to the cultivation of the tubercle bacillus, the bacillus of glanders, and some other pathogenic micro-organisms.

Boiled potato is a medium of great value in the determination of bacteria. No medium, however, requires greater care in preparation and after-treatment than this, in order to obtain satisfactory results. Any sound potato *which does not become mealy, or crack open on boiling*, will do for the purpose; it is first thoroughly washed and brushed, and all defective spots and deep eyes being removed, it is placed for one hour in a 5 to 1000 solution of bichloride of mercury, then in a steam sterilizer for one-half an hour to one hour. In the mean time the damp chamber is sterilized, and the bottom lined with filter-paper wet with sublimate solution, 5 to 1000. The potatoes are, while hot, removed from the sterilizer with sterilized forceps, cut into halves with a cold sterilized knife, and placed directly upon the sublimate paper (the cut surface up) and the cell closed. Potato sections prepared in this way should remain unchanged indefinitely. When the potato has become cool, the cover of the cell is carefully removed, and the micro-organism which is to be cultivated is spread upon a space about as large as a dime, in the center of the section. Micro-organisms which morphologically, as well as in their reaction upon gelatine, agar-agar, and blood-serum, show no appreciable differences, may sometimes be easily distinguished by aid of the potato culture. The potato can seldom be used to prepare pure cultures. It is chiefly used as a reagent in distinguishing between growths already in pure culture. For example, all comma bacilli yet discovered grow on potato, except the one found by Deneke in old cheese, which does not develop at all on potato, and is thereby at once distinguished as an entirely different bacterium.

Eggs may often be used to great advantage. They are prepared as follows: The *fresh* egg is placed in sublimate, 5 to 1000, for ten minutes, then in the steam sterilizer for one hour. The cell for eggs is prepared as for potatoes, except that a sterilized glass plate, resting on a glass bench, is placed in the bottom to support the egg sections. As the egg must be handled with the fingers, the hands must be thoroughly washed, then soaked in sublimate, 5 to 1000, and then washed again in absolute alcohol, to remove the sublimate. The eggs are shelled while still hot, and cut into two, three, or four sections. They are vaccinated in points, upon the white; the yellow is not so well adapted to culture experiments, since it cannot be cut with a smooth surface.

I always keep on hand sections of potato and egg, also tubes of gelatine, agar-agar, and blood-serum; and when in my practice particularly good material, or anything uncommon, presents itself, a portion of it is at once transferred to these different culture media, so that it is pretty sure to develop in one of them at least. For example, I have several times met with a bacterium in the human mouth which produces a yellowish coloring-matter, and which absolutely refuses to grow on anything which I have tried, except potato.

Liquid Media.

For studying the various processes of decomposition, fermentation, putrefaction, etc., brought about by bacteria, a great variety of liquid media have been employed. One which I have used extensively consists of water 100.0, peptone 2.0, sugar 1.0, beef extract 1.5, with occasional additions of starch. This I have found very well adapted to the culture and study of many oral bacteria. Other media are milk, urine, bread-juice, juice of fruits, decoctions or watery extracts of various plants or grains, saliva (to which, however, nutrient material must be added), etc. These may also be combined with each other in various proportions.

Application of the above Methods to Cultivations from the Human Mouth.

For general work on the bacteria of the oral cavity the best medium, in my opinion, is presented by neutral beef-water-peptone-sugar-agar-agar. On this medium I first make line cultures (which may be supplemented by dilution cultures at the same time), and then for the further study of the micro-organisms cultivated I make dilution cultures on gelatine, etc. It often happens, however, that bacteria which we have obtained on agar-agar do not grow at all on gelatine, because of the low temperature at which it must be kept, just as it may also happen that cultures made from the saliva on gelatine may develop nothing whatever, although the saliva at the time may have contained bacteria enough. If, therefore, I wish to obtain cultures from the deposits or accumulations, secretions, etc., of the human mouth, I make line cultures on agar-agar, either alone or supplemented by dilution cultures on gelatine. For particular purposes, as in the attempt to cultivate the Spirillum sputigenum, etc., I would of course employ various other materials.

Pure cultures of the bacteria of tooth-decay I obtain by the following method, which varies somewhat, according to whether we wish to secure cultures from the surface or from the deeper part of the dentine: In the former case, after having removed the remains of food from the cavity of decay, I scratch out a small portion of the decomposing dentine with a sterilized excavator; this is then transferred to a plate of agar-agar in the manner above described. To obtain a pure culture from the deeper parts of the dentine, I first wash the tooth in a stream of pure water and place it for some minutes in a 5 per cent. solution of carbolic acid, also brushing carefully with the same solution, so as perfectly to remove all traces of food and to destroy those bacteria which are found only on the surface. I then dry the tooth with sterilized bibulous paper, and remove the outer layers of decayed dentine with a sterilized, spoon-shaped excavator. With a second excavator I remove a second layer, with a third a third layer, and so on, till I arrive near to the border of the sound dentine; or, I undercut the decayed dentine at one side of the cavity with a sharp instrument, and, grasping the detached edge with a strong pair of pliers, I shell out the largest part of the decayed matter in one piece. In either case I then detach a small portion of the decayed dentine from the bottom of the cavity, and place it in a drop of sterilized water, where it is torn to pieces with two stiff needles, or fine excavators. With these pieces, and with the water, the agar-agar plate is then inoculated.

At the same time dilution cultures may be made upon plates of nutritive gelatine. These must of course be kept at a lower temperature, in consequence of which the bacteria do not develop so rapidly as they do on the agar-agar plates; sometimes no development whatever takes place. The thought naturally presents itself to every one, that the bacteria growing in the deeper parts of dentine may not develop under free access of air. Accordingly, small pieces of decayed dentine should be placed in tubes of melted gelatine or agar-agar, and allowed to sink to different distances from the surface, where, on the medium becoming solid, they obtain but a very limited supply of air.

To obtain a pure culture from a gangrenous pulp, I carefully cleanse and sterilize the tooth as before, so as to be absolutely sure that no living germs are present upon the surface; I then split the tooth by means of a pair of sterilized incising forceps. Very often the tooth may be split without the forceps coming into contact with the pulp, in which case the pulp, or portions of it, may be lifted from its bed by means of a nerve-needle, and transferred to a drop or two of water or gelatine. It is then torn or picked to pieces so as to liberate the bacteria, after which it may be drawn several times across the surface of the agar-agar, or the inoculations may be made from the water.

For such micro-organisms as grow at low temperatures, gelatine forms a much more convenient material than agar-agar; furthermore, differences of growth are much more readily recognized on gelatine than on agar-agar. Consequently, we should not rely upon cultures on agar-agar alone, but all of the bacteria which we succeed in cultivating on agar-agar we should likewise attempt to cultivate on gelatine. The majority of them will grow, though by no means all of them.

The great advantage possessed by the solid culture media over liquid media, consists in the fact that each germ must remain at the point where it is at the time the media becomes solid. A number of different kinds of micro-organisms, therefore, on a plate of gelatine, may develop without mixing together, each one remaining as a pure culture, whereas in liquids they would naturally mix, thereby causing an impure culture.

Preparation of Nutrient Gelatine, or Agar-Agar.

Having prepared the solution which we wish to make the base of our nutrient gelatine, we add to 100 grams of the solution 5 to 10, or even 20 grams, of the finest gelatine cut into small pieces, and allow it to stand one-half hour to one hour, when the gelatine should be completely dissolved by gently warming the solution, and carbonate of sodium carefully added until the reaction becomes neutral, or very slightly alkaline. It is then boiled for about an hour, in order to effect a complete precipitation of the salts and coagulable substances (otherwise the medium when done will appear cloudy), and while hot filtered directly into test tubes, or into flasks from which it may subsequently be transferred to the tubes, each tube receiving about one and one-half to two inches. The tubes are then exposed to steam at a temperature of 100° C. in the steam sterilizer for one-quarter to one-half hour. Twelve hours later they are again exposed for the same length of time, which will usually suffice to effect a complete sterilization of the contents.

A solution which I have used very frequently consisted of water 100.0, peptone 2.0, sugar 1.0, beef-extract 1.5, to which five to twenty grams of gelatine is added, according to the strength required. In summer 20 per cent. will often be found necessary to prevent melting of the cultures at room temperature. The beef-water-peptone-gelatine now so extensively used is made in the following manner: "One-half kilogram of good, finely minced meat, is covered with 1 liter of distilled water, well mixed and left for twenty-four hours in the refrigerator. It is then pressed through gauze, and enough distilled water added to bring the quantity up to 1 liter. To this water we add 10 grams of dry peptone, 5 grams of table-salt, and 50 to 100 grams of gelatine" (Hüppe). As a universal culture material for oral bacteria this is improved by the addition of 10 grams of sugar. The further preparation is conducted in the manner described above.

Nutrient agar-agar is prepared in the same way as nutrient gelatine, except that only 1 to 2 per cent. of agar-agar is added, instead of 5 to 20 per cent.

Naturally, every intelligent experimenter will be able to vary the culture medium according to the circumstances, bearing in mind that for many bacteria it is absolutely necessary that the character of the artificial culture medium be very similar to that of the substratum in which they are naturally found.

There are many kinds of bacteria which have not yet been cultivated, and which are therefore styled strictly obligatory parasitic, which I doubt not would grow well enough if we were able to prepare a medium for them identical with their natural nutriment.

Except for especial purposes, I would not advise any one whose time is so limited as that of a dentist or medical practitioner to attempt to make his own gelatine or agar-agar, as he will save much time in purchasing it already made.

Having obtained a pure culture of any given micro-organism, the further study of it is to be directed to the following points:

1. Its morphology, development, etc., as revealed by high powers of the microscope.
2. The characteristics of its growth on different nutrient media.
3. Its behavior in regard to atmospheric oxygen.
4. Its physiological action (fermentation, putrefaction).
5. Does it possess diastatic, hydrolitic (inverting), or peptonizing action?
6. Does it form coloring-matter?
7. How is it affected by various antiseptics?
8. Does it possess pathogenic properties, and if so, what are they?

The first question is answered by direct microscopical observation of stained and unstained specimens, with the help of good, homogeneous immersion lenses, particular attention being paid to the production or non-production of spores, since this is a matter not alone of botanical, but also of great hygienic interest, inasmuch as the resistance of a bacterium to devitalizing agents is to a great degree determined by the presence or absence of spores. A knowledge of the morphology and development of a bacterium is not, however, essential to the study of questions 2 to 8. Pure cultures may be obtained and all desirable experiments made without a knowledge of the form of the given bacterium.

Question 2 is to be answered by examining the pure culture on various nutrient media with the naked eye, or under weak magnifying power.

Question 3 is most easily answered by placing a thin glass plate or sheet of mica, on the plate culture; if the bacterium be aërobic, it will flourish only till the oxygen in the gelatine is consumed; the colonies will consequently present a stunted appearance. If it be anaërobic, the colonies under the mica will grow faster than the uncovered ones. The experiment may also be made in vessels from which the air has been exhausted, or in which it has been replaced by hydrogen.

Question 4 is decided by cultures on different media, principally on carbohydrates, then on albuminous substances, or in mixtures of both, as they generally occur in the mouth.

In order to answer question 5, cultures are made (*a*) in amylaceous substances, which, when the culture has obtained its full growth, are to be tested for sugar; (*b*) in solutions containing cane-sugar, which are tested for dextrose, levulose, etc., or as to a change in their rotatory power; (*c*) in solutions of albumen, which are then tested for peptone, or on coagulated albumen, which liquefies when the bacteria have a peptonizing action. We must watch the course of the fermentation, its duration, and especially note whether acids are generated or not, and what they are.

Question 6 is naturally decided by ocular inspection.

Question 7 by the usual disinfecting experiments, some of which may be found described in full in Chapter IX.

The pathogenesis (question 8) must be determined by experiments on living animals, for which purpose mice, rabbits, and guinea-pigs are most commonly made use of; less frequently dogs, fowls, or even sheep, calves, etc.

The material may be introduced into the animal body—

1. In form of powder, by inhalation.
2. With the food.
3. By cutaneous inoculations (performed by slightly scratching the purified skin with a sharp instrument charged with the material to be tested).

4. By subcutaneous inoculations. The hair is shaved or cut off and the skin cleansed at some point which cannot be licked or scratched by the animal, a fold of skin pulled up with the pincette, and a slight incision made with a pair of sterilized scissors. The skin is then loosened from the subcutaneous tissue so as to form a small pocket, into which the material is brought on the point of an instrument or platinum wire.

5. By intravenous inoculations, best made in rabbits by injecting the large vein at the base of the ear.

6. By injecting the material directly into the pleural or the abdominal cavity.

Less frequently, more difficult operations are undertaken for injecting or applying the material to various internal parts of the body,—for example, into the duodenum, to avoid the action of the gastric juice.

Examination of Micro-organisms under the Microscope.

Bacteria are frequently examined in a fresh (living) condition, in order to determine whether they are motile or not, but more particularly to study their mode of development. A small quantity of the material to be examined is brought upon a glass slide in a drop of pure water, and covered with a cover-glass, when it is ready for examination under the microscope. For a more careful study the method of hanging-drops is used. A drop of bouillon on a cover-glass is inoculated with a very minute quantity of the material (pure culture), and the cover-glass placed with the drop on the under side upon the concavity of a hollow object-glass (Fig. 18 *a*), the sides of the cover being

Fig. 18 *a*.

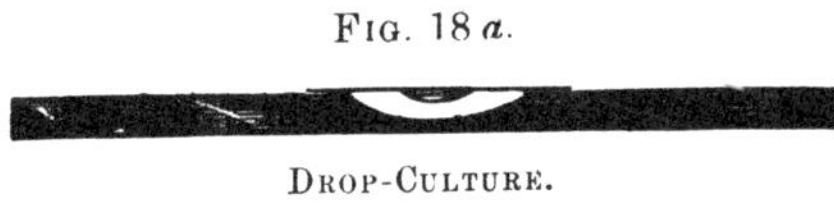

Drop-Culture.

then fixed to the slide (object-glass) by means of wax, fat, or paraffine, to prevent evaporation. The development of the bacteria may be observed for hours in succession. If it is desired to maintain a constant temperature above that of the room, the heatable object-table may be used.

The study of bacteria in an unstained condition is, however, always attended with considerable difficulty, and their detection and differentiation in tissues, or when mixed with various organic matters, is sometimes impossible. These difficulties are in a great measure, and in fact usually, entirely overcome by first properly staining the micro-organisms with some one of the basic aniline stains above mentioned.

For examining bacteria in liquids we employ the

Cover-Glass Preparations.

A minute quantity of the material to be examined (pure culture, or any soft substance supposed to contain bacteria) is spread over the surface of a cover-glass in a small drop of water and allowed to dry in the air (or the material is crushed in water between two cover-glasses, which are then pulled apart so that each receives a coating). The glass is then slowly passed three times through the flame of a spirit lamp or Bunsen burner, to *fix* the material, and two to three drops of the stain (aqueous solution) applied by means of a glass rod. The staining requires from thirty seconds to ten minutes; by tilting the glass to one side it is easy to see when the preparation has taken on the coloring-matter. The excess of staining matter is then removed with a gentle stream of water, or by floating the cover-glass in a vessel of pure water, when the preparation may be placed upon a slide and examined under the microscope. For permanent preparations the cover-glass, after washing, is dried and mounted in Canada balsam.

In order to stain the spores, float the cover-glass from ten minutes to one hour on a hot concentrated solution of fuchsine in aniline water, wash off the excess of coloring-matter, and treat the preparation for a few seconds or minutes with absolute alcohol containing a trace of fuchsine. Then stain in the usual manner with methylene blue (Hueppe). The bacilli appear blue, the spores red. Instead of fuchsine and methylene blue, methyl violet and vesuvine may be used.

Tissue Preparations.

It would lead us too far to attempt to give an idea of all the many methods employed in staining bacteria in tissues. I refer accordingly to only one or two:

Löffler's method. The sections are brought for a few minutes into the strong alkaline solution (concentrated alcoholic solution of methylene blue 30 c.cm., caustic potash (1 : 10,000) 100 c.cm.), then they are washed in 0.5 per cent. acetic acid, dehydrated in absolute alcohol, cleared up in oil of cedar, and mounted in Canada balsam.

Gram's method. Sections are placed first in alcohol, then in the aniline water-gentian violet solution a few minutes, then in the iodine solution for one to three minutes, then in absolute alcohol till they lose all visible color. Clear up in oil of cloves, and mount in Canada balsam; or, better, after *Günther*, stain one minute, the iodine solution (page 51) two minutes, alcohol one-half minute, 3 per cent. hydrochloric acid in alcohol exactly ten seconds, then alcohol, oil of cloves, etc.

To obtain double coloring, bring the sections, stained in gentian violet, from the alcohol into an aqueous solution of vesuvine for some minutes, then again into absolute alcohol, clear up, and mount in Canada balsam.

CHAPTER IV.

BIOLOGICAL STUDIES ON THE BACTERIA OF THE MOUTH.

IF we compare the life-conditions of bacteria as described in Chapter I. with the conditions prevailing in the human mouth, it becomes evident that the oral cavity must be an excellent breeding-place for these organisms. It is equally clear that both their number and variety are continually being augmented by new germs which enter with the air, food, and drink. In the course of a few years hundreds of kinds of bacteria would therefore become established in the mouth, if the majority of them did not perish, sooner or later, in the struggle for existence. Any one, therefore, who continues the search for oral bacteria, by means of the modern culture-methods, for a long period of time, will continually meet with new kinds, until at last all cultivable micro-organisms, whose germs occur in the air, in food and drink, will have been found in the oral cavity. Within the last few years I have isolated more than one hundred different kinds of bacteria from the juices and deposits in the mouth. A number of these were identical with well-known and widely distributed species (for example, hay bacillus, potato bacillus, lactic acid bacillus, bacillus of green pus, Micrococcus tetragenus, Mycoderma aceti, Staphylococcus pyogenes aureus and albus, etc.), while others appeared to be new kinds, although I was not able, on account of the great number, to attempt in every case to establish the identity or non-identity with known species.

It must be supposed that the occurrence of many of these bacteria in the mouth was purely accidental, that they had entered the oral cavity but shortly before the examination was made, and disappeared again soon after. Some years ago, I found in the mouth of a patient suffering from acute gingivitis, a spirillum very similar to, if not identical with, the bacillus of Finkler-Prior. Repeated efforts, made a few days later, to obtain this bacterium from the same mouth, proved futile. In a like manner I was able to isolate the vinegar bacterium from my own saliva, after having drank a glass of beer in which this particular organism was present in large numbers; on the following day my endeavors to find it failed, doubtless because this bacterium cannot bear the high temperature of the mouth for any length of time.

There are, however, a number of bacteria which almost invariably occur in every mouth, and which may be termed

Mouth Bacteria Proper.

These are:

1. Leptothrix innominata.
2. Bacillus buccalis maximus.
3. Leptothrix buccalis maxima.
4. Jodococcus vaginatus.
5. Spirillum sputigenum.
6. Spirochæte dentium (denticola).

These bacteria occur in every mouth; sometimes even an almost pure culture of No. 5 is found. They all have the peculiarity that they will not grow on any of the usual culture media. All endeavors at cultivation—and thousands have been made—proved unsuccessful. I have myself made hundreds of attempts to cultivate them on all the various solid and fluid media. For these experiments I had excellent material. My errand-boy had a very carious right inferior molar, covered with tartar and deposits, the surrounding gum being slightly inflamed. In the cavity I found an almost pure culture of Spirillum sputigenum, and on the margin of the gum one of Spirochæte dentium. During several months I made cultures almost daily; first, I tried the usual Koch nutrient media, beef-water-peptone-gelatine, blood-serum, agar-agar, potato, etc. These experiments not succeeding, I varied the media by adding different substances, such as sugar, starch, etc., and by using saliva instead of water as a solvent. I also employed weak alkaline and acid, as well as neutral media. Finally, I adapted my experiments to the boy's food, and made up a mixture whose composition showed the greatest possible similarity to the contents of the cavity. I furthermore tried dentine glue instead of gelatine, which I procured by boiling decalcified teeth. Nevertheless, all these attempts remained fruitless. Only line cultures afforded a very limited growth, but the colonies never developed more than fifteen to twenty cells, and a transference to a second plate proved futile, no further growth taking place. Vignal's experiments in reference to this question will be mentioned later.

It is very easy, as has been done by a writer in the October number of the *Oest. Ungar. Vierteljahrsschrift für Zahnheilkunde*, 1889, who signs himself π, to account for the failure to cultivate these micro-organisms on the assumption that they are strictly parasitic (*vide* page 17), and consequently cannot, under any condition, grow when separated from their host. I find it, however, more reasonable to explain the failure on the simple ground that these bacteria are very sensible to slight changes in the culture media, and that no one has yet succeeded in constructing an artificial medium sufficiently similar to that found in certain mouths to admit of their cultivation. I have by no means given up the hope of yet obtaining cultures of these most interesting forms.

We must guard against the very common error of considering every thread-forming organism which occurs in the oral cavity, or is obtained in pure culture from the juices of the mouth, as "Leptothrix buccalis," inasmuch as threads are formed by various micro-organisms.

Leptothrix buccalis.

Leptothrix buccalis is a name chosen by Robin[55] for those organisms in the human mouth which were formerly described as animalcula, tooth-animalcules, Bühlmann's fibers, denticolæ, etc. Almost every living organism occurring in the mouth was designated by this common name.

Hallier,[57] and many of his successors up to the present time, adopted this view. The motile bacteria of the mouth were regarded as the swarm-spores of Leptothrix buccalis, the immotile (cocci, etc.) as the spores at rest. "Elements of Leptothrix buccalis" were found everywhere.

Leber and Rottenstein[58] considered "a beautiful violet color produced by iodine and acids" as characteristic of Leptothrix buccalis, but we may easily convince ourselves that several bacteria possessing this reaction occur in the mouth, and consequently this does not especially characterize any particular kind.

Leptothrix buccalis is now usually described as long, thin, apparently inarticulate threads, etc., while mouth-bacteria which show the iodine reaction are distinctly and regularly articulated.

Vignal[59] has obtained in pure culture from the mouth a bacterium which he calls Leptothrix buccalis. It is characterized by "*la présence à l'intérieur des bâtonnets de cloisons transversales sur les préparations colorées avec les couleurs d'aniline.*" Robin,[55] on the contrary, writes, "*On ne remarque pas trace d'articulation dans toute leur longueur.*" It is not stated whether this micro-organism cultivated by Vignal shows the iodine reaction or not. In short, the name Leptothrix buccalis designates no particular organism possessing peculiar characteristics, and the name deserves to be retained as little as "denticola," "Bühlmann's fibers," etc.; the more so, since it has always been the expression for an obscure and erroneous conception. Morphologically, as well as physiologically considered, Leptothrix buccalis has been regarded as a veritable wonder. It has been said to perforate and split up teeth, its elements to cause all kinds of diseases in the oral cavity, to penetrate into the lungs, the stomach, and other parts of the body, and everywhere to manifest a destructive influence. As absolutely nothing was known concerning the biology and pathogenesis of this organism, all sorts of wonderful properties were ascribed to it. It is therefore high time to banish this confusing name from bacteriological writings.* For those bacteria growing in threads, whose biology is too little known to define their relation to other mouth-bacteria, or to form a

* Equally objectionable is the inclination of some observers to class everything showing a slight contraction in the middle as Bacterium termo. This is also a term which, on account of its application by different authors to very different organisms, might well be dispensed with.

separate group with distinct characteristics, I propose the provisional name of

Leptothrix innominata.

Leptothrix innominata in this sense is found in the soft, white deposit on the teeth (Leeuwenhoek's materia alba). It invariably occurs in every mouth, but by no means always in the same numbers. In one case it may be found in masses, in another but very sparingly. If a portion of this white deposit mixed with water be brought under the microscope, we see different sized heaps, apparently consisting of small, round granules, from whose margins thin, more or less zigzagged threads project (Fig. 19). These granular masses form the so-called "matrix of Leptothrix buccalis," and were formerly regarded as its spores; they are, however, partly micrococci, which have no genetic connection with the threads, and partly only crossings of the threads themselves. The length of the threads varies considerably; they are from 0.5 to 0.8μ broad, twisted and tortuous, immotile, inarticulated; they generally show an irregular course, and often appear degenerated, or even lifeless. Many shorter threads or rods will also be found, that resemble fragments of the threads, and may be regarded as such, or as younger cells.

FIG. 19.

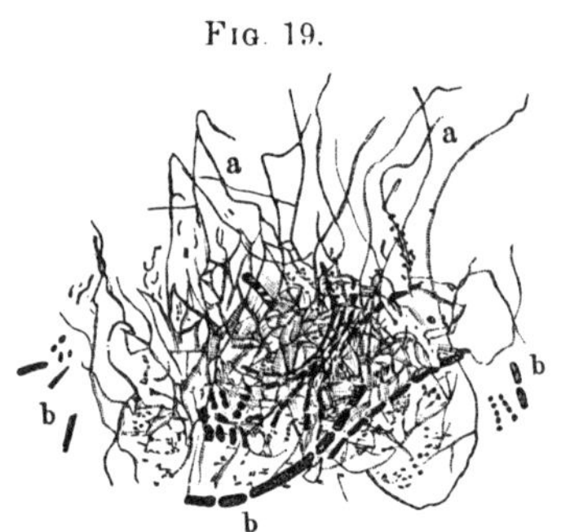

GROUP OF BACTERIA FROM THE HUMAN MOUTH.
a, Leptothrix innominata; *b*, Various Rod- and Coccus-forms.

If a small quantity of the white deposit is brought into a drop of a solution of iodine in iodide of potassium slightly acidulated with lactic acid, it will be observed (under about 350 diameters) that the larger part of this substance, consisting of epithelium, masses of micrococci, and diverse rod- and thread-shaped organisms, assumes a faint yellowish or yellow color, as do also the irregular projecting threads of Leptothrix innominata.

As a rule, however, we find also chains of cocci, either scattered or in small groups, and thick bacilli, distinctly colored blue violet. These two kinds, which I have entitled Jodococcus vaginatus, and Bacillus buccalis maximus, I shall now describe more at length. Other mouth-bacteria with a similar reaction are mentioned below.

Fig. 20.

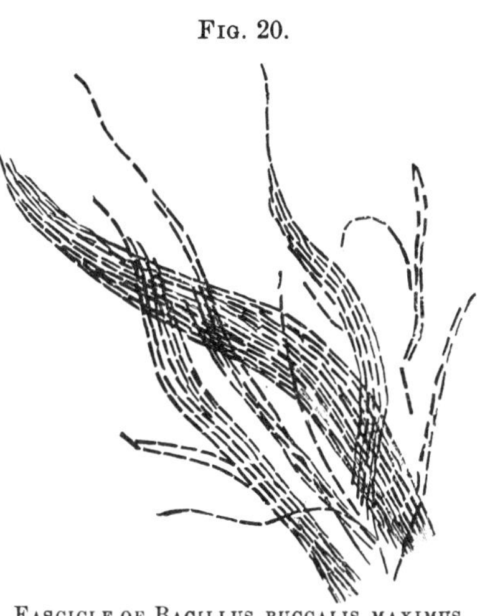

Fascicle of Bacillus buccalis maximus.
Colored with the iodine solution. 400 : 1.

Bacillus buccalis maximus

appears in the shape of isolated bacilli or threads, but much oftener as tufts of threads, parallel to or crossing each other, from 30 to 150μ long, and distinctly articulated (Fig. 20). The rods are from 2 to 10μ long, sometimes even longer, and from 1 to 1.3μ broad. This bacterium is therefore the largest occurring

Fig. 21.

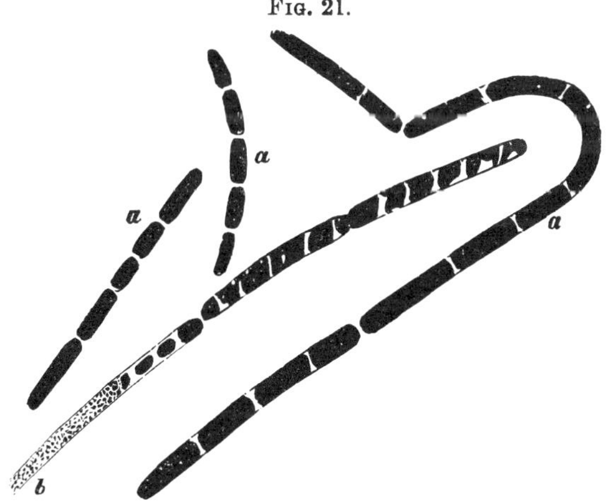

Bacillus buccalis maximus.
After treatment with iodine solution. 1800 : 1.

in the mouth; it has a very regular contour, and usually the same thickness throughout. (*b*, Fig. 21, is an exception.)

Not all the cells of this bacterium show the iodine reaction, a statement which applies equally well to most bacteria that turn blue on the addition of iodine. The majority of them, however, respond very distinctly to the test, becoming stained brown violet, either throughout (Fig. 21, *a*) or only in isolated places (Fig. 21, *b*). I have not observed this bacillus in the dentinal tubules; indeed, its size would seem to oppose a barrier to its entrance into the tubules. The size, the distinct and regular articulation, the absence of the zigzag windings, as well as the iodine reaction before mentioned, hinder me from admitting this micro-organism into the cyclus of the above-described Leptothrix innominata.

Leptothrix buccalis maxima.

There is also found in the mucous deposits upon the teeth quite a large number of long, thick, straight, or curved filaments, which show a marked resemblance of form to Bacillus buccalis maximus, except as regards the joints, which are, perhaps, somewhat shorter in the latter. These cells do not give the iodine reaction. Whether they are, therefore, to be regarded as a different variety, or as cells of the same variety, in which the substance which assumes the blue color is not yet formed (possibly younger cells), must for the present remain undecided. I have called this organism Leptothrix buccalis maxima.

Jodococcus vaginatus.

Fig. 22.

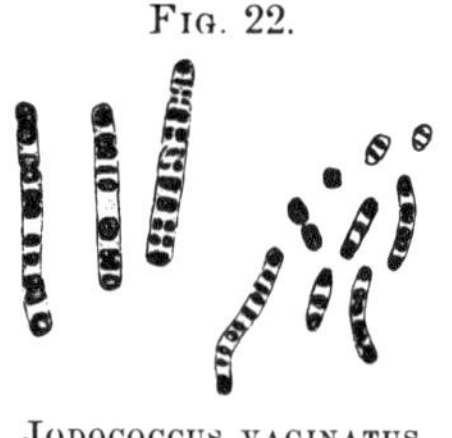

Jodococcus vaginatus. 1100 : 1.

This micro-organism occurs in considerable numbers in all unclean mouths. Only in the case of two children, aged five and eight years respectively, have I failed to find it. It appears singly or in chains of from 4 to 10 cells, longer being rarely seen. The chains are furnished with a sheath in which the cells appear as flat disks, or as more rounded, even square shapes, which sometimes show a great likeness to tetrads (Fig. 22). The chains have a diameter of 0.75μ. Occasionally chains are found in which one or more cells are missing, *i.e.* have escaped from the sheath; others again, whose sheaths have burst, while the separate members have not entirely severed their connection with the chain. Sometimes the remains of the broken sheath may be easily detected; it does not show the iodine reaction, but remains colorless, or becomes yellowish after the continued action of the reagent. The contents of the cells are always stained dark blue to violet by iodine.

Spirillum sputigenum.

Spirillum sputigenum also occurs in every mouth, but in varying proportions. In mouths properly cared for it will be found only in very small numbers; in neglected mouths, however, it often exists in enormous masses. If a small quantity of the soft deposit on the margin of the inflamed gums is taken from an unclean mouth and brought under the microscope, we sometimes find an almost pure culture of Spirillum sputigenum, or of Spirochæte dentium. The former occurs in the shape of rods, curved like commas, which show very active spiral movements.

By the growth of the rods, where fissation does not occur, or when the separate rods remain connected with each other, S-forms and short spirals are produced. (See Figs. 23 to 29.)

This bacillus was regarded by Lewis, Klein, and others as identical with the cholera bacillus, a view which a more careful study of these two morphologically similar organisms will show to be incorrect. I have given an exposition of the real relation of the curved bacilli in the oral cavity to the cholera bacillus, in the *Deutsche med. Wochenschr.*[60] From this source I quote the following: Prof. Lewis's communication on comma bacilli in the human mouth has added extraordinary interest to the study of the fungi of the oral cavity. As is known, Lewis[61] discovered(?) a curved bacillus in the mucus of the mouth, which in form, size, and color-reaction is said to correspond to the cholera bacillus and consequently to be identical with it. Its occurrence in the mouth is, however, by no means a discovery of Prof. Lewis's, but a long-known fact. I mentioned it in the Transactions of the Botanical Society, 1883, p. 224, and expressed the opinion that it belonged in the cyclus of development of Spirochæte dentium, since I was able now and then to find cells of this organism, which were composed of a series of short comma-like joints, in my own specimens.[62] The fact that the comma bacilli of the mouth take up coloring matter so much more easily than do the Spirochætes, does not, however, favor this supposition. I have also referred to this spirillum in Klebs's Archives for 1882, Vol. XVI, where a diagram of it will be found on Plate VII, Fig. 2. Furthermore, F. Y. Clark regarded it as the cause of dental caries as early as 1879, and called it "dental bacterium." He describes it as "half U-shaped, having screw-like movements." According to my experience it is to be found in every mouth,

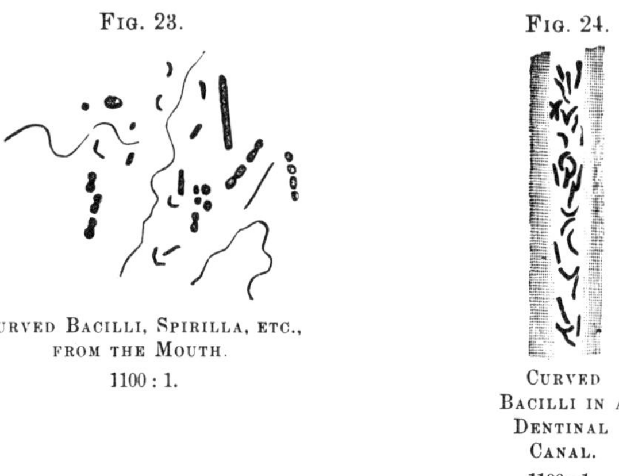

FIG. 23.
CURVED BACILLI, SPIRILLA, ETC., FROM THE MOUTH.
1100 : 1.

FIG. 24.
CURVED BACILLI IN A DENTINAL CANAL.
1100 : 1.

mixed with numerous other bacteria (Fig. 23). It frequently occurs in extraordinary numbers, exceeding all other forms put together, especially in cases where for some reason or other a slight hyperæmia of the gums has supervened. If a pointed instrument be introduced under the reddened gums, any desirable quantity of comma bacilli and Spirochætes may always be obtained. Between the teeth and in cavities of decay I have found it much more rarely. Now and then variously curved and twisted micro-organisms are met with in the dentinal tubules; the irregularity of the curves leads us to the inference that in most of such cases they are due only to the contracted space which does not admit of the organisms growing in straight lines (Fig. 24). Although I obtained nearly pure material in several cases, and used all possible kinds of nutrient media, I did not succeed in producing the slightest growth of this fungus. On gelatine and agar-agar with beef-extract, calf's broth, and beef-water-peptone, saliva, etc., also in fluid media at various temperatures, no development ever took place.

This fact alone is quite sufficient to establish the total difference of the organisms under consideration from the cholera bacillus, which, as is well known, grows very well on artificial culture-media. It is, however, to be hoped that a pure culture may yet be procured, since it is in itself an organism of great interest. But Spirillum sputigenum is not the only fungus occurring in the human mouth which produces curved rods. Another kind, not difficult to cultivate, occurs in short, plump, tapering rods, generally united in pairs, some of which show a slight curvature (Fig. 41); this is particularly observed in rods undergoing fissation. This bacterium is motile, grows well at room temperature, and quickly liquefies the gelatine.

FIG. 25.

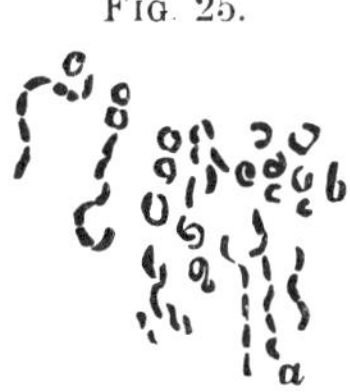

HALF-CIRCULAR RODS FROM A CULTURE OF THE ε-BACILLUS OF MILLER. 1100 : 1.

A third mouth-bacterium, which I have already described in the *Independent Practitioner*[63] and in No. 36 of the *Deutsche med. Wochenschr.*, 1884, occurs in the form of delicate rods of varying length, sometimes straight and sometimes so curved as to form the arc of a circle, two rods together making the letter O (Fig. 25). The cells vary in form to such an extent that I first supposed I had an impure culture before me; the attempt to separate them, however, did not succeed. Later, on observing various forms on one thread (Fig. 25, *c*), I became convinced that they belonged to the same fungus. The rods show every degree of curvature, from the straight to the semicircular. Two united rods sometimes form an S-, more frequently an O-shaped figure; in some cases the rods are so combined that they are scarcely distinguishable from cocci (Fig. 25, *b*). By the fissation of the rods, chains of cocci are formed, as is best seen in old cultures. No formation of spores was observed, and, examined in a hanging drop of bouillon, the rods displayed no motion.

On account of its slow growth on gelatine, its pure culture from saliva or dentine is connected with many difficulties. Cultures made of microscopically pure material offer nothing remarkable, as I have stated in a former communication. No growth occurs on the surface, nor does a liquefaction or evaporation of the gelatine take place. Its identity with the cholera bacillus is, therefore, quite out of the question. A true spirillum which possesses much more similarity to the comma bacillus of cholera asiatica, both morphologically and in the manner of its growth, I obtained from the human mouth in pure culture some five years ago. The isolation of this bacterium was accomplished in two cases by the use of coagulated beef-blood serum. The

FIG. 26.

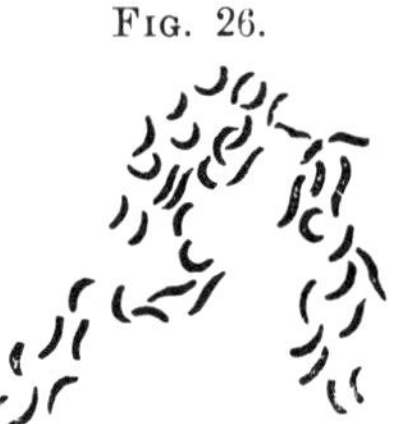

COMMA- AND S-FORMS FROM A PURE CULTURE OF A BACILLUS FOUND IN THE HUMAN MOUTH, PROBABLY FINKLER-PRIOR BACILLUS. 1100 : 1.

FIG. 27.

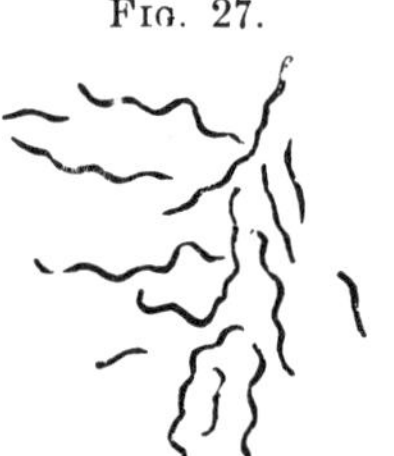

SPIRILLUM FORMS OF THE BACILLUS REPRESENTED IN FIG. 26. 1100 : 1.

material from which the cultures were made was, in each case, found under the margin of inflamed gums, in unhealthy mouths. Morphologically, this bacillus is very similar to the other well-known comma bacilli, occurring as commata, either singly or in twos (Fig. 26), or in spirillum form (Fig. 27). In old cultures on gelatine, all the commata sometimes grow out into spirilla, giving a pure spirillum culture. Cultivated on plates of beef-water-peptone-gelatine, at 20° C., they appear after twenty hours (in the second dilution), under a power of 100 diameters, as perfectly round, finely granular colonies, with a smooth border and brown color; in the same time the first dilution will be completely liquefied. They liquefy coagulated blood-serum with great energy, as do the other comma bacilli. On the surface of agar-agar they form a yellowish coating, and convert the medium, superficially only, into a paste. They grow slowly on boiled potato. I have, consequently, not yet been able to establish any definite peculiarity of growth. The reactions of this bacillus are such as at once establish the fact that it is altogether a different organism from the comma bacillus of Koch. It possesses, on the other hand, many of the peculiarities of the Finkler-Prior bacillus. Whether it is identical with this organism has never been determined beyond all doubt, though most bacteriologists believe it to be so.

It must be remarked that this organism is not the one which is constantly to be found in every mouth. This grows rapidly on ten per cent. gelatine, while the latter appears to be unable to grow at all on the same medium.

Not one of the many forms of micro-organisms, curved or otherwise, which I have obtained in pure culture from the human mouth, is for a moment to be mistaken for the bacillus of Koch.

I have before shown that micro-organisms occur in the mouth, which are not destroyed by a solution of artificial gastric juice, so that they may pass through the stomach into the intestines and still retain their power of reproduction.

That this should also be the case with curved bacilli occurring in the mouth, is not at all impossible. On the contrary, it is to be expected that, under certain conditions, they will be able to proliferate in abnormally large numbers in the intestines.

Fig 28.

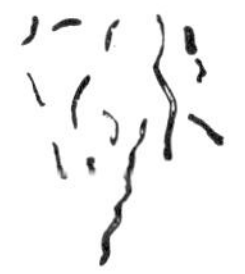

Curved Bacilli and Spirilla from the Fæces. 1100 : 1.

In my own fæces, during a slight diarrhœa, curved bacilli, as well as Spirochætes, were found in small numbers (Fig. 28), but they proved as uncultivable as the similar bacilli of the mouth. As a matter of course, the simple occurrence of a curved rod in the evacuations will not prove its specific character.

The above examples will suffice to demonstrate the existence of various screw-forms, which bear no more relation to each other than do the various species that occur in the form of cocci. They further show that the form of a fungus alone by no means always entitles us to draw conclusions as to its specific character. In doubtful cases this point can be decided by pure cultures alone.

Spirochæte dentium.

Spirochæte denticola (Spirochæte dentium, tooth spirochæte) is not found in decaying dentine, but in the same places in which Spirillum sputigenum is found, *i.e.*, under the margins of the gums, when they are covered with a dirty deposit and slightly inflamed,—in other words, in cases of gingivitis marginalis. This bacterium exhibits spirals from 8–25μ long, of very irregular windings and unequal thickness, which manifest a great difference in their affinity for coloring-matter. The thicker ones usually take it up much more readily than the thin ones; they also have fewer and broader windings (Fig. 29).

FIG. 29.

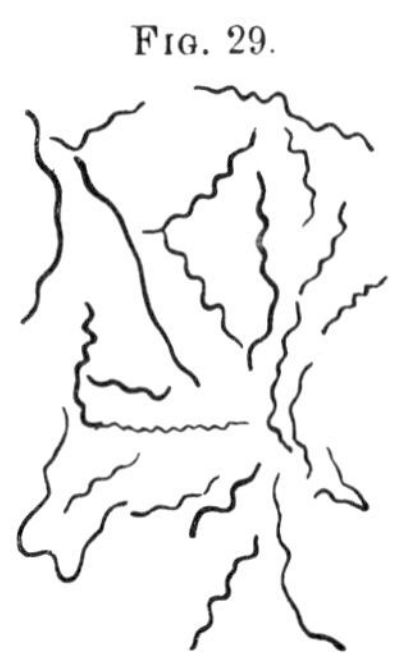

SCREW-FORMS (SPIRILLA AND SPIROCHÆTES) FROM THE MOUTH. 1100:1.

It is a question whether we have not to deal with two different organisms, the thicker of which may possibly represent a stage of development of Spirillum sputigenum. The development and pathogenesis of Spirochæte dentium is as obscure as that of the other above-mentioned uncultivable mouth-bacteria. Neither do we know anything definite as to their vital conditions and manifestations (fermentation, pathogenic action, etc.).

MOUTH-BACTERIA WHICH ARE UNCULTIVABLE AND WHOSE PATHOGENESIS IS UNKNOWN.

Under this head belong all the mouth-bacteria proper, as well as a bacterium of enormous dimensions which I discovered in great numbers in the mouth of a dog suffering from pyorrhœa alveolaris, and which I have designated by the name *Leptothrix gigantea* (Fig. 30). It appears in forms of tufts or fascicles whose threads diverge from a point of adhesion in different directions, somewhat like those of Crenothrix. It forms cocci, rods and threads, and therefore belongs to the pleomorphous bacteria. The threads of the same tuft may vary considerably in thickness, some relatively very thin, others very thick. The larger threads often show a difference in diameter between the

Fig. 30.

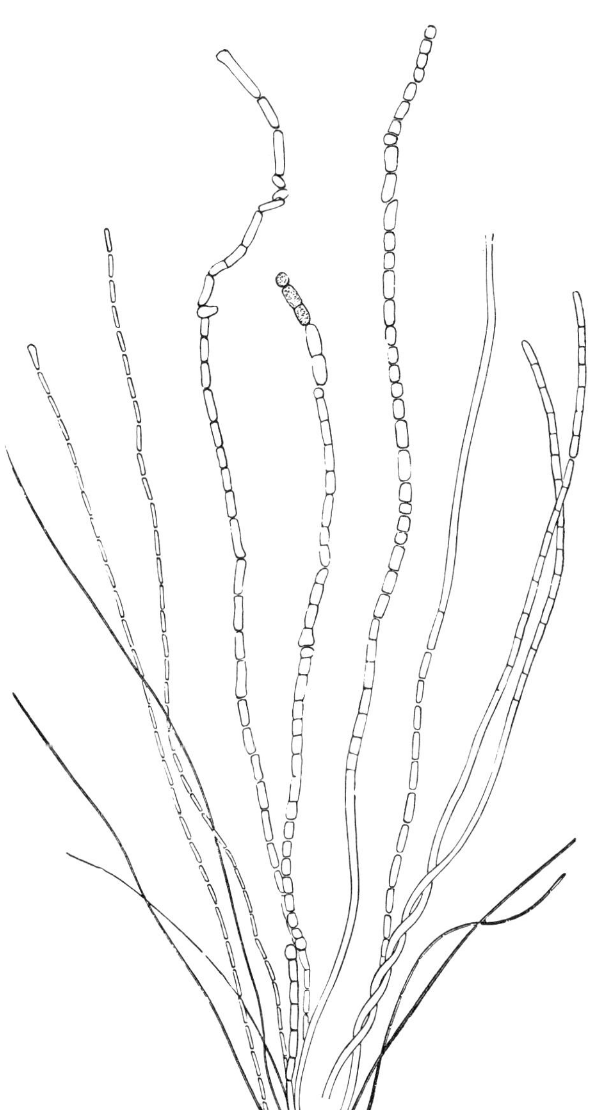

Leptothrix gigantea.
From the mouth of a dog suffering from pyorrhœa alveolaris.
540 : 1.

base and point; they sometimes appear straight, sometimes irregularly curved, sometimes twisted in regular spirals either throughout or only at the point or base. Now and then a spirulina may be observed. I have not been able to determine whether this fungus has any causal relation to the disease.

The question arises whether this organism may not also occur on the teeth of other carnivora, or even of phytophagous mammals. In order to determine this point, I examined the teeth of various animals and found very frequently leptothrix-like fungi in the mouths of sheep, cattle, pigs, horses, and so forth.

It can be determined by pure culture alone whether these species of Leptothrix, occurring in different animals, are identical or not. Some of them, at least, show morphologically great similarity; in general, however, those of the cat and rabbit seem to be more delicate and thin than those of the dog.

Mouth-Bacteria which give a Blue or Violet Reaction with Iodine.

Besides the Bacillus buccalis maximus and Jodococcus vaginatus, the following mouth-bacteria may be mentioned which give the iodine reaction described above:

a. A micro-organism which I shall for the present term *Jodococcus magnus;* large cocci or diplococci of different sizes (Fig. 31). I first succeeded in obtaining a pure culture of this micro-organism on a medium composed of equal parts of agar-agar gelatine and a solution of dentine glue sufficiently thick to become stiff at room temperature. In addition to these ingredients, the medium contained 1.5 per cent. of sugar and 1.5 per cent. of starch. If a small quantity of the soft deposit upon the necks of teeth be brought upon this medium after the manner employed in making line-cultures, a copious growth of different micro-organisms will be observed in twenty-four to forty-eight hours, if kept at the temperature of the human body. We now pour a slightly acidulated solution of iodine in iodide of potassium upon the plate. The culture-medium itself becomes bluish, most of the colonies yellowish; some individual points, however, often

Fig. 31.

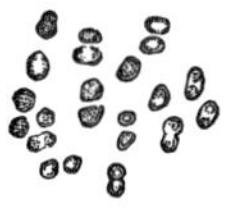

Jodococcus magnus. 800 : 1.

display a violet color, and if the latter are immediately transferred to a new plate a pure culture of the given bacterium may be easily obtained. The brief period of action of the iodine solution does not destroy these organisms, at least not all of them, and consequently its application affords an excellent means of determining and isolating them. They also flourish on ordinary nutrient agar-agar, but not on gelatine at room temperature. The reaction is best observed in media containing sugar, less plainly in amylaceous media. When cultivated on the latter, the colonies often show concentric variously-colored rings, thereby giving rise to very delicate and pretty patterns.

In form and in reaction this micrococcus exactly coincides with one which is found in carious dentine, and which produces the violet color characteristic of decayed dentine on addition of the iodine solution. The same has hitherto, without any definite reason, been considered as "elements of Leptothrix buccalis." The cells of the Jodococcus magnus are on the average larger than those of the coccus occurring in dentine; yet the difference is not so great that it may not be explained by the great dissimilarity in the conditions of growth.

b. A small micrococcus, of which I have succeeded in obtaining a pure culture recently, which, however, I have not more closely examined. It also gives a blue to violet color with iodine.

c. A micrococcus which gives a beautiful pink color under the action of iodine. I have observed a slight development of this bacterium on nutrient agar-agar, but have not been able to perpetuate it in pure culture.

Other bacteria, which are colored slightly blue or violet by iodine, also occur in the mouth. Their reaction is, however, too slight to justify a further examination in this connection.

I have furthermore obtained in pure cultures two yeast-fungi from the mouth, which show characteristic reactions with iodine.

Cultivable Mouth-Bacteria, partly Non-Pathogenic, partly of Unknown Pathogenesis.

The great number of different kinds of bacteria which have been obtained in pure culture from the mouth has hitherto made their classification impossible. We are also unable, with few exceptions, to state which of these bacteria occur most frequently in the mouth, or under what conditions the different kinds develop best. Any one who makes an extensive series of culture experiments will soon be overwhelmed with such a quantity of material that it will be impossible for him to work it up with the desired thoroughness. I have myself made the mistake, which I think others have made, of attempting the impracticable

FIG. 32.

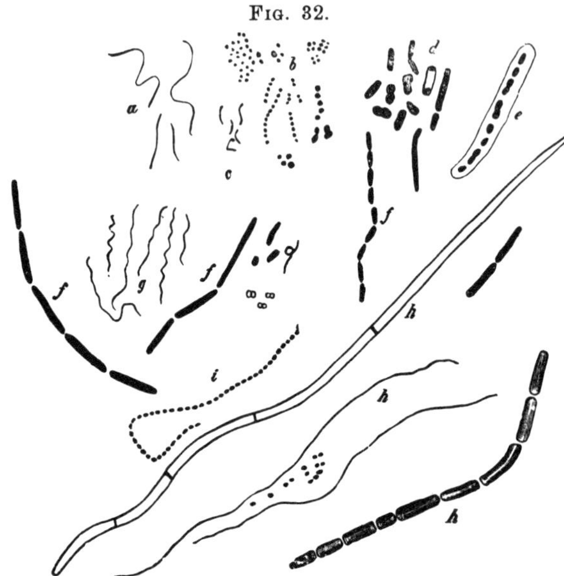

VARIOUS FORMS OF BACTERIA FROM THE MOUTH.
a, c, g, Screw-forms; *b*, Cocci; *d*, Rods; *e*, Coccus-chain with sheath; *i*, Coccus-chain (Streptococci); *f*, Rod-chains; *h*, Various thread-forms.

task of examining all the species which I have isolated, instead of concentrating my attention upon individual cases and studying them thoroughly. Consequently only general results have been obtained, and the researches of different authors have repeated, instead of complementing each other. Some confusion therefore exists in our conceptions of mouth-bacteria, which can only be cleared up by an enormous amount of labor.

With the exception of Cladothrix and Beggiatoa, all of the most common species of bacteria have their representatives in the oral cavity (Fig. 32).

Up to 1885, I had isolated twenty-two different kinds of bacteria from the human mouth. A number of these are represented in Figs. 33 to 44. In these figures *b* represents the form of the respective colonies, on 10 per cent. gelatine, slightly magnified.

Ten of the twenty-two kinds mentioned appear in the form of cocci; four of these are reproduced in Figs. 33–36: they are of different dimensions, from very small, round cells (Fig. 33) to remarkably large cocci, "macrococci" (Fig. 36).

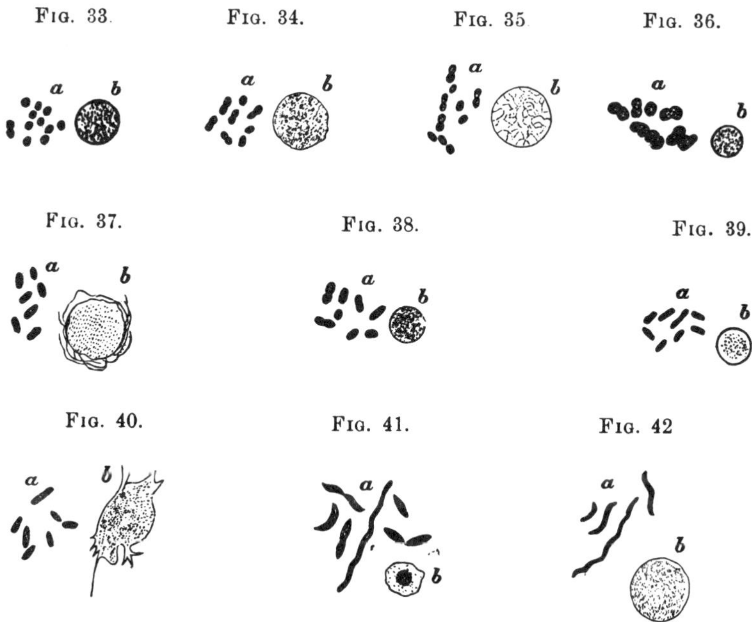

Fig. 33. Fig. 34. Fig. 35. Fig. 36.

Fig. 37. Fig. 38. Fig. 39.

Fig. 40. Fig. 41. Fig. 42.

Five appeared as short rods (Figs. 37, 38), six as somewhat longer rods (Figs. 39, 40). A curved species, which liquefied gelatine and produced a green coloring-matter, was designated by the name *Vibrio viridans* (Fig. 41). One species (Fig. 42) formed spirilla, another developed into long threads (Fig. 43). One again formed long jointed threads, some of which were furnished with sheaths (Fig. 44). Of thirty species cultivated later, eighteen were cocci, eleven rods, while one grew into threads.

In liquids three developed into rather long articulated or inarticulated threads, one kind occurred in spirillum form, eight were motile, fourteen immotile.

Formation of spores was observed in three cases only, the others appearing to develop by fissation alone; eight liquefied gelatine. Fourteen were cultivated on slices of potato, five of them growing rapidly, one in particular soon spreading over the whole surface of the slice and liquefying it completely to a depth of one to two millimeters. The others did not thrive well on potato. Of fifteen kinds which were cultivated on the white of egg, four grew well, evolving considerable quantities of sulphuretted hydrogen (H_2S) and later ammonia (NH_3). The white of egg was converted into a semi-transparent pasty mass, which

FIG. 43. FIG. 44.

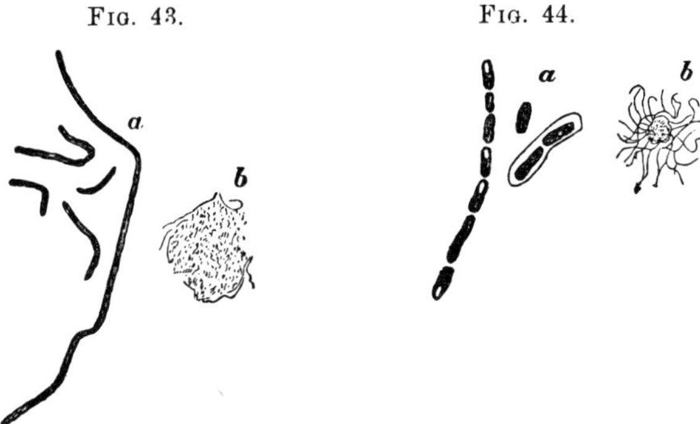

gradually disappeared. Seven grew slowly, and four not at all. On sections of normal undecalcified dentine certain bacteria seemed able to exist for some days, presumably till the organic substance exposed on the surface of the section was consumed. No growth occurred on enamel.

These bacteria showed, as far as they were examined, differences in relation to the action of atmospheric air. Ten of them were strictly obligatory aërobic, growing only with free access of air; four were not strictly obligatory aërobic, growing better, but not exclusively, when air was admitted; eight were facultative aërobic, that is, they seemed to grow equally well with or without oxygen.

If from the deposits about the necks of the teeth we make line-cultures on beef-water-peptone-sugar agar-agar, certain bacteria will develop with tolerable regularity. Of these I think the following worthy of mention:

1. A micro-organism occurring in somewhat irregular cocci or diplococci, singly or in chains (Fig. 45). It produces small, prominent, shining colonies resembling in older cultures tiny glass beads; these colonies are further characterized by their cartilaginous consistency, and by the fact that they cannot be taken up with the point of the needle, but run ahead of it on the surface of the plate. Under a low power the colonies appear roundish, very dark, lustrous, frequently having a villous margin and a black pattern within (Fig. 46). These two last characteristics are not, however, constant.

Fig. 45.

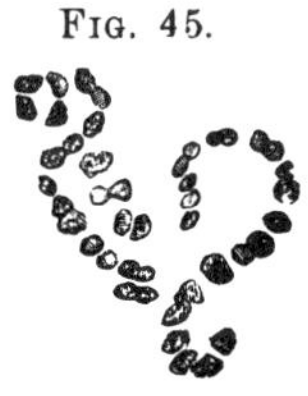

ASCOCOCCUS BUCCALIS. 1100 : 1.

2. A bacterium which appears in the form of unequally large cocci (Fig. 47). It forms small round or roundish, very thin colo-

Fig. 46. Fig. 47. Fig. 48.

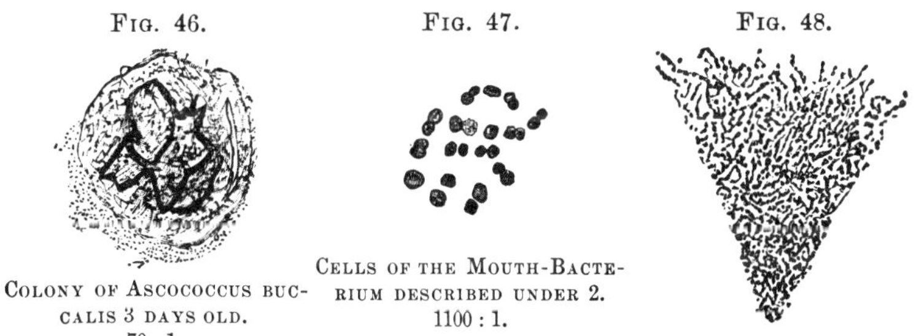

COLONY OF ASCOCOCCUS BUCCALIS 3 DAYS OLD. 70 : 1.

CELLS OF THE MOUTH-BACTERIUM DESCRIBED UNDER 2. 1100 : 1.

SECTOR OF A COLONY OF THE MOUTH-BACTERIUM DESCRIBED UNDER 2. 3 DAYS OLD. 200 : 1.

nies, without a distinct margin, which are quite colorless or tinged but faintly yellowish-gray when examined under the microscope. The separate cocci are visible under a power of about 200 diameters, the whole colony appearing coarsely granular, and the short chains of cocci or separate cocci protruding over the margin. Fig. 48 shows the sector of a colony under about 200 diameters.

3. A third bacterium appears as oval cocci, mostly in pairs or chains (Fig. 49). It also forms thin, small colonies, hardly

visible to the naked eye; under weak power without distinct outlines or wholly transparent at the margin, becoming denser toward the center, which has a grayish color. Under 320 diameters the sector of a colony has the appearance represented in Fig. 50. I have named this bacterium *Micrococcus nexifer* on account of the loops formed by the chains of cocci in pure culture.

4. A bacterium somewhat less frequent, which appears under the microscope as scattered, unequally large, irregular colonies, composed of a few cells. These colonies are without distinct form, dark gray: micrococci.

5. The bacterium which I mention as the fifth is conspicuous to the naked eye for the size of its colonies. It appears in almost all cultures, but in comparatively small numbers. To the naked eye the colonies appear milky-white; under the microscope they show a gray margin and a yellowish to dark-brown center wholly opaque. The margin of the colony is occasionally indented and strongly refractive. Morphology: beautiful round cocci in dense masses.

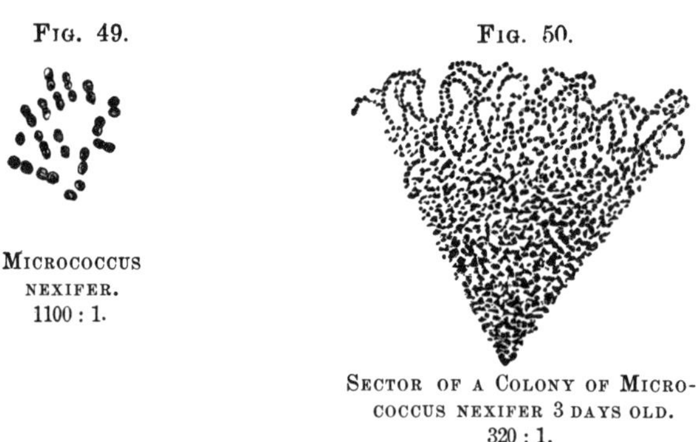

FIG. 49.

MICROCOCCUS NEXIFER. 1100 : 1.

FIG. 50.

SECTOR OF A COLONY OF MICROCOCCUS NEXIFER 3 DAYS OLD. 320 : 1.

6. A micro-organism which is remarkable for its very characteristic growth may often be found on culture-plates, whether inoculated from the secretions of the oral cavity or from decayed dentine. It forms colorless, transparent, prominent colonies, which obtain a height of 1.5 millimeter and a breadth of from 2.5 to 4 millimeters, having the consistency of paste. Under the microscope the separate cells in form of chains of cocci are distinctly visible, lying scattered in this paste.

7. I have found the *Jodococcus magnus* in almost all cases in which I have particularly searched for it in the secretions of the mouth.

These bacteria, cultivated in saccharine solutions, bring about fermentation, accompanied by a strong acid reaction. Experiments undertaken for the purpose of determining their other physiological characteristics are not yet concluded. Various other coccus and bacillus kinds are less constant; some of them are shown in Figs. 33 to 44. Colonies of yeast-fungi may almost invariably be found on plates inoculated from the human mouth. I have, however, made no attempt to examine them more closely. (See Chapter XII.)

W. Vignal ("Recherches sur les microorganismes de la bouche," *Archives de Physiologie norm. et pathol.*, 1886, No. 8) has made very extensive and exact experiments upon the bacteria of the mouth. In his communication, which is accompanied by very instructive illustrations, he describes seventeen different kinds of bacteria found in the mouth and obtained by him in pure culture. Some of these were identical with well-known species, while others were new to him.

Concerning the frequency with which the various bacteria examined occur in the human mouth, Vignal makes the following determination, for which, however, he claims only approximate accuracy. Most frequently of all he found Bacterium termo, then Bacillus e (Bacillus ulna?) etc., in the following order:

1. Bacterium termo.
2. Bacillus e (Bacillus ulna?).
3. Potato bacillus.
4. Coccus a (δ of Miller?).
5. Bacillus b.
6. Bacillus d.
7. Bacillus c (Bacillus alvei?).
8. Bacillus subtilis.
9. Staphylococcus pyogenes albus.
10. Staphylococcus pyogenes aureus.
11. Bacillus i.
12. Bacillus f.
13. Bacillus j.

14. Bacillus g.
15. Bacillus h.
16. Leptothrix.

Vignal's table is characterized by the predominance of bacilli. With the exception of the two pyogenic bacteria, he met with but a single coccus form (Coccus a), while other investigators—Black, Biondi, Gysi, and myself—found a preponderance of coccus forms. An examination of a few preparations derived from mucous tooth deposits or carious dentine will, as a rule, show a prevalence of micrococci.

This difference in the results of different investigators can be explained, I think, by the circumstance that Vignal cultivated all of his bacteria on gelatine. Since, however, very many mouth-bacteria do not grow on gelatine, cultures made upon agar-agar may lead to different results.

In America, Black[64] has entered upon the study of the micro-organisms of the human mouth with great zeal. He describes among others *Streptococcus continuosus*, *Staphylococcus medius*, *Staphylococcus magnus*, *Coccus cumulus minor* (probably Sarcina or Micrococcus tetragenus), and a "gelatine-forming" organism, Bacillus gelatogenes. (See page 22.)

Chromogenic Mouth-bacteria.

It needs scarcely to be remarked that many theories have been proposed to account for the various colors presented by decayed dentine. The best known is that of Watt,[65] which attributes these colors to the action of various mineral acids, supposed to be concerned in the production of caries. Another view assigns the chief rôle to articles of food, drink, etc., which do certainly sometimes produce discoloration of the decayed as well as of the healthy tooth-tissue.

Others, again, would have us believe that the color comes from within and is one of the results of the vital reaction of the tooth-substance itself. Black seeks to account for the discoloration by the impregnation of the carious tissue with sulphides, while, finally, the view has not been wanting in advocates that certain bacteria which possess the property of forming various coloring matters are the chief factors in bringing about the pigmentation in question.

The following presentation of the characteristics of the color-forming bacteria of the human mouth, as far as they have as yet been revealed to us by actual research, is undertaken in the hope of determining how far they are accountable for the work which has been assigned to them.

Chromogenic bacteria are widely distributed in nature. A plate of gelatine exposed to impure air for a short time will almost invariably develop one or more colored colonies; green, various shades of yellow, brown, red, being sometimes represented on the same plate. Such being the case, it must naturally happen that these bacteria often find their way into the human mouth with food, drink, and chiefly with the air. As a matter of fact, they are by no means seldom met with in the oral cavity.

As a rule, the colorless bacteria predominate in the human mouth to such an extent that the chromogenic bacteria, if present, cannot be detected; occasionally, however, they may be easily recognized even by the naked eye. I have observed a brick-red color more frequently than any other, on the lingual surface of the lower front teeth and on the buccal surface of the molar teeth.

When this organism has once become established in the mouth, it does not readily allow itself to be expelled. I have in my practice a number of patients in whose mouths I have watched its growth for six to eight years. One case which particularly interested me was that of four children, brothers and sisters, aged about ten to seventeen years, for whom I repeatedly removed the brick-colored deposit on the lower incisors only to see it faithfully return in the course of a few weeks. Having recently had occasion to examine the mouth of the mother, I found the same deposit, from which I conclude that there is some constitutional peculiarity about these children, inherited from the mother, which renders the secretions of their mouths peculiarly adapted to the needs of this organism.

Attempts to cultivate the bacterium of brick-colored deposit have been unsuccessful, although I did succeed in isolating from the mouth an organism which produces about the same color

(Fig. 1, Plate III). My present opinion, however, is that the one I obtained is not the one I have been seeking.

A number of times I have found cavities of decay, usually dark brown, in which the surface of the dentine was colored with a bright yellow mass of cheesy consistency. I have not been able to obtain a pure culture of this bacterium on gelatine, though I have repeatedly observed a slight growth on potatoes.

Any one who will keep a lookout for the two appearances just described will certainly see them. A case which was interesting in more than one respect occurred at the polyclinic of the Dental Institute at Berlin, some time ago. A man presented himself, having a swelling on the right side of the face, almost as large as a man's fist, connected with the inferior wisdom-tooth (impeded eruption). The larger portion of the surface of the mouth and tongue was covered with a canary-yellow deposit, which could not be accounted for by anything that the patient had taken into his mouth.

I found a bacillus in the pus which was evacuated upon the extraction of the tooth, and also in the yellow layer upon the surface of the cheeks and gums, which reproduced the same color in pure cultures, and besides showed considerable pathogenic action. I had no opportunity to see the patient again, consequently do not know the result of the infection. A pure culture of this micro-organism on gelatine is seen in Fig. 2 of the plate.

I have found in the human mouth and isolated no less than eight different kinds of bacteria which produce a yellow pigment, not including the well-known yellow sarcina. These bacteria are themselves yellow, but do not impart any color to the culture-medium.

I have made a great many attempts to cultivate the supposed bacterium of greenstain, but so far without success. I have indeed isolated five different species of bacteria from the mouth which *impart a green color to the culture-media*, although themselves colorless, and all of which grow well on the usual media, but I do not bring any of them into causal connection with the greenstain, since, as far as my observation goes, the bacterium of greenstain, if there be such a thing, does not grow on gelatine.

I found one of these in the contents of an alveolar abscess; it grew with tolerable rapidity, liquefying the gelatine. If cultivated without the presence of oxygen, no color is developed, but if the culture is shaken with air, it will in a few seconds assume a beautiful green color. I found the second in a cavity of decay, and the other three in my search for the supposed bacterium of pyorrhœa alveolaris; they are colorless, but impart a beautiful opalescent color to the gelatine, one of them having at the beginning a decidedly bluish tinge. A pure culture of one of these is seen in Fig. 3 of the plate. It is, however, impossible in the lithograph to reproduce the beautiful opalescent color of this growth. The cultures of one bacterium obtained from the mouth have a red color on the surface, but are colorless beneath the surface (Fig. 1, plate); the protoplasm of the living cells contains the coloring-matter, and no color is imparted to the gelatine. Another has a reddish color, also confined to the bacteria themselves. Cultures of still another have a decided brownish color (Fig. 4, plate); it liquefies the gelatine, and sinks to the bottom as a brownish irregular mass.

I have recently isolated a bacterium from the mouth occurring in form of long large rods and jointed threads, which, cultivated on the surface of nutritive agar-agar, imparts to the medium, in the course of a few weeks, a yellowish-brown color which gradually darkens and extends deeper into the substratum as the age of the culture increases. To this bacterium, whose characteristics I have not yet sufficiently investigated, I have assigned the name, *Bacillus fuscans.*

I shall not enter into a discussion of the biology of these bacteria. At present we are interested in the question as to what part they may take, if any, in the production of the various colors or shades of color in carious dentine.

Of all the chromogenic bacteria above referred to, only the ones represented in Fig. 4 of the plate and the one described as Bacillus fuscans could be looked upon as taking any direct part in the pigmentation of carious dentine. These, however, as far as we know at present, do not occur with sufficient constancy in the mouth to admit of assigning an important rôle to them.

The green-producing bacteria, which I have named *Bacteria*

viridantia, are excluded, because green dentine does not occur. Those which assume a yellow color (*Bacteria flavescentia*) cannot be looked upon as the direct cause of the yellow shade of carious dentine, because the color is confined to the micro-organisms themselves, the medium on which they are cultivated becoming very little, if at all, stained. In the case of dentine, the relations are exactly the opposite; the dentine becomes stained, while the micro-organisms remain colorless (white). This is probably well known to those who have made a few sections of carious dentine.

The following experiment may serve to furnish an idea of the manner in which the pigmentation of the carious tooth-tissue may be brought about.

I inoculated a tube of culture-gelatine with a bacterium obtained from decayed dentine; almost any bacterium which liquefies the gelatine would, however, have served the same purpose. In about two weeks the gelatine was completely melted and a white mass of bacteria lay on the bottom of the tube.

At the beginning of the experiment the gelatine had only the slight yellowish tinge often present in culture gelatine. Soon, however, a yellowish-brown color made its appearance, which gradually became darker even after all life had disappeared from the culture, until at the end of ten weeks the whole mass of melted gelatine had a deep brownish color.

A very old dry culture presented about the color of the black spots (so-called caries nigra) often seen on the approximal surfaces of teeth where caries once began and then ceased after the removal of the approximating tooth. Organic matter undergoing decomposition assumes, as is well known, a dark color, and the same is true of decaying dentine. The colors characteristic of decaying dentine do not exist in the very beginning of the decay, but appear subsequently. The more recent or acute the decay, the less the discoloration; the older or more chronic the decay, the deeper the color.

There is, however, another factor which may play a part in the discoloration of dentine, more particularly in teeth containing dead pulps; the latter sometimes become intensely black, and it is to these in particular that the following suggestion refers. My attention was some time since called to the fact that recent experiments had demonstrated the presence of iron in a variety of tissues where it had not previously been detected. This discovery led to the thought that iron might be present in the dental pulp, and that in such case the black color of the putrid pulps might be accounted for by the formation of the sulphide of iron. I made a few preliminary experiments relating to this question, the results of which I here give. The tests were made in the following manner: A tooth was cracked in a porcelain mortar, so as to thoroughly expose the pulp, and then placed in a mixture of dilute hydrochloric acid, to which was added a small proportion of a 10 per cent. solution of ferrocyanide of potassium. The hydrochloric acid, as well as the water used for diluting it, must be free from iron; neither must any iron instrument be brought in contact with the freshly-broken surfaces of the tooth. Those parts of the tooth containing iron, even in minute quantities, will, after an exposure of from one to sixty minutes, assume a blue color—Prussian blue being formed. One source of error is introduced in the necessary use of an iron instrument in extracting the tooth, but this will only affect those points on the external surface of the tooth with which the forceps come in contact, and may therefore be easily eliminated.

I have found iron (1) constantly in Nasmyth's membrane (probably only as a deposit from external sources); (2) in the dental pulp, though not constantly; (3) in carious dentine almost constantly, a bright blue line often forming on the border between the decalcified and normal tissue,—a rather remarkable appearance for which I can at present attempt no explanation; (4) in enamel, particularly around the margin of cavities of decay.*

It seems, consequently, not impossible that the sulphide of iron which would be formed during putrefaction of the pulp may have something to do with the discoloration of the same. Whether sulphide of iron may be formed through decay of the dentine or enamel in sufficient quantity to aid in discoloring the same, I cannot say; at present I doubt it. Further experiments may furnish an answer to this question.

---

* Traces of iron have been detected (as is well known) by chemical analysis in both dentine and enamel.

THE BACTERIA OF DISEASED PULPS.

In the mouth we find certain conditions which are presented by no other part of the human body, in that a direct way is furnished for parasites through the medium of root-canals and diseased tooth-pulps into the deeper parts (Fig. 51).

The question arises, Is this way equally passable for all bacteria and under all circumstances, or are there only certain kinds which find a suitable culture-medium in different conditions of the pulp, and are thereby enabled to effect the passage through it to the apex of the root or to the periapical tissue?

FIG. 51.

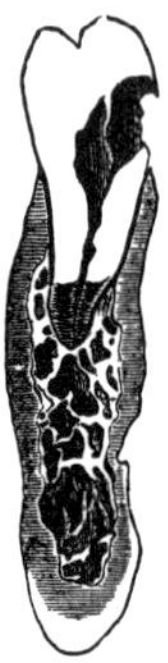

CROSS-SECTION THROUGH THE LOWER JAW WITH HALF OF A DECAYED PREMOLAR IN SITU, showing how germs of infection may pass from the mouth directly into the spongy portion of the bone.

As far as I know, nothing has as yet been ascertained in regard to this point, and I can here only communicate the results of my own investigations, which have, in fact, as yet but begun.

We have reason to suppose that in the living pulp, for instance in the case of chronic pulpitis, as well as in all suppurative inflammations of the pulp, chiefly bacteria of a pathogenic nature may obtain a footing, since in such cases these find the most suitable nutrient medium, and that the more harmless parasites of the human mouth, on the other hand, would prefer the dead organic matter of the oral cavity. It has, moreover, appeared to me that in cultures from such pulps I have not, as a rule, found the large number of different kinds of bacteria which may usually be found in the mouth.

Again, since the access of air, particularly in case of closed pulp-chambers, is very limited, we would expect to find a preponderance of anaërobic or of facultative anaërobic bacteria. In regard to this point, also, experimental evidence is wanting.

In the third place, in case the pulp-chamber has not been opened, the entire store of nutrient material being soon consumed, the bacteria may perish from want of nourishment, or even be destroyed by their own products, or finally they may enter upon the state of spores.

It may, therefore, readily occur that a putrid pulp does not contain a single bacterium capable of development.

Of seventeen necrotic tooth-pulps which I have examined with reference to this question, I found seven without living (at least without cultivable) bacteria. Attention has already been called to the fact that the dental pulp presents in a high degree the conditions essential to the formation of spores; and since spores possess high power of resistance, the antiseptic treatment of root-canals is thereby rendered more difficult.

In order to determine whether a necrotic pulp contains living bacteria or not, we proceed in the following manner. Taking a freshly extracted tooth (the best are such whose pulp-chambers have not been opened), we first cleanse it by placing it for a short time in a solution of sublimate 5 : 1000; then carefully wash it with sterilized water to remove the sublimate, dry it with sterilized paper, and split it with sterilized forceps. The pulp is then removed with a sterilized needle and brought into the culture-medium, in which it is crushed, the solution being repeatedly shaken in order to distribute the organisms equally throughout. From this a second or even a third dilution is made, and the number of colonies determined in the usual manner.

Experiments 1 to 5 were made on gelatine, the others on agar-agar at a temperature from 37° to 38° C.

From Pulp 1	4800	colonies developed.
" " 2	4800	" "
" " 3	235	" "
" " 4	0	" "
" " 5	0	" "
" " 6	275	" "
" " 7	0	" "
" " 8	3	" "
" " 9	0	" "
" " 10	4	" "
" " 11	250,000	" "
" " 12, dry, black, foul-smelling .	0	" "

From Pulp 13, moist, bad-smelling	2050	colonies developed.
" " 14, almost dry, black	0	" "
" " 15, suppurating	405	" "
" " 16, black, liquefied, very bad-smelling	512	" "
" " 17	0	" "

The fourth case is that in which the pulp-chamber is widely opened, so as to permit the entrance of new culture-material from the mouth. Processes of putrefaction or fermentation here continually take place. In the lower part of the canal, at least, the same organisms are present which are found in the other part of the oral cavity, with the exception of such whose growth depends upon the presence of more or less inflamed gums.

The subject of the bacteria of the diseased pulp is one which has as yet but little occupied the attention of bacteriologists, consequently little definite is known about them; nor has any classification of them been made. A series of experiments which I myself began in this direction had to be broken off on account of want of time.

The general infections which are brought about by inoculation with the bacteria of diseased tooth-pulps will be treated of in Chapter XI.

It often happens that a tooth, which has occasioned no disturbance for years, in spite of a necrotic pulp, will exhibit a severe inflammation of the pericementum a few hours after the pulp-chamber has been opened for the purpose of removing the remains of the pulp and filling the root-canals.

An attempt has been made to ascribe this very unpleasant result to an infection of the pulp occasioned by germs from the air. When the pulp-chamber is opened, air is supposed to rush in, carrying bacteria along with it. These excite decomposition of the contents of the root-canal, thereby giving origin to an inflammation of the pericementum. This idea deserves to be ranked among the many other wonderful theories of olden times.

Every practitioner in dentistry knows very well that air or

gas often enough *escapes* as soon as an opening is made into a pulp-chamber containing a gangrenous pulp. No one, however, as far as I am aware, has observed that the air *enters* the pulp-chamber under such conditions.

It would indeed be difficult to explain how a vacuum could exist in the canal of a root. Granted, however, that a partial vacuum did exist at the time the pulp-chamber was opened, and that ten cubic millimeters of air were admitted into the pulp-chamber (which is a large estimate), how many organisms would likely be introduced with it?

The number of micro-organisms in a given quantity of air depends of course upon the purity of the air, and consequently varies according to the locality. Pure air in Berlin was found to contain, on the average, 0.1 to 0.5 bacteria per liter, and the air in hospital wards, with seventeen or eighteen beds, to contain 2.4 and 2.7 per liter respectively.

Now, if we suppose the air of a dental office to contain double the amount represented by the largest number found in pure Berlin air, there will exist in one liter, that is, in one million cubic millimeters, one germ. Ten cubic millimeters would then contain $\frac{1}{1000000} \times 10 = \frac{1}{100000}$ germs.

The chances would then be that in one hundred thousand operations of this kind the success of one would be endangered by the entrance of one germ into the pulp-cavity. Whether this one germ in such case could produce any disturbance, would depend upon the existing circumstances.

The appearance of pericementitis after opening into a pulp-chamber is due solely to the carelessness or helplessness of the operator. He either forces particles of the putrid pulp through the foramen apicale, or introduces new infected fermentable matter into the root-canal from without, or occasions an infection by means of unclean instruments.

The Relation of Mouth-Bacteria to the Formation of Tartar.

Since the discovery of the existence of great numbers of microscopical organisms in the human mouth, repeated efforts have been made to make them responsible for the formation of tartar. Lebeaume compared tartar to coral; Mandl supposed it to be caused by the accumulation of calcareous remains of vibrios; Klebs, Galippe, and others express the opinion that tartar is to be regarded as an excretion of micro-organisms.

There is such a vast difference between tartar and coral, as well as between bacteria and coral-forming polyps, that Lebeaume's comparison is certainly unwarranted, while the theory of Klebs is an apparent contradiction of facts known to every practitioner. As is well known, tartar is formed chiefly, sometimes exclusively, where the salivary glands discharge their products into the oral cavity, particularly on the lingual surfaces of the lower incisors. In no other locality of the mouth have the bacteria so little opportunity of gaining a foothold as at this particular point, since the tongue keeps these surfaces nearly free from bacteria and soft deposits.

Moreover, the amount of tartar in a given mouth is in no wise proportional to the number of bacteria contained in the same, nor am I aware that calcareous deposits anyway resembling tartar have been observed in pure cultures of mouth-bacteria.

Other considerations also seem to me to render this explanation untenable. Tartar contains about 25 per cent. of organic matter and 75 per cent. of salts (almost exclusively lime-salts; bacteria, on the other hand, contain about 0.5 per cent. of ashes, consequently the percentage of ashes in bacteria is equal to but $\frac{1}{150}$ of that in tartar; a formation of tartar, therefore, by an accumulation of the calcareous remains of bacteria appears to me to be out of the question.

Normal saliva contains calcium phosphate as well as carbonate; these are held in solution in the blood and in the glands by carbonic acid. When the saliva enters into the mouth, the carbonic acid escapes and the lime-salts are precipitated. The following experiment will demonstrate this process:

Small quantities of calcium phosphate and calcium carbonate are brought into water charged with carbonic acid (a bottle of soda-water serves the purpose very well), shaken at brief intervals, and left standing until the water becomes quite clear. On opening the bottle very carefully and permitting the carbonic acid slowly to escape, the precipitation of the salts held in solution will produce a distinct cloudiness.

At the June meeting of the Odontological Society of Great Britain, 1889, Cunningham and Robinson presented impure cultures of bacteria partly from the mouth, in which well-formed crystals might easily be seen with the naked eye. The analysis proved these crystals to consist of the double ammonium-magnesium phosphate or triple phosphate ($NH_4,Mg,PO_4,2H_2O$). The authors were of the opinion that "the deposition of tartar on the teeth and the formation of some calculi in other parts of the body may be due, in part at least, to this action." On a visit of Dr. Cunningham to my laboratory a short time ago we examined a number of pure cultures from the mouth and found in three cases, all from two to three months old, distinct crystalline formations not imbedded in the growth, but projecting from it into the pure gelatine or agar-agar.

As stated to Dr. Cunningham at the time, I am not quite prepared to believe that this process has much to do with the formation of tartar. Of course it remains for him to show whether such crystals really are found in tartar, and whether tartar actually contains the above-mentioned triple phosphate in any considerable quantity.

A communication on the subject of salivary calculus by A. C. Castle, in the January number of *The Forcep*, 1855, may be of interest in this connection. He writes, "Microscopic examination discovers that this calculus exists in a crystalline state, and by its irritating effects frequently causes what are supposed to be neuralgic pains.

"The next form of salivary calculus is of a soft, friable, pulverant nature. It is of two kinds, the simple *phosphate of lime*, and the *ammoniaco-magnesia phosphate of lime*, with the usual combinations of animal matter, and *oxalate of lime* upon investigation will be found to exist in large quantities in those subjects where the oxalates exist in excess."

CHAPTER V.

MOUTH-BACTERIA AS EXCITERS OF FERMENTATION.

General Remarks.

Numerous experiments and investigations from the time of Schwann to the present day, and particularly the exact methods of bacteriological research employed within the last few years, have demonstrated beyond all doubt that all processes of fermentation and putrefaction depend upon the presence of microscopically small living organisms. Nevertheless, certain authors, not in dental literature alone, are in the habit of completely disregarding all the facts established in the last fifty years, putting themselves back into the first half of the century and speaking of putrefactive processes which are supposed to arise in some inexplicable manner without the aid of micro-organisms, and to yield certain products, among which bacteria themselves are not unfrequently reckoned.

It is actually astonishing that the question, which is first, the bacteria or the fermentation? can still claim the attention of any mind, and that irrefutable facts can be entirely overlooked, although handbooks of bacteriology are so numerous and widely circulated that ample information may be easily obtained in regard to these fundamental questions. We are constantly confronted by the statement that the decomposition of certain substances may be effected by means of finely divided platinum, that alcohol may be directly oxidized to acetic acid. Many dentists also continue to refer to the possibility that acids may develop during the putrefaction of organic substances in the mouth without the participation of micro-organisms, and obstinately ignore the fact that without micro-organisms the putrefaction of organic substances is altogether impossible. Others, again, settle the question in a manner which they think should be satisfactory to every one by the stereotyped assertion, "Bacteria are not the cause, but the result of fermentation."

Whoever is at all versed in the fundamental principles of bacteriology will regard it as a matter of course that the process of fermentation going on in the oral cavity offers no exception to the rule that all fermentative and putrefactive processes are conditioned by the presence of living micro-organisms. This fact may be established experimentally by the following simple tests:

Exp. 1. Add 2 per cent. of sugar or starch to fresh saliva, and keep the mixture at blood temperature. It invariably becomes acid in four to five hours; or fill a glass tube two cm. long and three mm. wide with starch, sterilize it, and fasten it to a molar tooth in the mouth on going to bed; next morning the contents of the tube will have a strong acid reaction. A cavity in a tooth, or a piece of linen, which may be saturated with a solution of starch, will answer the purpose as well as the glass tube.

Exp. 2. Keep the mixture of saliva with starch or sugar for one hour in the sterilizer at 100° C., and then place it in the incubator; it does not become sour in four, nor in twenty-four hours; in fact, not at all. We conclude that the agent which caused the mixture in 1 to become sour (*i.e.*, the ferment) is rendered inactive by a temperature of 100° C.

Exp. 3. Heat the starch alone to 150° C. before mixing with the saliva; the solution still becomes sour. Heat the saliva alone, and the mixture does not become sour. Conclusion: the ferment exists, not in the starch, but in the saliva.

We have now to determine the question, Is it an organized ferment (micro-organisms), or is it an unorganized ferment (ptyaline)?

This question is determined by the following experiments:

Exp. 4. From six to eight grams of saliva are agitated in a test tube with as much sulphuric ether as it will take up, starch added, and the whole put in the incubator. On examination after a few hours, we will find sugar in the solution, but no acid;

in other words, the acid-forming ferment has been rendered inactive, but the unorganized, sugar-forming ferment, not.

Exp. 5. Instead of ether, enough carbolic acid is added to make the solution one-half per cent. strong; the result is the same. These two experiments show that the ptyaline of the saliva (which was not injured by the presence of the ether or the carbolic acid, as proved by the fact that it retained its diastatic action) is not the cause of the acid reaction.

Exp. 6. According to Paschutin, ptyaline is devitalized by an exposure of twenty minutes to a temperature of 67° C. Organized ferments could not be killed by the same means. We accordingly subject a mixture of saliva and grape-sugar to the given temperature for twenty minutes. We thereby destroy the ptyaline; the mixture, nevertheless, becomes sour if allowed to stand in the incubator for twenty hours.

This experiment confirms the result of experiments 4 and 5, and we begin to suspect that we have to deal with an organized ferment. This supposition is confirmed by the following experiment:

Exp. 7. A small quantity of a perfectly sterilized solution of sugar in saliva (1–40), in a test tube with cotton cork, is infected from the mouth, or with carious dentine, as described above; in twenty-four hours the solution will be acid; with a fraction of a drop of this solution a second tube is infected; it will likewise become acid; from this a third, etc.; each becomes acid in turn, while the control tube (containing the same solution, not infected) remains neutral.

The conclusion is plain that we have to do with a ferment which is capable of reproducing itself; in other words, the agent giving rise to acid fermentations in the juices of the human mouth exists in the form of living organisms.

I have examined twenty-two different species of bacteria which up to the year 1885 I had isolated out of the secretions, etc., of the human mouth, in reference to their fermentative action; and although, as may readily be seen, it was impossible with so large a number of different organisms to carry out the experiments to the desired degree of completion, I have nevertheless obtained some results which may be of interest and may somewhat contribute to our knowledge of the different fermentative processes in the human mouth and the diseases consequent upon them.

The chief source of nourishment for micro-organisms in the human mouth is furnished by two groups of substances, the carbohydrates and the albuminous substances. Both are almost invariably present in the human mouth in depressions, in fissures of the teeth, or in the spaces between them, or finally upon their free surfaces.

The carbohydrates undergo fermentations which lead to an acid reaction of the medium, while decompositions of albuminous substances are accompanied by an alkaline reaction. As a rule, mixtures of both produce an acid reaction. The reaction, which may be observed in any hidden recess of the human mouth, depends, consequently, partly upon the nature of the food present at the time, partly upon the kind of bacterium.

In the case of one bacterium which I examined with particular reference to this question, I found that it caused a neutral reaction when cultivated in a 3 per cent. solution of beef extract in the presence of $\frac{1}{10}$ per cent. of sugar, while the reaction became acid on increasing the quantity of sugar and alkaline upon diminishing it. I shall revert to these facts in Chapter VIII, inasmuch as they explain a number of phenomena accompanying dental caries.

A. Action of Mouth-Bacteria upon Carbohydrates.

1. *Lactic Acid Fermentation.*

The action of bacteria upon carbohydrates is of the greatest importance to the dentist in particular, to the medical practitioner, and, in fact, to every one, inasmuch as the origin of decay, with its evil consequences, depends upon it. Of the twenty-two kinds of mouth-bacteria already mentioned, sixteen soon brought about an acid reaction when cultivated in beef-extract-peptone-sugar solutions, four produced an alkaline reaction under the same conditions, while in case of two only the reaction remained neutral.

In a later series of experiments, twenty-five mouth-bacteria, thirteen stomach-bacteria, and fourteen bacteria from the intestines were examined in regard to the reaction which they produce in saccharine solutions. Of the mouth-bacteria, sixteen occasioned acid reaction, four alkaline, while five yielded inconstant results; the corresponding numbers for the stomach-bacteria were nine, two, and two; for the intestine-bacteria, six, five, and three. The number of acidifying bacteria is therefore comparatively larger in the stomach and mouth than in the intestines. Whether these relations are constant could, of course, be established only by a larger number of experiments than I am as yet able to record.

Cultures on sterilized milk give slightly different results. It was furthermore found impossible to draw a sharp line between those bacteria which produce an acid reaction and such as cause an alkaline reaction, because in some cases the reaction was very weak and changed during the course of the experiment, while in others it was materially influenced by change in the amount of sugar.

In consequence of the large number of bacteria experimented upon, it was naturally not possible to undertake for each one a qualitative determination of the acid which it produced. In the case of eighteen different bacteria, however, the examination was made, and in ten cases out of these eighteen lactic acid was found. It was formerly believed that the lactic acid fermentation could be brought about by only one specific micro-organism, which was designated as the lactic-acid fungus (Bacterium acidi lactici). Some years ago I called attention to the fact that many different bacteria are found in the human mouth which are capable of forming lactic acid out of sugar, and it has now been established by various investigators that this property, as well as the inverting and peptonizing property, is very widely distributed among bacteria. This fact offers an easy explanation for the long-known constant presence of lactic acid in the stomach and intestines.

The determination of the acid was made partly by analysis, partly by crystallization tests, and partly by the color test of Ewald.*

* Five to ten cc. of water plus one drop of chloride of iron plus two drops carbolic acid gives a violet color, which becomes yellow on addition of lactic acid even in very minute quantities.

By this simple reaction the detection of lactic acid, which is otherwise often extremely difficult, is very much facilitated. Unfortunately, however, it cannot be applied under all conditions, since not only lactic acid and its salts, but also tartaric acid, malic acid, acetic acid, oxalic acid and its salts, as far as I have examined them, and possibly some other substances not yet examined, give the same reaction. In order to produce the yellow color, it is, in fact, only necessary to add to the violet solution a small piece of fruit (apple, grape, plum, tomato), a few drops of white wine (Mosel, etc.). All these acids must, of course, be first excluded before the presence of lactic acid can be assumed with absolute certainty.

In order to determine more accurately the acid formed in a mixed fermentation of carbohydrates, as it occurs in the mouth, a chemical analysis was made.

The method of carrying out such an analysis will now be given: Two hundred cc. of fresh saliva are mixed with 2.0 starch and allowed to stand forty-eight hours at blood temperature; the mixture is then filtered, and heated to 100° C., to stop the fermentation. This process is repeated until about a liter of the solution has accumulated. It is then placed in a retort and reduced to a volume of about 75 cc. It will be very strongly acid. A few drops of this liquid added to a very thin solution of methyl-violet, leave it unchanged; from this we conclude that we have to deal with an organic acid, as an inorganic acid would turn it first blue and then green. Since the acid did not distill during the prolonged boiling, we may set it down as non-volatile, hence a non-volatile organic acid. The distillate was very slightly acid; we will call it distillate No. 1, as we wish to refer to it again.

The solution was further reduced in volume to about 40 cc. over the water-bath, and then transferred to a large glass vessel, briskly shaken with one and one-half to two liters of sulphuric ether, and allowed to stand until the ether became perfectly transparent. This was then filtered into a large retort and distilled, proper precautions being observed to prevent accidents. When the volume had been reduced to about 50 cc., the solution was filtered into a porcelain vessel, and still further reduced over the water-bath. A portion of the solution tested in the short tube of a Mitscherlich double-shadow polaristrobometer gave, as a mean of nine readings, a rotation of the plane of polarization equal to 0.015 degree, or 0° 0.9′. In other words, the solution was optically inactive, the 0° 0.9′ being far within the range of the error of experiment, especially as the solution was not absolutely transparent.

An excess of freshly prepared oxide of zinc was then added to the solution, and the whole slowly and carefully boiled, water being added as it was found necessary, till the reaction became neutral, or nearly so, filtered into a large glass evaporating dish, and put away at the temperature of the room for the salt to crystallize. A drop of this solution placed upon a glass slide gave, upon crystallization, the forms seen in Fig. 52, which are at once recognized as crystals of lactate of zinc. In a few days a quantity of a whitish crystalline powder had formed. This was placed upon a filter, the mother-liquid squeezed out, washed in absolute alcohol, dissolved in hot water, recrystallized and dried over sulphuric acid; it then weighed 0.343. After exposing to a temperature of 100° C., or a little more, till the weight became constant, it weighed 0.2816; it lost accordingly 17.9 per cent.* of water of crystallization, corresponding to three molecules of water. The salt was then dissolved in water, the zinc precipitated as carbonate and burned. The burned mass (zinc oxide) weighed 0.0970. We have, consequently,—

Fig. 52.

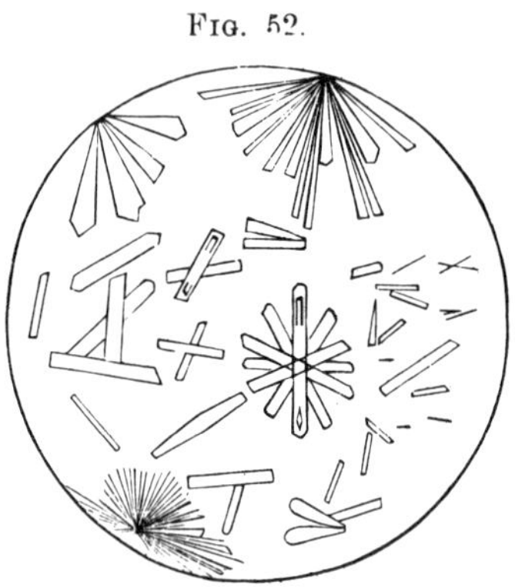

Crystals of Lactate of Zinc.

Substance analyzed (a zinc salt)	= 0.343
Oxide of zinc	= 0.097

The zinc oxide is seen to be equivalent to 28.2 per cent. of the substance analyzed.

* Theoretically 18.2, or 0.3 per cent. more.

The formula for the inactive ethylidene lactate of zinc is—

$$\left.\begin{matrix} C_3H_5O_3 \\ C_3H_5O_3 \end{matrix}\right\} Zn + 3H_2O, = 243 + 54.$$

Dried at ordinary temperature it contains 27.3 per cent. zinc oxide. The result obtained from the analysis differs, therefore, from that deduced from the formula by less than 1 per cent., and settles beyond doubt the fact that the substance analyzed was the lactate of zinc, or that the acid generated by the fermentation is lactic acid, or, more exactly, inactive ethylidene lactic acid, since, as shown above, the acid solution was optically inactive, and the zinc salt contained three molecules of water of crystallization. The salt was furthermore soluble in sixty-two parts water at 14° C.

I repeated the analysis with the following solution:

Water, 1000 cc.
Saliva, 300 cc.
Bouillon, 200 cc., made by boiling 125 grams of beef ten minutes in 300 cc. of water.
Sugar, 10.0.

This solution being slightly acid was neutralized with the carbonates of lime and sodium, sterilized, and infected from a pure culture of the bacterium in question. It was treated throughout exactly as above described, except that the zinc salt was converted into the sulphide instead of the carbonate, and burned with powdered sulphur in a stream of hydrogen. The result was:

Substance analyzed = 1.0540
Zinc sulphide = 0.415
Zinc = 26.38 per cent.,

instead of 26.74 per cent., as deduced from the formula, a difference of only one-third of one per cent.

In this case the substance was dried at 100° C. before weighing, and the formula becomes—

$$\left.\begin{matrix} C_3H_5O_3 \\ C_3H_5O_3 \end{matrix}\right\} Zn = 243.$$

One more analysis was made, using—

Water, 1000 cc.
Liquid beef extract, 20 cc.
Sugar, 10.0.

The result was the same, and need not be given; the two analyses above described being abundantly sufficient to show that the acid generated by the fungus in question is the common ferment lactic acid. Distillate No. 1, referred to above, owed its slight acidity, we now know, in part at least to lactic acid, since, when an aqueous solution of lactic acid is boiled, a small fraction of the acid goes over with the water. To ascertain, however, whether any other acid, especially volatile, was present, the distillate was boiled with carbonate of lime, filtered, evaporated to dryness, a small amount of dilute sulphuric acid added, and heated in a retort over the water-bath; a few drops of an oily acid came over, which, when taken upon the fingers, smelled like butyric acid; the amount, however, was so small that no attempt could be made to analyze it.

Among the products of fermentation of these bacteria I have also found formic,* acetic, and butyric acids, the latter, however, only in very small quantities. The greatest amount of acid which I have as yet observed in lactic acid fermentation is 0.75 per cent. Although the coefficient of separation of lactic acid is very small compared to that of the inorganic acids, it is, nevertheless, rather large when compared to that of other organic acids. My investigations have convinced me that it is considerably increased in syrupy solutions, so that instead of 10, the coefficient for aqueous solutions, a multiple of 10 must be taken, large quantities of ether (one and a half to two liters) being necessary to effect even an approximate extraction of the acids.

Formation of Gas in Lactic Acid Fermentation.

The fermentations which are brought about by different lactic acid bacteria show great differences in respect to the amount of gas evolved. I have already called attention to the fact that the fermentations of carbohydrates frequently proceed without generating the least trace of gas. On the other hand, some of the bacteria more recently examined formed very large quantities of gas (CO_2 and H), so that the gelatine in the culture-tubes was

* The distillation with phosphoric acid was made very carefully over the water-bath.

completely torn to pieces, or a part of it even driven out of the tube (Fig. 53). In some cases the pressure was even great enough to burst the tube.

From this violent evolution of gas the conclusion was drawn that it was not a pure lactic acid fermentation, corresponding to the equation $C_6H_{12}O_6 = 2C_3H_6O_3$, a conjecture which was verified by the analysis, which revealed the above-mentioned by-products, formic, acetic, and butyric acids. During the fermentation of half a liter of beef-extract-sugar solution I collected two hundred and fifty cubic centimeters of gas (CO_2 and H) in three hours.

Fig. 53.

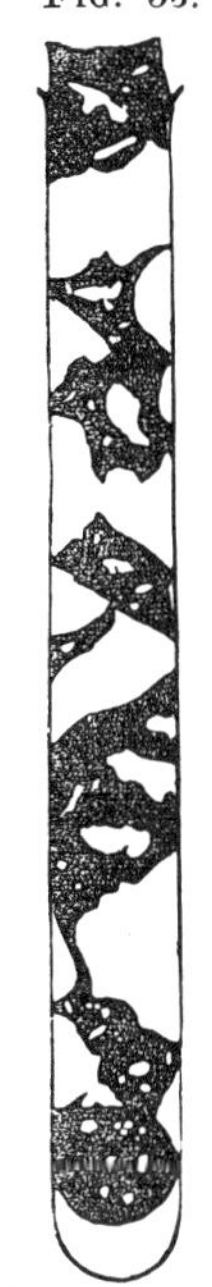

Culture of a Gas-forming Bacterium from the Stomach, in Bread-Sugar Gelatine. One day old. ½ : 1.

I would call especial attention to five different gas-forming bacteria, which invariably form large gas-bubbles in the gelatine or tear it to pieces, as is represented in the figure. One of these bacteria, which generates considerable quantities of gas also in albuminous substances, I found in the human fæces as well as in a gangrenous tooth-pulp. Its appearance in the latter place may help to explain the frequent occurrence of dental abscesses. If a tooth be filled before removing the necrotic pulp and sterilizing the root-canals, the gas formed will force itself through the foramen in the apex of the root, or carry particles of the putrid pulp along with it, causing irritation, if not immediate inflammation, of the pericementum.

It was formerly customary in such cases to bore into the tooth at the neck in order to "ventilate the nerve," that is, to permit the gases or other products of putrefaction to escape. Several of these bore-holes, which continually discharge pus, stinking gases, etc., may sometimes be found in one mouth.

Of the other gas-forming bacteria I found three in the stomach and one in the fæces; and it may be readily seen what unpleasant results might accompany their profuse development in the stomach or intestines.

These results of my investigations, which I published in 1884 and 1885, have been verified by different investigators. Vignal[66] investigated the action of seventeen different mouth-bacteria cultivated on various nutrient substances, particularly on such containing carbohydrates. Seven of these micro-organisms dissolve albumen, five cause it to swell up or make it transparent, ten dissolve fibrin, four cause it to swell up and become transparent, nine dissolve glutine, seven coagulate milk, six dissolve caseine, three transform starch, nine convert lactose into lactic acid, seven invert crystallized sugar, seven ferment glucose and partially convert it into alcohol.

Hueppe[67] also calls attention to the presence of lactic acid in the oral cavity. He isolated two different micro-organisms (one of which seems to be identical with one described by me), which formed lactic acid in saccharine solutions.

As already mentioned above, by-products, such as butyric acid, formic acid, acetic acid, etc., are often produced in lactic acid fermentation of carbohydrates. But, as far as my observation goes, these by-products are produced in comparatively very small quantities, so that they perform no important rôle in the various processes in the human mouth. Moreover, direct statements as to the detection of these acids in the human mouth are entirely wanting in the literature of this subject. A great deal has been said about butyric and acetic acids as causes of dental decay. These statements, however, have no scientific foundation whatever. Any other proof of the presence of these acids in the human mouth than that which I myself have produced has not been given.

2. *The Spontaneous Butyric Acid Fermentation*

does not appear to take place in the human mouth; at any rate, the Bacillus butyricus has not been detected in it; furthermore, the free access of air is not favorable to the development of this bacterium. Whether other kinds of the butyric acid forming bacteria, which are tolerably widespread in nature, occur in the human mouth and there cause their characteristic fermentation, is not known; the possibility is not to be excluded. I only affirm that as yet the occurrence of butyric acid fermentation in the human mouth has not been proved.

3. *The Acetic Acid Fermentation*

certainly does not occur in the oral cavity, for the simple reason that this fermentation cannot take place at a higher temperature than 35° C.; besides, the necessary quantity of alcohol and of acid essential to this fermentation is wanting. Escherich[68] discovered in the intestinal tract of a child a micro-organism called by him *Bacterium lactis aërogenes*, to which he ascribes the pure lactic acid fermentation. According to Baginsky,[69] however, it develops only minute quantities of lactic acid and profuse quantities of acetic acid. Nothing is known as to its occurrence in the mouth. Among seven of the bacteria which Vignal examined, he found one which brought about a fermentation of carbohydrates, by which, in addition to other products, alcohol and carbonic acid were formed.

4. *Diastatic Action of Mouth-Bacteria.*

The bacteria which I examined very seldom displayed a diastatic action. Indeed, out of nine different kinds I found but one possessing a pronounced saccharifying action. This bacterium formed from starch a kind of sugar having the power of reducing the oxide of copper, and then further decomposed the same under development of an acid reaction. It is frequently asserted that a bacterium possesses a diastatic action, simply because it grows on slices of boiled potato. This assumption, however, is inadmissible, inasmuch as the micro-organisms are by no means restricted to the potato starch alone, but may also derive nourishment from the albumen, sugar, etc., of the potato.

5. *Inverting Action of Mouth-Bacteria.*

Cane-sugar, $C_{12}H_{22}O_{11}$ (which is unfermentable, does not reduce oxide of copper in alkaline solutions, and turns the plane of polarization to the *right*), treated with a ferment, soluble in water and contained in beer-yeast, higher plants, and apparently also in many fungi, will, on the addition of water, be converted into invert-sugar. The latter is a mixture of grape- and fruit-sugar, which turns the plane of polarization to the *left*, reduces cupric to cuprous oxide, and is directly fermentable.

$$\underset{\text{Cane-sugar.}}{C_{12}H_{22}O_{11}} + \underset{\text{Water.}}{H_2O} = \underset{\text{Grape-sugar.}}{C_6H_{12}O_6} + \underset{\text{Fruit-sugar.}}{C_6H_{12}O_6}$$

The ferment which occasions this conversion of cane-sugar, designated as a hydrolytic decomposition, seems to be produced by many mouth-bacteria, since under their action cane-sugar very soon acquires the properties of invert-sugar.

That this conversion is really due to the action of an enzym formed by and separable from the bacterium, I have, as I think, proved in one case by the following experiment. A number of cultures in Florence flasks having been made at the same time, I was able after forty-eight hours to obtain the bacteria which had collected at the bottom of the vessels in considerable quantity. In this way I obtained about 10 c.cm. of a rather thick pap. The organisms were then devitalized by 90 per cent. alcohol, dried in a porcelain bowl, rubbed with sand, thoroughly soaked in water, and filtered. The filtrate, or watery extract, which must be clear, was added to a cane-sugar solution at room temperature; this solution then showed in the long tube of a Mitscherlich double-shadow polaristrobometer a rotation of 5.19 as the average of nine readings. The solution was left standing in a damp chamber for four hours at 39° C., whereupon it produced a rotation of 4.98. There was consequently a decrease of two-thirds of a degree, indicating a corresponding inversion of the cane-sugar solution. The solution also caused a slight reduction of an alkaline solution of sulphate of copper.

Many ferment bacteria of the mouth do not seem to be dependent upon the presence of free oxygen for their fermentative action. I have made cultures in which (1) the air was excluded by a thick layer of oil; (2) in vessels from which the air had been exhausted by a mercury air-pump; (3) in vessels which had been freed from oxygen by an alkaline solution of pyrogallic acid. It was ascertained that as much acid was generated in these cases as when the air had free access. We must conclude from the above that *fermentation* itself is not a process which requires oxygen, since the traces of oxygen still present in these experiments were entirely out of proportion to the acids formed.

B. Action of the Mouth-Bacteria on Albuminous Substances.

By far the majority of mouth-bacteria, in fact of all bacteria, possess an action similar to pepsine, in converting (peptonizing) coagulated albumen into soluble modifications. The essential difference, however, consists in this: that, while pepsine exerts its peptonizing action only in the presence of acids (especially muriatic), bacteria exert it in neutral or alkaline media also. The albuminous substances, therefore, even when insoluble, offer an excellent nutrient medium for bacteria. The products arising from the development of mouth-bacteria in albuminous media are the same as those arising from putrefaction of organic substances in general. These are chiefly bad-smelling gases, sulphuretted hydrogen (SH_2), ammonia (NH_3); further, CO_2, H,N, sulphide of ammonia and the products mentioned on page 28. The resultant reaction of all the products of any process of putrefaction is, as far as my observations go, invariably alkaline.

In my experiments the albumen was so congealed in the test tubes as to expose the largest possible surface, *i.e.*, the tubes were prepared in the same way as tubes of beef-blood serum. If kept in a damp chamber to prevent drying up, the material may be held ready for use for any desired length of time. Four of the bacteria examined would not grow on this medium, six exhibited but limited growth, while the others developed comparatively well, in some cases completely liquefying the albumen. Whether these bacteria produce more peptone than is necessary for their own nutrition, and whether and to what extent they might thereby benefit the human body, is a very difficult problem. In a large quantity of coagulated white of egg inoculated with a bacillus from the mouth, which showed intense putrefactive properties, I was able on the third day to detect traces of peptone by means of the biuret test.

In the presence of small quantities of sugar the characteristic phenomena of putrefaction are much less pronounced, or are altogether wanting. No bad-smelling products are formed, or, if formed, they immediately undergo further changes, and an acid reaction takes the place of the alkaline. I found that a bacterium, tested particularly in reference to this point, occasioned a neutral reaction in the presence of $\frac{1}{10}$ per cent. of sugar when cultivated in a 3 per cent. beef-extract solution. Increase of sugar caused acid reaction, while a diminution rendered it alkaline.

The products arising from the process of assimilation and growth of the living cells, or, in other words, their waste products, are such as impart an alkaline reaction to the medium; those arising from the fermentation of sugar are acid. The resulting reaction depends upon the predominance of the former or the latter. In my opinion, no sharp distinction can be drawn between fermentative and putrefactive bacteria, since many of the former possess also a ferment which decomposes albumen under formation of the characteristic products of putrefaction, while, on the other hand, there are fungi which, though regarded as putrefactive, when cultivated in saccharine solutions cause them to ferment without displaying the slightest signs of putrefaction.

One of the mouth-bacteria I examined rapidly dissolved boiled white of egg, forming bad-smelling products, among which sulphuretted hydrogen and ammonia were easily detectable. It also showed an inverting action, transforming cane-sugar into dextrose and levulose; in the third place it decomposed fermentable sugars into lactic acid with generation of carbonic acid; it, fourthly, caused an acid reaction in an amylaceous beef-extract solution, investing this solution at the same time with a slight power of reducing cupric oxide; in other words, it exerts finally a diastatic action also.

By-products presumably also arise in the last stages of these various fermentations, making the transformations caused by one and the same organism and the substances produced by it very numerous. This fact explains the profusion of products which may arise in putrefying mixtures, and makes the supposition somewhat doubtful that the number of kinds of bacteria in a fermenting mixture coincides with that of the products of fermentation. The twenty to thirty different substances which may be formed in an exposed putrefying mixture are not produced by one organism alone; it is, however, not in accordance with the facts to assume that each product or each stage requires a different organism.

Pure putrefactive processes are found in those localities of the oral cavity where no carbohydrates exist, or where their amount is very insignificant as compared to that of the albuminous substances,—for example, in gangrenous pulps, also when particles of meat decompose between the teeth. Pledgets of cotton pressed slightly against the gums absorb the albuminous secretion of the inflamed gums and very soon emit the disagreeable odor of putrefaction. Ulceration or sloughing of the gums (stomacace, stomatitis ulcerosa, etc.) is, as is well known, likewise accompanied by marked signs of putrefaction. It cannot be doubted that putrefaction alkaloids, ptomaïnes, must be formed in considerable quantities during the intense putrefactive and fermentative processes which are too often observed in very unclean mouths, but what part they play and what influence they have on the local and general state of the body has not yet been fully ascertained. (See Chapter XI.)

C. Fermentation of Fats and Fatty Acids in the Oral Cavity.

Whether and under what conditions the fermentation of fats and fatty acids (mentioned on page 26) takes place in the human mouth I am not at present able to state. Since, however, the salts most liable to cause fermentation (lime-salts, especially lactate of lime) are constantly being formed, we have every reason to suspect that such fermentations do there occur.

D. Nitrification and Denitrification in the Mouth.

On page 30 I gave an account of various experiments which have shown that fermentation processes in the soil, as well as in artificial media, where there is free access of air, may lead to the formation of nitrates from organic matter, and that, on the other hand, nitrates may be reduced to nitrites or to ammonia when the air is excluded. The formation of nitric acid in the human mouth has, as will be known to many, been advocated by Watt, the ammonia, undoubtedly formed in the mouth in certain quantities by the putrefaction of albuminous substances, becoming, according to his view, oxidized to nitric acid. This assertion of Watt is, however, not based upon experimental evidence. The question now arises whether, in the light of the facts recorded above, such a process can occur in the mouth by the agency of a "ferment nitrique"? This question can be solved by experiment only. The fact that nitric acid does not occur in the mouth in appreciable quantities speaks against it. Furthermore, the process of nitrification demands an abundant supply of air, while the centers of fermentation in the mouth are but sparingly supplied. The assumption that not oxidations but reductions may take place in the human mouth to some extent is much more in accordance with our knowledge of the conditions under which oxidizing or reducing processes may be effected by bacteria.

The nitrous acid compound found with tolerable constancy in mixed saliva we may presume to be formed by the reduction (denitrificatión) of nitrates contained in water and in vegetable nutrients.

It is, to say the least, very doubtful whether the fermentations mentioned on page 27, in which lactic, acetic, butyric, and propionic acids, etc., are formed, take place in the oral cavity to any considerable extent. No experiments have been made relating to this matter.

CHAPTER VI.

ACTION OF THE PRODUCTS OF FERMENTATION ON THE DIFFERENT STRUCTURES OF THE MOUTH.

It might appear from a superficial observation that the products formed by the above-mentioned fermentations, of which one or more is constantly going on in the mouth, do not exert any, or at most but a slight deleterious influence on the soft tissues. Considerable quantities of food may remain in contact with the mucous membrane of the gums and cheeks for some length of time without exciting any apparent local disturbances, which might not be explained by the mechanical irritation caused by them. A more thorough examination, however, will enable us to trace serious local and general diseases to the influence of parasites in the mouth. These disorders will be discussed at length in Part II. For the present I propose to consider that particular action of the parasites and their products which has as its result the most frequent and widespread of all diseases of the human body,—

THE DECAY OF THE TEETH.

The destruction of the hard substances of the teeth, commonly known as caries of the teeth, decay of the teeth, tooth-rot, etc., has, more than any other topic in the domain of dentistry, continued to excite the scientific interest of dentists and physicians for more than two thousand years. The numerous theories which have been held at different times concerning the origin of dental decay prove that the problem is no easy one. Not one of them has as yet been universally accepted. Among the causes which have been assigned for decay of the teeth the following are the most important:

1. Depraved juices accumulated in the teeth.
2. Disturbances of nutrition.
3. Inflammation.
4. Worms.
5. Putrefaction.
6. Chemical dissolution.
7. Parasites.
8. Electrolytic decomposition.
9. Diverse causes.
10. Chemico-parasitic influences.

THE STAGNATION OF DEPRAVED JUICES IN THE TEETH

was first designated by Hippocrates (456 B.C.) as the cause of toothache.

Kraütermann[70] (1732) gives a similar explanation of caries: "The teeth are corroded by the great influx of the lymphæ acrioris. The fermento acri rodente in the hollow tooth reappears, after being removed by the application of remedies."

This theory was held for many centuries. Bourdet[71] (1757) also accepted it: "When the juices contained in the vessels of the teeth are too thick, they stagnate, decay, and soon attack the tooth."

Benj. Bell (1787), Serre (1788), Kappis (1794), and others[72] accuse the juices carried to the teeth of playing an important part in the origin of decay.*

DISTURBANCES OF NUTRITION AS CAUSE OF DECAY

are alluded to by Galen (131 A.D.). He says, "The lack of nutrition makes the teeth weak, thin, and brittle. An excess of nutrition excites a kind of inflammation similar to that of the soft parts." A deficiency of nourishment not only causes the tooth to die away, but also enlarges the cavities. Crumbling, cor-

* A detailed treatise of the old literature on diseases of the teeth is found in Schlenker[72] and Carabelli.[73] From these authors some of the following references were obtained.

roded teeth are to be treated with astringents. Galen explained the loosening of the teeth "by an excess of moisture, which impairs the nerves."

This view is also held by Aëtius of Amida (550), partially, too, by Ebn-Sina (Avicenna, 978–1036), and Serapion[73] (1002).

Inflammation Theory of Decay.

A great number of writers even up to the present time have regarded tooth-decay as a process of inflammation. As early as 131 A.D., Galen mentions a kind of inflammation which is called forth in the tooth by excessive nourishment. Eustachius[74] (1574) expresses himself more definitely: "*Redundantia, quamvis dentes substantiam duram habeant ac prope lapideam, similem in eis affectionem excitat cujusmodi est circa carnosas partes inflammatio quod sane ut admiratione dignum sit tamen ex alimenti copia accidere posse et Galenus testatur et ratio ipsa confirmat.*"

John Hunter[75] (1778) approaches the inflammation theory when he says (after having designated caries as mortification), "I am apt to suspect that during life there is some operation going on which produces a change in the diseased part."

Kappis (1794) expresses the same views.

Joseph Fox[76] (1806) says, "The diseases to which the teeth are subject have their origin in inflammation."

Thomas Bell[77] (1831) characterizes caries of the teeth as gangrene, and says, "The true, proximate cause of dental gangrene is inflammation."

E. Neumann,[78] Hertz,[79] Koecker,[80] and others entertained the same views.

Koecker writes, "Caries, in fact, is that state of the tooth in which mortification has taken place in one part and inflammation in the part contiguous to it, the former originally produced by the latter, and the latter continually kept up by the former."

In more recent times the inflammatory theory of dental decay has derived its chief and almost only support from the contributions of Frank Abbott, Heitzmann, and Boedecker.[81] These authors have strenuously advocated the view that "there occurs a primary inflammation in dentine independent of pulpitis or pericementitis, running its course in the middle of the dentinal tissue and leading, as all inflammatory processes do, either to a new formation or to destruction by suppuration." "Inflammation causes first a solution of the lime-salts, and afterward a liquefaction of the basis-substance both in bone and dentinal tissue. The result will be the appearance of globular spaces or bay-like excavations which exhibit medullary corpuscles or sometimes clear protoplasmic masses corresponding to the embryonal stage of the inflamed tissue." . . . "By the breaking apart of these medullary corpuscles pus may be formed in the middle of the dentine, thus representing an abscess independently of the pulp-tissue," or, on the other hand, a healing process may take place through the redeposition of lime-salts. The reasons given in support of this view do not appear to me to be such as admit of a very close examination. The first reason is simply the assertion that the hardening or consolidation, sometimes believed to take place under fillings, is "the consequence of an inflammatory reaction of the dentine," and further, "instances are not rare in which the insertion of an oxyphosphate, oxychloride, or a gold filling gives rise to excruciating pain. . . . The latter result is due to intense and acute inflammation of the dentine."

It is not quite clear to me how the cases stated by Heitzmann and Boedecker justify the conclusions which they draw from them. We might say that the consolidation of the dentine is due to a continued or even increased functional activity of the dentinal fibrils; a number of facts might be, and have been, brought forward in support of this statement, though some oppose it; but to jump at once to inflammation of the dentine, is making rather free with logic, to say the least.

Again, pain following the insertion of fillings may be due to the mechanical or chemical insult to the exposed dentinal fibers, or it may be due to the insult to the pulp itself. I cannot help thinking that it is here also perfectly gratuitous to speak of inflammation of the dentine. It is not proved by the cases referred to.

The second argument of Heitzmann and Boedecker is based upon the utterly mistaken idea that the ivory of elephants' tusks has the property of healing wounds and of encapsuling musket-balls without the intervention of the pulp or pericementum. In regard to this point they write, "The present writers have had no chance to study an elephant's tusk immediately after its injury, but the illustrations, as given by Carl Wedl, are sufficient for the assertion that all changes in the ivory are produced by an inflammatory reaction around the foreign body driven into it."

Against this view, obtained from the examination of four woodcuts, we have the unanimous voice of Cuvier, Owen, Goodsir, Murie, Tomes, and all the most recent writers on this subject. I personally have examined not less than fifty-two cases of gunshot and lance wounds of elephants' tusks, and well-nigh one hundred abscess-cavities, and, without entering into a discussion of the question here, will simply state that not a single one of all these cases affords the slightest indication of any inflammatory reaction on the part of the ivory.

In the third place, Heitzmann and Boedecker attempt to establish their views of inflammatory action in dentine through microscopical investigations. They have found and illustrated in the articles above referred to "excavations of the dentine which are identical with those seen in the process of absorption of the dentine of temporary teeth, and those of secondary dentine in the neighborhood of an inflamed pulp." The thought naturally occurs to every one that the authors have simple cases of absorption before them. They affirm, however, that the "diagnosis of primary eburnitis was established by the presence of such excavations in the middle of the dentine, without any connection with the surface or the pulp-chamber of the tooth."

Fig. 53 *a*.

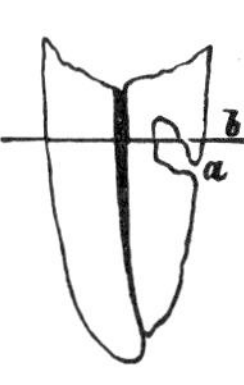

It must be supposed that the connection or non-connection of the excavation with the surface of the tooth or pulp-chamber was established by macroscopical examination of the tooth before cutting or by serial sections, since the occurrence of absorption lacunæ in the middle of a preparation would, of course, not exclude the possibility or probability of an outlet on some other plane. For example, in the accompanying diagram (Fig. 53 *a*), a root in which absorption is going on at *a*, a section through the plane *b* would show excavations in the middle of the dentine without connection with pericementum. If primary inflammation of the dentine occurs as often as we are to infer from the communications of Heitzmann and Boedecker, then it is very strange that their observations have not been confirmed by other investigators. One might think, too, that by placing their preparations before the many competent microscopists in various parts of America the question could be very soon settled beyond all doubt.

It is certainly owing to the authors to examine their preparations from a perfectly objective stand-point, and they also owe it to us to place their preparations before us in order finally to dispose of a subject of controversy which has already taken up enough of the time of the profession. For my own part, having spent not a little amount of time in the study of pathological conditions in human dentine and in ivory, I am forced to accept the eburnitis theory of Heitzmann and Boedecker (the inflammation, suppuration, and healing of dentine without the intervention of the pericementum or pulp) with a great deal of reserve. Not, however, having had the opportunity of examining a preparation from these gentlemen, I cannot give any definite opinion as to my idea of the nature of the processes which they have styled eburnitis, though I cannot get rid of a lurking suspicion that it is nothing more than absorption.

Heitzmann and Boedecker[82] also claim that the views commonly held regarding the development of dentine and enamel are false. Neither the odontoblasts nor the ameloblasts take part directly in the formation of the dentine and enamel, but these bodies first break up into medullary corpuscles, between which the dentinal fibers are formed. It is not the place here to discuss these views. They still await confirmation.

Abbott[83] describes decay of a living tooth as "an inflammatory process which, beginning as a chemical process, in turn reduces the tissues of the tooth into embryonic or medullary elements evidently the same as, during the development of the tooth, have shared in its formation; and its development and intensity are in direct proportion to the amount of living matter which they contain as compared with other tissues."

"Micrococci and leptothrix by no means produce caries; they

do not penetrate the cavities in the basis-substance of the tissues of the tooth, but appear only as secondary formations, owing to the decay of medullary elements."

Abbott's communication, from which these statements are taken, is accompanied by a number of illustrations, of which one is reproduced in Fig. 54, together with the explanation accompanying it.

FIG. 54.

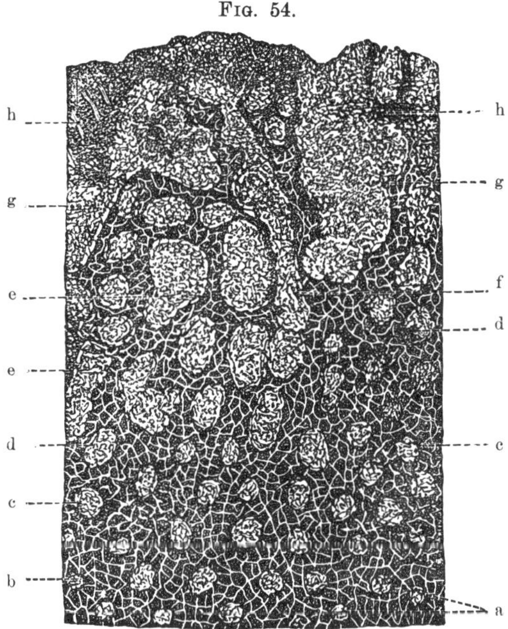

CROSS-SECTION OF CARIOUS DENTINE. After Abbott.

"At a certain distance from the decay the canaliculi look unchanged, and each contains the central transverse section of the dentinal fiber, with its delicate radiated offshoots (Fig. 54, *a*). Nearer to the decay we meet with moderately enlarged canaliculi, the center of which is occupied by a cluster of protoplasm, the granules and threads of which have readily taken up the carmine (Fig. 54, *b*). One step farther we find the canaliculi considerably enlarged, to double or treble their original size, and they are filled with yellow protoplasm, plainly exhibiting the net-like arrangement of the living matter (Fig. 54, *c*, *c*). The most peripheral granules send delicate conical offshoots through the surrounding light space toward the unchanged basis-substance. In some of the enlarged canaliculi, accumulations of living matter are seen fully in the shape of nuclei. Sometimes two or more such nuclei may be seen surrounded by a varying amount of protoplasm (Fig. 54, *d*, *d*). Still nearer to the decay the canaliculi are enlarged to ten or fifteen times their original diameter, and the cavities thus produced are all filled with a partly nucleated protoplasm (Fig. 54, *e*, *e*). Between the roundish cavities we meet with longitudinal cavities, arisen from the confluence of several cavities in one main direction (Fig. 54, *f*). The cavities continue increasing in size, and form large spaces, with rounded, bay-like boundaries, between which only scanty traces of unchanged basis-substance are left (Fig. 54, *g*, *g*). Lastly, the basis-substance has entirely disappeared, and only protoplasm is visible in its place, either in the shape of multinuclear layers or of irregular so-called medullary elements, with rather faint marks of division (Fig. 54, *h*, *h*)."

So much for Abbott's explanation of the figure. But what, in reality, are those cellular elements, clusters of protoplasm, medullary elements, etc.? *They are masses of micro-organisms mixed with the débris of the decomposing dentine.*

The discoveries of Abbott have received no confirmation, whereas, on the other hand, the untenableness of the inflammatory theory has been exposed by various authors. It is not necessary therefore to call especial attention to the many points of Abbott's argument, which, in my judgment, are at variance with indisputable facts. I will accordingly content myself with a recital of the following oft-repeated facts, which cannot be made to tally with the postulates of the inflammatory theory of decay.

1. The elements which appear in inflammation of other tissues of the animal body cannot be found in decayed dentine. Among the thousands of preparations of decayed or decaying dentine that I have examined, I have not found there anything which I could identify with the process of inflammation, suppuration, etc., illustrated by Heitzmann and Boedecker. The appearances represented by these authors either do not occur at all in

decay of the dentine, or so very seldom, that we could not for a moment think of connecting them with the process of decay. The mere detection of swelling or tumefaction of the dentinal fibrils is no evidence that decay is the result of inflammatory action. The custom of certain dental pathologists to assume that every variation from the normal detected in the tissue is of an inflammatory nature is about as rational as it would be for the general histologist to ascribe the many post-mortem changes which take place in delicate tissues, while being prepared for examination, to inflammation.

I do not say that changes of a vital nature may not take place in the dentinal fibrils as a result of the action of the decay-producing agents, or in connection with inflammation of the pulp. Indeed, it would be strange if the acids penetrating the dentine and bathing the fibrils did not produce some change in them. But it remains to be shown that in either case these changes either produce decay or accelerate the process when once established.

Heitzmann's[84] attempt to explain the inability of others to see things under the microscope just as he sees them, on the ground that they work with inferior lenses or that their eyes have not been properly educated, can scarcely be said to meet all the requirements of a final argument. Anyone disposed to make use of the same sort of argument might be led to inquire whether Heitzmann and some of his followers have not sometimes seen just a bit too well.

2. It is not possible to produce decay of the tooth, or anything resembling decay, by means of any or all of those mechanical or chemical agents which invariably produce inflammation in other tissues.

We all know very well that we may file, grind, saw, bore, and pound the living dentine, may break away large portions with the forceps, or subject it to the action of the most irritating substances; indeed, we may do what we please with it, we cannot produce in this way a trace of caries.

The operation of filling teeth is of itself a continued testimonial to the inconsistency of the inflammatory theory of decay; for we know very well what would result if we should bore a hole in any tissue capable of inflammation (bone) and pound it full of gold.

3. The liquefaction of the basis-substance, the melting together of the tubules, the production of caverns, etc., characteristic of decay, cannot be found when bacteria are not present.

4. Pulpless teeth and dead teeth worn on plates or as pivot teeth are subject to decay in the same degree as teeth with living pulps: they show also the same microscopical changes in the structure.

5. It is possible to produce artificial changes of the dentine, or, in other words, artificial decay, which under the microscope cannot be distinguished from natural decay.

These facts are not here brought to notice for the first time, and are probably well known to the advocates of the inflammatory theory; they ignore them, however, completely, and thereby admit their inability to answer them.

Worm Theory of Caries.

For many centuries worms were regarded as an essential factor in the origin of caries, and all sorts of remedies were employed to drive them out. Thus, *e.g.*, Scribonius[73] used fumigations against them; Ebn-Sina recommended for this purpose seeds of henbane, leek, and onions. Musitanus[73] (1114), Kräutermann[70] (1732), Ringelmann (1824), Kremler, and many others took similar measures to get rid of the worms. Even to this day the worm theory is not entirely abandoned. Among the lower classes in many countries the belief prevails that worms are the source of toothache, and Chinese dentists especially are said to understand how to make superstition pay. When a patient with the toothache presents himself, they are in the habit of making an incision into the gums "to let the worms out." For this purpose they employ an instrument which has a hollow handle filled with artificial worms. When the incision is made, the operator, by a dextrous turn of the instrument, drops the worms into the mouth; the excitement of the patient and the loss of blood cause at least a temporary relief. The worms are collected, dried, and are then ready to be taken out of the next patient's gums. The Japanese term for tooth-decay, or rather for a hollow tooth, is "mushi ba" —mushi = worm, ba = tooth, therefore a worm-tooth.

In Chinese, a hollow tooth is called "chung choo," which has exactly the same meaning.

The existence of tooth-worms was called in question by Hollarius as early as 600. According to his idea, the worms are nothing else than "particles of the henbane which fly off during the fumigations."

It is rather difficult to understand how the first authorities in the dental art should for so many centuries go on accepting burnt particles of henbane or other vegetable substances for worms.

Peter Fauchard[85] (1728) also made futile efforts to discover the worms. Pfaff[86] (1756) saw worms on the gums, "particularly in the case of very common people who are in the habit of eating decaying cheese." He was "not able, however, to observe that such worms had produced toothache by gnawing," although he is willing to admit such a possibility.

Putrefaction as Cause of Decay.

Putrefaction was specified as the cause of decay by Pfaff[86] (1756). "Remains of food which undergo putrefaction between the teeth occasion decay of the teeth." At the present time even, many designate decay simply as tooth-rot (Zahnfäule) and regard it as a process of putrefaction, overlooking the fact that an extracted tooth may be left an indefinite length of time in a putrefying mixture without showing any trace of decomposition.

Some years ago Mayr and Stockwell attempted to establish the putrefaction theory of decay on a new basis. Bacteria were said to grow into the tubules and to destroy or absorb the basis-substance, whereupon the lime-salts fall apart. In conformity with this theory, the analysis of carious dentine should not reveal a decrease, but rather an increase of lime or a loss of organic substance. In reality, the very reverse is the case, so that this theory soon had to be abandoned.

CHEMICAL THEORY OF DENTAL DECAY.

Up to very recent times no theory of dental decay has enjoyed the approbation of so large a number of distinguished odontologists as the chemical.

Paul of Ægina[73] (636) advises, "in order to preserve the teeth, to take precautions against the spoiling of food in the stomach (indigestion), since the frequent vomiting resulting from it is very injurious to the teeth."

According to Carabelli, the first experiments on the action of acids on the teeth were made by Berdmore (1771), who tested the action of nitric and sulphuric acids. Pasch (1767), Bücking (1782), Becker (1808), and Ringelmann (1824) attribute injurious effects to sour food and acids. Linderer[87] (1837) characterizes caries as a purely chemical process. Robertson[88] combated the inflammation theory. According to him, caries is a chemical decomposition of the dental tissues by means of acids; the latter are formed in the mouth by the dissolution of food-particles. Rognard[89] follows Robertson, and particularly mentions sulphuric and nitric acids as products of the decomposition of vegetable and animal substances. These acids are the cause of the decay of the teeth.

Magitot[90] writes, "*Les considérations qui précèdent tendent à établir que la carie dentaire résulte d'une altération purement chimique, exercée sur l'émail et l'ivoire des dents,*" etc. Wedl[91] also defends the chemical theory; he regards the action of an acid as the chief cause of caries in all cases where even the slightest traces of decalcification are discernible.* The acid secretion of the gums, especially in the cases of children and of women during pregnancy, and the acidity of the saliva accompanying disorders of the digestion, deserve special mention. Leptothrix bears no direct relation to the origin of caries.

Tomes[92] (1873) concludes "that caries is the effect of external causes in which so-called 'vital' forces play *no* part; that it is due to the solvent action of acids which have been generated by fermentation going on in the mouth, the buccal mucus probably

*In my opinion, decay without decalcification, which Wedl here seems to assume, does not occur.

playing no small part in the matter; and when once the disintegration is established in some congenitally defective point, the accumulations of food and secretions in the oral cavity will intensify the mischief by furnishing new supplies of acids." In the last edition of Tomes's work the phrase "organisms having no small share in the matter" takes the place of "buccal mucus probably playing no small part in the matter."

Watt has also made himself conspicuous by his obstinate defence of the chemical theory. He refers the different colors of carious dentine to the action of various mineral acids.

J. Taft[93] also favors the chemical theory. "Acid mucus and saliva, vitiated secretions, products of decomposition of animal and vegetable matter in the mouth, and galvanic action, mineral and vegetable acids," are, in his opinion, the chief causes of dental decay.

Schlencker[72] writes, "Dental caries is therefore a purely chemical process. Be it repeated, where there is no acid, no caries is possible."

Baume adheres to the chemical and opposes the parasitic theory. "*The fungi are the result of the caries*" (!)

Comparative microscopical examinations of decayed dentine and dentine simply decalcified by acids, and even a macroscopic comparison of decayed teeth with teeth which have been acted upon for a certain length of time by acids only, furnish sufficient proof for the untenableness of the purely chemical theory. The microscopic changes characteristic of decayed dentine as represented in Figs. 58–88 cannot be produced by any acid or acids.

It is not to be denied that such changes as the swelling or tumefaction of the fresh or living dentinal fibrils may be brought about by the action of acids, since all delicate organic tissues suffer more or less change when acted upon by external agents. But the enlargement of the dentinal tubules, the liquefaction of the basis-substances, the confluence of the canals, and the formation of cavities in the dentine are absolutely inexplicable by the action of acids in such a diluted state as they occur in the mouth.

By the action of sugar, as well as of various acids, Magitot[94] succeeded in producing cavities in the dental tissues which were very similar to those formed by decay. It is not difficult by the action of almost any acid to produce cavities especially in enamel, since by the decalcification the entire tissue of the enamel is destroyed. Moreover, when the experiment is made in the air, more or less discoloration appears. By such experiments, however, nothing more is proved than the universally recognized fact that acids exert a decalcifying effect on dental tissue. The identity of a destructive process in the tooth with decay itself can be established by the microscope only.

But the untenableness of the purely chemical theory of decay has been so strikingly and repeatedly demonstrated within the last few years that it seems unnecessary to enter upon a closer consideration of the subject here.

Parasitic Theory of Dental Decay.

It is not quite certain who was the first to accuse micro-organisms of being concerned in the production of tooth-decay. The credit of having originated this view is generally given to the Dresden physician, Ficinus.[53] Prof. Erdl,[52] however, seems to have been two years in advance of Ficinus. Erdl regards the "caries materie" as parasites. This on its first appearance forms upon the crown a delicate, colorless membrane composed of cells; later these cells become more irregular and their nuclei more distinct. But since Erdl employed muriatic acid to isolate his "caries matter," it is quite probable that the delicate membrane which he obtained was nothing else than Nasmyth's membrane. In order to destroy these parasites and thereby hinder the progress of the decay, Erdl recommends creasote and nitric acid. He first applies creasote until the "caries matter" is impregnated with it, then nitric acid, which immediately produces violent and complete decomposition of the creasote, as well as of the parasites saturated with it.

Ficinus[53] attributes decay to the action of his "denticolæ." These proliferate in the enamel-cuticle, which they decompose; they then attack the enamel, destroy the connection between the enamel-prisms, and thus penetrate to the dentine, which they cause to decay in the same manner.

Klencke[56] also describes a parasite, Protococcus dentalis, discovered by him in the human mouth, which liquefies dentine and enamel in pretty much the same manner as the fungus *Merulius lacrymans* softens the wood of houses or furniture (?).

"We have, consequently, in this process, which I shall call for sake of brevity destructio dentis vegetativa, a fungus which softens and destroys dental substances and is nourished by their chemical elements; this parasite is a true Protococcus dentalis."

Klencke assumed "four kinds of tooth-decay, viz: (1) central decay, destructio sive dissolutio dentis centralis—s. inflammatoria; (2) peripheric vegetative decay (caries acuta), destructio dentis vegetativa, caused by the tooth-fungus Protococcus dentalis; (3) peripheric putrid decay, destructio s. colliquatio dentis putrida—s. infusoria (caries acuta), caused by infusoria (dental animalcula, denticolæ hominis); (4) disintegration of the tooth, destructio dentis chemica (caries chronica)."

Leber and Rottenstein[58] deserve the credit of having placed the parasitic theory of caries on a more solid basis. They regarded the commencement of caries as a purely chemical process; but as soon as the dentine is superficially decalcified the elements of the fungus Leptothrix buccalis penetrate the dentinal tubules, enlarge them, and thereby facilitate the rapid penetration of the acids. These authors discovered a reaction which for a long time was thought to be characteristic of Leptothrix buccalis. The elements of this fungus, treated with a slightly acidulated solution of iodine in iodide of potassium, show a violet color. Sections of carious dentine exhibit the same reaction. But, as I have explained on page 71, Leptothrix buccalis, treated with iodine, gives no, or at most a yellowish, color. The violet reaction of the accumulations in the mouth, as well as of decayed dentine, is occasioned by an entirely different organism.

The communication of Milles and Underwood[95] presented before the Dental Section of the International Medical Congress in London, 1881, served to revive the interest in the parasitic theory of dental decay, which at that time appeared to be on the wane. They noted the constant presence of micro-organisms in decayed dentine, and the widening of the tubules produced by them. They rejected the chemical theory of decay, and stated their conviction that in the decay of the hard tooth-structures "two factors have always been in operation: (1) the action of acids, and (2) the action of germs." "This theory—which for the sake of distinction may be called the septic—is rather an amplification of the chemical theory than a contradiction of it. Most probably the work of decalcification is entirely performed by the action of acids, but these acids are, we think, secreted by the germs themselves, and the organic fibrils upon which the organisms feed and in which they multiply are the scene of the manufacture of their characteristic acids, which in turn decalcify the matrix and discolor the whole mass." It need not be said that the investigations of Milles and Underwood marked a great step in advance of anything hitherto accomplished in this direction.

Ad. Weil[96] writes, "Decay generally begins from without, and must, therefore, first make its way through the enamel-cuticle. . . . I regard it as highly probable that this fungus (Leptothrix buccalis) bores directly through it. The fungi now proceed farther into the enamel and force apart its prisms, gradually breaking up its structure. From the enamel they penetrate into the tubules of the dentine, which they often enlarge to three times their natural size, at the same time extracting the lime-salts."

Arkövy[97] describes caries as "a breach of continuity of the hard dental substance brought about by chemical action, in which the invasion of nosogenous fungi play an essential part."

Baštýr[98]: "As long as it cannot be shown that the appearances observed in the decay of living teeth, decay of dead teeth in the mouth, and artificial caries show any appreciable differences, so long will every attempt to explain decay as a vital process be very difficult."

Alfred Gysi[99]: "As all my experiments and investigations on this subject have presented facts which are consistent with this theory (the chemico-parasitic), I accept it as a satisfactory explanation of dental caries."

Sudduth[100] says, "Dr. Miller's theory of the formation of cavities by the action of a digestive ferment upon the basis-substance of dentine has been the only theory ever advanced that explains the formation of cavities."

Peirce[101]: "I am a firm believer in the fact that dental caries cannot progress without these low forms of life."

Allan[102]: "The germ theory is the only one so far that clearly and satisfactorily accounts for the acid." "The germ theory fully explains the distended tubules and the broken-down basis-substance."

Black[103]: "In this way the tubules become packed full of organisms, and the surrounding dentine is always decalcified in advance of the growth of the fungus by the lactic acid produced. That this is the true explanation of the etiology of dental caries, there is no longer a reasonable doubt."

Electrical Theory of Decay.

A theory making decay of the teeth dependent upon galvanic action was promulgated by Bridgman[104] in a prize essay before the Odontological Society of Great Britain. The human mouth is to be regarded as a galvanic battery; the individual teeth represent the different elements, and the secretions of the mouth a common electrolyte. Under normal conditions the crowns of the teeth are electro-positive, the roots electro-negative. When, however, the roots become exposed by recession of the gums, the exposed portion must be electro-positive. In like manner the pulp is electro-negative to the dentine and to the enamel of the crown. To be consistent, Bridgman should have gone further and pronounced the dentine negative to the enamel, the cement negative to the dentine, and the enamel positive to the cement. The electric current generated between the two parts produces an electrolytic decomposition of the fluids of the mouth; the acids (electro-negative) are given off on the surface of the crown of the tooth (electro-positive) and cause decalcification. Furthermore, inasmuch as the "formation of the dentine is due to electro-voltaic action," so, too, the dentine may be directly pulled down electrolytically and decomposed by the same force.

Bridgman's treatise won the prize offered by the Odontological Society for the best essay on dental decay; it naturally excited some notice at the time, but was not accepted with confidence. We will not stop to consider the forty-five theses of Bridgman separately; very few of them would bear a careful analysis, not being based upon direct proof but upon certain principles or beliefs which, in themselves doubtful enough, become still more so when applied to the teeth. For example, he says, "The condition and arrangement of the several layers (composing the skin) are incontestably those of an electro-voltaic series," consequently the pulp-vessels, together with the dentine and enamel, also form an electro-voltaic series.

At present the electric theory is to be regarded rather as a curiosity than as a theory of dental decay. Its promulgation had, however, a secondary action which for a time was very strong, and which is still felt to some extent at the present day; it may consequently not be out of place to consider it at some length. Prompted by Bridgman's exposition, experiments were undertaken to determine the position of dentine in the electro-chemical series. These experiments resulted in the establishment of the following scale: Electro-negative—gold, amalgam, tin, gutta-percha, dentine, oxychloride of zinc+electro-positive. From this it follows that the highest electro-motive force, or the strongest electrical action, is generated by a combination of gold and dentine; combination of amalgam and dentine yields a weaker force; still weaker is that produced by a combination of gutta-percha and dentine. On the strength of these and similar experiments Chase[105] maintained that a tooth filled with gold would necessarily soon become carious again on the margins of the cavity, wherever the acid secretions of the mouth constantly bathe the filling and the bordering tooth-substance. A tooth filled with amalgam succumbs to this electro-chemical process less rapidly, while one filled with tin still longer escapes destruction. The comparative rapidity with which teeth filled with gold, amalgam, and tin are destroyed is expressed by the numbers 100, 67, and 50. On the other hand, a tooth filled with oxychloride of zinc becomes electro-negative by contact with this material, and is therefore protected from the effects of acids (which are also electro-negative).

Chase also succeeded in obtaining experimental evidence in support of these calculations. He prepared pieces of ivory of equal shape and size, bored a hole in each, and filled the holes with different materials. After these pieces had been exposed to the action of an acid for a week, he found that they had decreased in weight in the following gradation:

The piece filled with gold . . .	0.06
" " " " amalgam . .	0.04
" " " " tin . . .	0.03
" " " " gutta-percha . .	0.01
" " " " wax . . .	0.01
" " " " oxychloride of zinc	0.00

From these results Chase concluded that gold is the worst of all filling-materials, and laid down his notorious proposition, "Every tooth filled with a metal is a galvanic battery which begins its work as soon as the surrounding liquid has an acid reaction." Practitioners of repute actually discarded gold as a filling-material on the strength of this unfounded statement.

It is necessary to grasp two fundamental facts in order to understand the arguments upon which the electrical theory is based.

1. When two heterogeneous metals (in general two chemically dissimilar conductors) touch one another, a difference of potential is produced between the two conductors, charging one of them (electro-positive) with positive electricity, and the other (electro-negative) with negative electricity in exactly equal amounts. In this state, the former, the electro-positive, has an increased affinity for electro-negative or acid bodies. The charge of electricity so developed, as well as the increased chemical activity resulting from it, is, however, very small.

2. In any cell of a galvanic battery acid is set free at the positive pole and alkali at the negative, and so long as the current continues to flow, the positive pole (when not a noble metal) continues to be acted upon by the acid so liberated.

Therefore, if we were to take a piece of zinc or a zinc model of a tooth and make a gold filling in it or attach a piece of gold to it, the zinc would be more rapidly attacked when immersed in any electrolyte than when no other metal was in contact with it, and for two reasons: (1) because the whole surface of the zinc would become electro-positive by contact with gold, and would therefore more rapidly decompose a solution and take the acid constituents to itself. This action is inconsiderable as compared with the following, (2) because the electric current generated between the two metals would liberate acid over the whole surface of the zinc, by which the action upon the zinc would be still much more increased. We see, then, if teeth were made of zinc, what disastrous results would follow their filling with gold.

But can we, without further question, assume that the same takes place even to a limited extent, or to any extent whatever, when a natural tooth is filled with gold or any other metal?

In other words, do any two substances when brought into contact assume a difference of potential, or can any two substances act as the generating plates of an electric element? An article in the *Correspondenz-Blatt für Zahnärzte*, translated from the *Practitioner*, contains the statement that a galvanic battery may be constructed with almost any two different substances whatever. It is only necessary that one of them be more readily acted upon chemically than the other.

A stick of wood and a piece of mica are two substances which fulfill the above condition, but we would try in vain to form an electric element by use of them; we would equally fail with sealing-wax and glass, or with gold and glass, even though both substances might be entirely consumed in the attempt. But what condition necessary to the production of an electric current is wanting in the above cases?

Conductivity.—When two chemically dissimilar substances are made to touch one another, they do not assume a difference of potential or become charged with electricity if one (or both) of them is a non-conductor, and no electric current can be produced by the use of any two chemically dissimilar substances if one (or both) of them is a non-conductor. Tooth-bone is a non-conductor, and consequently cannot become electro-positive, or be changed in potential by contact with gold, and cannot act as the pole of a cell when immersed in an acid or salt solution.

I say that tooth-bone is a non-conductor, though the fluids with which the tooth is permeated are conductors.

It is necessary that the difference be thoroughly understood. A silk thread, for instance, is a perfect non-conductor, but by dipping a silk thread in a salt solution, or in any liquid which conducts, we obtain a conductor. Now, it is not the particles of the thread which transmit the current, but the particles of the liquid; and if we were to bring a piece of metal in contact with this moistened thread, the potential of the particles of silk would not be changed.

This is what we have in the living human tooth,—a non-conductor permeated by a conductor. If we were able to construct a tooth of glass and fill the pulp-cavity, the canals, and tubules of that tooth with a 0.75 per cent. solution of table-salt (which has about the same specific resistance as the tissues of the body), then we would have an electrical instrument similar to a living human tooth. Such an instrument would transmit a current of electricity; in other words, it would be a conductor just as the wet silk thread is, but the substance of the tooth—the glass—could not receive any potential, even by contact with gold or any other metal.

It has just been stated that dry dentine, as well as enamel, is a non-conductor. Although the fact that the constituents of which dentine is composed are themselves non-conductors justifies this conclusion, it nevertheless appeared desirable to test the question by direct experiment. This test was made in the following manner:

A cross-section of dentine $\frac{1}{300}$ millimeter thick was inclosed in a circuit of three Siemen's cells. The galvanometer used had a multiplicator with 16,000 turns of wire and a resistance of 5000 Siemen's units. When the circuit was closed, not the slightest deflection of the needle could be observed. The section of dentine was placed between the ends of two wires which had a diameter of 1.9 millimeter under a pressure of about two grams to the square millimeter.

FIG. 55.

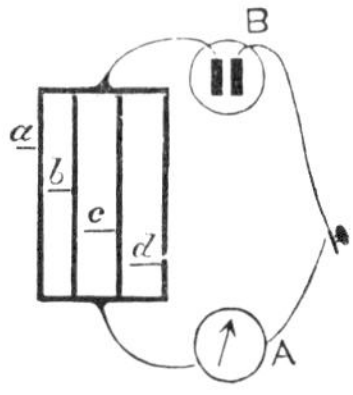

This experiment was then varied by inclosing three sections in a circuit in a manner illustrated in Fig. 55, so that the surface of contact was three times as great and the resistance consequently only one-third of that in the above experiment. The deflection remained, however, zero; in other words, the resistance was infinitely great.

If, as we have stated, the conductivity of the living tooth for electric currents depends entirely upon the liquids contained in its pores, then dentine, which is more porous than enamel, should show a less resistance than the latter; furthermore, a section of dentine which cuts the canaliculi at right angles or nearly so would have less resistance than one parallel with them, and finally the resistance would increase with that of the liquid with which the section is moistened.

In order to determine whether the resistances of dentine and enamel, of cross-sections and longitudinal sections, in reality bear the relations to each other demanded by the above condition, the following tests were made:

The section whose resistance was to be determined was held between the ends of two amalgamated zinc wires, which had a diameter of 1.9 millimeter, under a constant pressure of about two grams to the square millimeter. The section of dentine, $\frac{1}{400}$ of a millimeter thick, was moistened with a concentrated solution of sulphate of zinc.

FIG. 56.

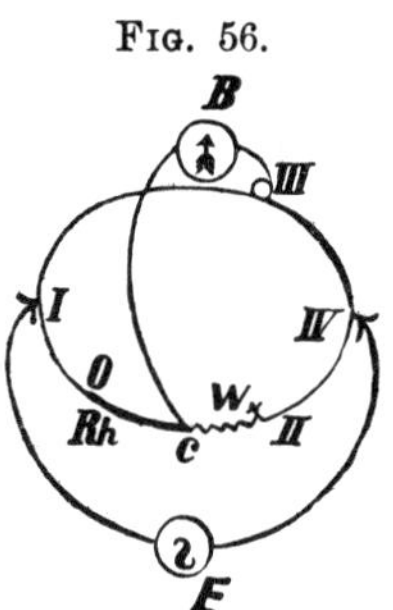

The arrangement of the apparatus for determining the resistance may be seen in the accompanying figure (Fig. 56).

Here *E* denotes two Siemen's elements; *B*, a mirror galvanometer after Wiedemann, with 16,000 turns of wire and a resistance of 5000 Siemen's units, having an aperiodized magnet ring after E. du Bois-Reymond; *Rh*, the rheostat; *Wx*, the resistance to be determined; *O*, *I*, *II*, *III*, *IV*, denote the connections with a round compensator after E. du Bois-Reymond with the modifications of Christiani.

As result of the large number of experiments, I found that a section of dentine $\frac{1}{400}$ millimeter thick, cutting the canaliculi at right angles, had a resistance of about 1700 Siemen's units; that a similar section, parallel or nearly so with the canaliculi, had a resistance at the beginning of about 8050 Siemen's units. As the piece began to dry, the resistance rapidly increased, till it soon became infinitely great.

When the same sections were moistened with water, the resistance was much greater; it could not, however, be definitely determined on account of the polarization.

It may be easily shown by the following simple experiment that the resistance of the enamel is much greater than that of the dentine. Place one pole of a battery consisting of four Siemen's cells upon the gums and the other upon the enamel of a sound tooth, not the slightest sensation will be produced; if, however, we place the second end upon the dentine or upon a metallic filling in contact with the dentine, we will at once experience a very unpleasant sensation.

There can be no doubt that there are electric currents in the mouth whenever there are teeth with metallic fillings. These currents do not, however, exist in such a manner between the filling and the tooth-substance that the latter could in any way be compared with the generating plate of a galvanic cell; they owe their existence alone to the heterogeneity of the metallic fillings.

Electric currents will be produced on the surface of every filling, even of a pure gold one, when the filling does not have the same density in all parts. They flow from the denser to the less dense points of the surface. If these currents were even strong enough and durable enough to be considered as anything more than infinitesimal, they still could have no injurious effect upon the tooth deserving of mention, since it could rarely happen that a great excess of them would be directed toward the margin of the filling.

When two fillings of different materials, in the same tooth or in approximating teeth touch each other, a current is produced, which flows from the more oxidizable (electro-positive) metal through the liquids of the mouth and tooth to the less oxidizable (electro-negative). These currents, by electrolytically decomposing the liquids of the mouth, may produce injurious effects upon the teeth. Through them acid will be set free on the surface of the electro-positive metal, which may attack the tooth at the margin of the filling. This action, however, is very slight at best, and appears to cease altogether as soon as the surface of the positive pole becomes oxidized; in short, we have not found in practice that such a process has any injurious effect upon the teeth.

When gold plates with clamps of baser metal are put into the mouth, a weak electric current is produced through which acid may be liberated upon the clamp. This, in course of time, may have a marked injurious effect upon the tooth with which it comes in contact. This action may be demonstrated by the following experiment: I attached a bicuspid by means of a platinum wire, twisted around the neck of the same, to the positive pole of a Siemen's battery of three cells, and a second bicuspid in the same manner to the negative pole. The teeth were then placed one in each arm of a U-shaped tube which was filled with a 0.75 per cent. solution of chloride of sodium. The circuit contained, for observing the current, a galvanometer possessing a multiplicator of 1000 turns and a resistance of 200 Siemen's units. On closing the circuit there followed a deflection of the needle amounting to thirty-one degrees; after two weeks, the deflection had decreased to eight degrees. On removing the teeth from the solution it was found that the wire, by virtue of the acid liberated upon its surface, had cut a groove about ½ mm. deep around the neck of the anode tooth. At the kathode tooth no change was observed.

Electric currents may therefore occur in the mouth (1) when a metallic filling has not the same density throughout; (2) when two fillings of different metals touch; (3) when a plate is composed of different alloys.

Dentine being, as shown by these experiments, an absolute non-conductor of electricity, all these electric currents between different parts of the teeth or between filling and tooth-substance can have only an imaginary existence, and the results obtained by Chase in the experiments referred to above must be erroneous. That they are utterly so may be easily determined by a few carefully made experiments of the same nature.

I have made in all over twenty such experiments, with different substances and under varying conditions.[106] The results of ten of these experiments are given below, and each one may draw his own conclusions from them. These ten were not selected from the whole number, but each alternate one was taken in the order in which they were made. The first series of experiments I made with ivory, the second with dentine taken from a fish tooth, the third with dentine from human teeth. The pieces of human dentine were made in pairs, both members of each pair being obtained from the same tooth by making a cross-section of a sound, large molar, removing all traces of pulp-cavity and of the enamel, and then dividing the section symmetrically into halves. In this way the two pieces of each pair were as nearly alike as they could well be made.

In some of the experiments the pieces were filled with different materials; in others they were suspended to equal depth in the solution by means of wires of different metals and of silk thread, the latter method being equivalent to making fillings of the same materials, the silk thread corresponding to a filling of wax; the wires were all of the same diameter. In the sixth column of figures I have given the results which would have obtained in accordance with the experiment of Chase, on the theory that if gold causes a certain loss in weight, amalgam will cause two-thirds the same; tin, one-half; gutta-percha, one-sixth; wax, one-sixth, while the piece filled with zinc-oxychloride suffers no loss in weight. The balance used was capable of noting a variation of two-tenths of a milligram.

I.

Substance.	Weight in Mgs.	Solution.	Time.	Suspended by	Loss in Weight.	Comparison.
1. Ivory	115.6	Sulphuric acid, 1 per cent.	Six weeks	Gold wire	30.6	30.6
2. "	"	Sulphuric acid, 1 per cent.	"	Silk thread	31.1	5.1

III.

Substance.	Weight in Mgs.	Solution.	Time.	Suspended by	Loss in Weight.	Comparison.
1. Ivory	204.0	Vinegar	Two weeks	Gold wire	76.0	76.0
2. "	"	"	"	Platinum wire	76.4	
3. "	"	"	"	Copper "	76.5	
4. "	"	"	"	Tin "	75.0	38.0
5. "	"	"	"	Silk thread	76.8	12.7

V.

Substance.	Weight in Mgs.	Solution.	Time.	Suspended by	Loss in Weight.	Comparison.
1. Dentine from fish tooth	912.0	Lemon-juice	Eight days	Gold wire	248.0	248.0
2 Dentine from fish tooth	"	"	"	Silk thread	244.0	41.3

VII.

Substance.	Weight in Mgs.	Solution.	Time.	Suspended by	Loss in Weight.	Comparison.
1. Dentine from human tooth	39.3	Acetic acid, 20 per cent.	Ten days	Gold wire	5.0	5.0
2. Dentine from human tooth	"	Acetic acid, 20 per cent.	"	Silk thread	4.6	0.8

IX.

Substance.	Weight in Mgs.	Solution.	Time.	Suspended by	Loss in Weight.	Comparison.
1. Ivory	201.5	Hydrochloric acid, ½ per cent.	One week	Gold wire	53.3	53.3
2. "	"	Hydrochloric acid, ½ per cent.	"	Silk thread	54.0	8.9

XI.

Substance.	Weight in Mgs.	Solution.	Time.	Suspended by	Loss in Weight.	Comparison.
1. Ivory	201.5	Sulphuric acid, 2 per cent.	One week	Gold	7.5	7.5
2. "	"	Sulphuric acid, 2 per cent.	"	Amalgam	7.3	5.0
3. "	"	Sulphuric acid, 2 per cent.	"	Tin	6.3	3.7
4. "	"	Sulphuric acid, 2 per cent.	"	Zinc-oxychloride	6.5	0.0

XIII.

Substance.	Weight in Mgs.	Solution.	Time.	Suspended by	Loss in Weight.	Comparison.
1. Ivory	195.5	Lemon-juice	One week	Gold	68.0	6.80
2. "	"	"	"	Amalgam	68.5	45.3
3. "	"	"	"	Tin	69.0	34.0
4. "	"	"	"	Zinc-oxychloride	70.4	0.0

XV.

Substance.	Weight in Mgs.	Solution.	Time.	Suspended by	Loss in Weight.	Comparison.
1. Dentine from human tooth	88.4	Acetic acid, 20 per ct.	Two weeks	Gold	13.5	13.5
2. Dentine from human tooth	"	Acetic acid, 20 per ct.	"	Zinc-oxychloride	14.9	0.0

XVII.

Substance.	Weight in Mgs.	Solution.	Time.	Suspended by	Loss in Weight.	Comparison.
1. Dentine from human tooth	70.9	Lemon-juice	Six days	Gold	49.6	49.6
2. Dentine from human tooth	"	"	"	Zinc-oxychloride	48.6	0.0

XIX.

Substance.	Weight in Mgs.	Solution.	Time.	Suspended by	Loss in Weight.	Comparison.
1. A sound bicuspid	885.0	Acetic acid, dilute	Three w'ks	Gold	79.0	79.0
2. A sound bicuspid	875 0	Acetic acid, dilute	"	Zinc-oxychloride	82.0	0.0

Diverse Causes of Caries.

Mechanical injuries, particularly such as are caused by sharp or rough particles of food (splinters of bone), sharp tooth-powders, sudden changes of temperature, climatic influences, humidity of the air, use of tobacco, medicines, mineral waters, mercury, mental exertion, the quality of the food, erosions, "salty, acid, pointed or rough particles which irritate the very delicate membranes of the alveoli or the nerve-filaments," etc., are mentioned by many as the cause of toothache.

Some also accuse sugar or strongly sugared beverages. Ovelgrün[72] (1771), Pfaff[86] (1756), directed attention to the bad teeth of confectioners, while Peter Forest[72] (1597) pointed out the occurrence of a similar malady in the case of apothecaries, "who ruin their teeth with licking the juices."

Westcott holds that sugar is injurious only on account of its fermentation products, viz, lactic and butyric acids. At present, sugar is universally regarded by dentists as well as laymen as injurious to the teeth. Many investigators, as Fauchard (1728), Angermann (1806), Guttmann (1827), Desirabode[72] (1846), etc., distinguish external and internal or local and general causes. Fauchard also mentions different forms of decay, such as scrofulous, scorbutic, moist, dry, superficial, deep, etc.

As external causes, were mentioned mechanical, chemical, etc.; as internal, bad juices, deformities, constitutional diseases, etc.

CHAPTER VII.

ORIGINAL INVESTIGATIONS ON THE DECAY OF THE TEETH.

INTRODUCTORY REMARKS ON THE HISTOLOGY AND CHEMISTRY OF THE TEETH.

THE peculiar structure of the hard dental tissues, especially of the dentine, not only determines to a great extent the manner in which the change designated as decay advances in the tissues, but also accounts for the microscopic appearances characteristic of this disease, and also greatly influences the spreading of caries in the tissues. I shall, therefore, as briefly as possible, call attention to those structural properties of enamel and dentine, which are of special significance.

Furthermore, an intimate knowledge of the chemical composition of the hard dental tissues is requisite to an understanding of the process of decay.

Dentine forms the chief constituent or fundament of the human tooth, and retains approximately the original form of the tooth after the removal of the enamel and cement. For our purpose, dentine may be defined as a dense, glue-giving basis-substance, impregnated with lime-salts and traversed by sheathed tubules radiating from the pulp-chamber. These, the dentinal tubules, have a diameter of 1.3–2.5μ; their average diameter is consequently greater than that of bacteria, with the exception of Crenothrix, Beggiatoa, and a few other species as yet not met with in the human mouth. They are straight or slightly undulating, and radiate from the pulp-chamber to the surface of the dentine. They are not empty, but contain living matter, and, by means of their many ramifications and anastomoses, form a delicate net-work, particularly on the border of the enamel. The quantity of organic substance near the enamel and cement may be increased by numerous small interglobular spaces (stratum granulosum) filled with protoplasm. Larger interglobular spaces are also often found in dentine, especially in teeth of poor structure.

The sheaths of the tubules are remarkable for their great power of resistance to acids and to putrefying agents. According to Hoppe-Seyler,[19] the tubules of many fossil teeth may be sufficiently isolated as to permit of examination under the microscope. The isolation is performed by extracting the lime-salts, washing carefully with water to remove the salt and acids, then boiling for a certain length of time in water.

The enamel covers the crown of the tooth somewhat like a thimble. At the margin, that is, at the neck of the tooth, it is very thin, thicker toward the grinding-surface, and thickest on the cusps of the molars, where it sometimes has a thickness of 2.5 mm.

It is the hardest tissue of the human and animal body. According to Hoppe-Seyler, only the siliceous urinary calculi which occur in ruminants, and, perhaps, the siliceous sheaths of bacillaria, exceed it in hardness.

In the fissures of molars and bicuspids, as well as in the foramina cœca of molars and superior lateral incisors, the formation of the enamel-cap is very imperfect. These localities consequently form loci minoris resistentiæ which but feebly resist the attack of caries. Indeed, they rather induce it by the retention of food-particles. The fissures, cracks, etc., of old enamel act in the same way, although in a minor degree.

Morphologically, enamel consists of four- to six-sided straight or undulating, usually parallel prisms, which are separated by an extremely thin layer of intervening substance (binding substance). The spaces between the prisms are, however, under normal conditions, by far too narrow to permit the entrance of micro-organisms.

The enamel-cuticle (Nasmyth's membrane) forms a thin, transparent, glueless layer on the crown of every tooth, in so far as the latter is not worn down by mastication. It resembles the sheaths of the dentinal tubules in the high power of resistance which it shows to the action of acids and putrefactive agents.

The structure of cement is similar to that of bone, from which it differs, however, particularly in the absence of Haversian canals, which, if present in the cement, would naturally render it far more susceptible to the action of external agents than it in reality is.

The relation of Sharpey's fibers to the progress of decay in the cement is very significant; they may accordingly claim especial mention. Without concerning ourselves about the genesis of these so-called penetrating fibers, or fibers of Sharpey, it may suffice to say that they indicate the presence of tubules or canals running perpendicular to the longitudinal axis of the tooth, present in all parts of the cement, but particularly numerous at the neck of the tooth. In case of decay, the micro-organisms are seen to penetrate these canals very much as they enter the dentinal tubules. They thereby facilitate the invasion of bacteria into the interior of the cement, often making the course of cement-decay very similar to that of dentine-decay.

Chemical Composition of the Hard Dental Substance.

Numerous analyses of the hard tooth-substance have been made by different chemists. Some of the older ones, however, are unreliable, and the results obtained are at variance with each other.

Dentine contains a quantity of organic substance which is subject to slight variations in different teeth; in very hard dentine it amounts to about 26 per cent., in very soft to 28.5 per cent. These variations, however, stand in no direct proportion to the hardness of the dentine; that is to say, we find much greater differences in the density of the dentine of different teeth than we do in the percentage of lime-salts which they contain. They probably do not relate to the normally formed intertubular substance, but depend upon the composition of the entire mass of dentine, including the tubules, interglobular spaces, etc. For example, a tooth with wide tubules and large interglobular spaces would, on analysis, give a higher percentage of organic matter than a tooth with narrow tubules and smaller interglobular spaces, even though the intertubular substance should have exactly the same composition in both cases.

In like manner, differences in the proportion of organic matter in the compact and spongy parts of one and the same bone are not to be attributed to the bony matter itself, but to the whole bone, including the contents of the lacunæ, Haversian canals, etc. (Hoppe-Seyler).

In the compact matter of the femur of women aged ninety-seven, eighty-eight, eighty-one, eighty, and twenty-two years respectively, Fremy found the same quantity of organic substance as in the case of a new-born female child.

In conformity with these and other similar results, Hoppe-Seyler maintains the unchangeableness of the combinations occurring in bone, dentine, etc. If Hoppe-Seyler's conception is correct, the small increase of inorganic matter supposed to occur in senile teeth is not to be explained by an increased amount of lime-salts in the dentine, but must be attributed to a decrease in the volume of the soft tissues of the dentine,—in other words, by a formation of basis-substance at the expense of the tubular substance. We shall recur to this question in our remarks upon the transparency of dentine.

The organic constituent of dentine yields glutine when boiled with water, and readily undergoes putrefaction.

The enamel contains but two to five per cent. of organic substance, and usually falls completely to pieces during decalcification, unless special precautions are taken. This remnant of the enamel-forming organ is of epithelial origin, and consequently yields no glutine when boiled in water.

According to Hoppe-Seyler, bone, dentine, and enamel all contain $(PO_4)_6Ca_{10}CO_3$, or $3[(PO_4)_2Ca_3]CaCO_3$,—that is, saturated calcium phosphate carbonate in a combination which corresponds to apatite $(PO_4)_6Ca_{10}Fl_2$.

The following analyses of the ashes of bone, dentine, and enamel gave values which conform with this view :

Bone.*		Dentine.†		Enamel.‡	
Ca	37.99	Ca	37.54	Ca	38.31
PO_4	54.91	PO_4	56.05	PO_4	56.20
CO_3	4.98	Co_3	4.79	CO_3	5.60
Fl	1.29(?)			Cl	0.47
Mg	0.83	Mg	0.38		

* According to Wildt. † Average of several analyses.
‡ According to Hoppe-Seyler.

Notwithstanding the very considerable difficulties attending the analysis, we notice a marked conformity between the values found and those calculated from the atomic complex $(PO_4)_6 Ca_{10}CO_3$, since the latter demands Ca 38.83 per cent., PO_4 55.34 per cent., CO_3 5.83 per cent.

The question whether this combination has been brought together by the glue-giving substance (glutine) had to be answered in the negative, as it also occurs in enamel which contains no glutine.

Another question which has been broached by Hoppe-Seyler now engages our attention: What is the relation of these salts to the glue-giving basis-substance? Are they precipitated in the cartilage according to physical laws, or are they held together by means of the organic substance, and do they enter into a chemical union with it? This is a matter of importance for the understanding of certain pathological phenomena exhibited by the teeth. As emphasized above, the variations in the amount of salts in the dentine are by no means great enough to explain the variations in hardness. But in the case of a chemical union between the organic and inorganic constituents of the tooth, we should expect to find dentine hard or soft according as the union is firm or unstable.

Unfortunately, our knowledge of the nature of the combinations occurring in teeth is as yet very incomplete, nor does it at present appear how we may approach this problem experimentally. "No affinities are known which might make a chemical union conceivable, nor do we know any physical conditions which could explain the impregnation of the organic substance with this calcium phosphate carbonate."

The density of the dentine cartilage is about 0.55, consequently about equal to that of bone; this, by the way, shows that the substance of the odontoblasts, as well as that of the osteoblasts, must undergo a very great condensation during or before calcification.

The density of the organic substance of enamel, on the other hand, is only about 0.075. Regarded from this point, the formation of enamel is a process which essentially differs from the formation of dentine and bone.

PHYSICAL PHENOMENA OF DENTAL DECAY.

a. Decay of Enamel.

In making a study of the phenomena of dental decay which is intended to be anywise complete, it will be necessary to subject the physical, chemical, and microscopical changes of the tissues involved to a rigid examination.

Let us begin with the *physical phenomena of dental decay*, in so far as they are revealed by inspection with the unaided eye or by examination with such simple instruments as excavators, probes, etc. A clear insight into the macroscopical changes which occur at the beginning of enamel-caries can be gained most easily from a freshly extracted molar or bicuspid, decayed on the approximal surface. Cases of fissure-decay are not serviceable for this purpose, because the appearance of the decaying enamel is here generally obscured by other processes occurring simultaneously (precipitates, discolorations, etc.).

Suitable material is not always easily obtained, because teeth showing the very first stages of decay are seldom extracted, and because caries on the approximal surfaces of unextracted teeth becomes apparent only after it has made considerable progress. The opportunity of observing decay at its beginning is therefore very rare.

As the first indication that the process of destruction has begun on the external surface of the enamel, we notice that it has lost its normal polish and transparency; then a *white* (not *black*) irregular spot of chalky color appears; a sharp instrument (*e.g.*, the point of a needle) will not easily glide over the surface, but will readily detect the presence of a slight roughness caused by a softening or disintegration of the enamel, by which it is gradually changed into a soft cheesy powder. This dissolution of the enamel may be best observed when decay advances from the dentine upon the inner surface of the enamel (secondary decay); here the broken-down enamel-prisms cannot be washed away, so that quite a thick layer of a perfectly *white* cheesy substance may often be found.

In primary decay the disorganized enamel-prisms are soon mechanically washed away, whereby an excavation or cavity is formed. The form of the cavity depends upon various circumstances, among others upon the breadth of the surface of contact with the adjacent tooth, also in a high degree upon the structure of the enamel; it is sometimes flat and broad with scarcely distinguishable margins, sometimes narrow and deep with sharp ragged margins. Soon after the commencement of decay, a more or less pronounced discoloration sets in. In my opinion the view held by some that this discoloration is to be regarded as the first sign of decay is based on an error which is to be explained only on the supposition that the advocates of this view have not examined decay in its earliest stages.

A discoloration of intact smooth enamel does not occur; some change or other must have taken place in the enamel before a discoloration can take place, and this change is nothing else than a softening or decalcification of it.

This discoloration appears in very different grades; when the decay proceeds very rapidly (caries acutissima), it is slight or wholly wanting (white decay). In other cases, only the margin of the enamel is colored brown to black while the center of the cavity remains white. When the decay proceeds very slowly, that is, when it is of long standing (caries chronica), the greater part of the affected tissue is deep brown or black. This is also the case where the progress of the decay has been interrupted, as is often observed on the approximal surfaces of teeth which have been exposed by extraction of the adjacent tooth. Such cases are usually designated as caries nigra (black decay). This badly-chosen term must, however, not mislead us to suppose that we have to do here with an especial form of decay. As a matter of fact, we are scarcely entitled to speak of such places as decay at all, any more than we are to say that a man with a pock-marked face has got the smallpox, because they do not indicate that the process of decay is going on at the time being. They are simply degenerated tissue which in the course of time has become discolored by oxidation, precipitation, or other processes of this nature. Decay-marks would be a much better name for such spots.

b. Decay of Dentine.

By the progress of the above-described process the destruction of the enamel spreads until the surface of the dentine is reached (Fig. 57). Here the disease takes on a very different form, inasmuch as we no longer find the tissue being changed into a soft cheesy mass, but into a tough cartilaginous substance which does not readily fall to pieces or yield to the slightest friction, as does the decayed enamel, but may retain its form for some time. This stage is designated as softening of dentine, and is conditioned, as will be seen below, by a more or less complete decalcification of the dentine. The softening spreads in all directions in the dentine, with a rapidity dependent upon the intensity of the fermentation processes present in the mouth and the physical and chemical constitution of the dentine.

Fig. 57.

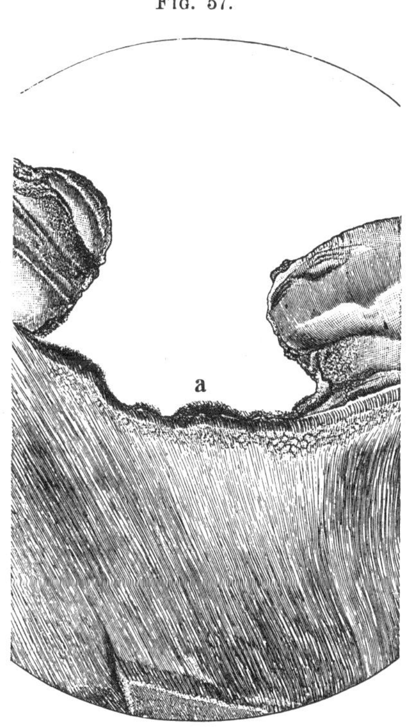

Undermining Enamel Decay.
a, Masses of bacteria lining the cavity. Circa 50 : 1.

The softened mass may be easily cut or peeled off with a sharp instrument; upon pressure, it discharges a small quantity of a liquid which in the great majority of cases will be found to redden blue litmus-paper, *i.e.*, to have an acid reaction.

The thickness of the softened layer varies considerably in different cases, for reasons which will be fully discussed in Chapter VIII. Very soon after the softening of the dentine its disintegration or dissolution begins, leading to the formation of a cavity in the dentine. The surface now appears uneven, soft, and porous, infiltrated and contaminated with particles of fermenting food, masses of bacteria, etc.

The discoloration of the dentine is brought about by the same causes as that of the enamel; it also shows the same variations in acute and chronic decay, and all shades, from the natural color of dentine to black.

As the destructive process spreads more rapidly in dentine than in enamel, the latter becomes usually more or less undermined, and the cavity may acquire a shape resembling a short-necked Florence flask (Fig. 58). The undermined enamel-margins become dry and brittle, and easily break off; it therefore not unfrequently happens, particularly in case of extensive decay on the approximal surface, that the cover of enamel breaks under the pressure exerted by mastication and reveals a large previously invisible cavity. Or, decay proceeding from the grinding-surface of molars destroys the greater part of the dentine, so that only a perforated enamel-cap remains; this finally breaks into pieces at the neck of the tooth, thereby completing the destruction of the crown. In rare cases, caries beginning on the grinding-surface seems to proceed particularly rapidly at the border between enamel and dentine. The bond of union between the two tissues is weakened or destroyed, the enamel-walls break away, while a large portion of the decalcified dentine remains (Fig. 59).

FIG. 58.

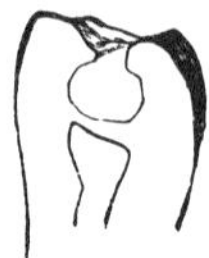

UNDERMINING DECAY. Flask-shaped cavity.

FIG. 59.

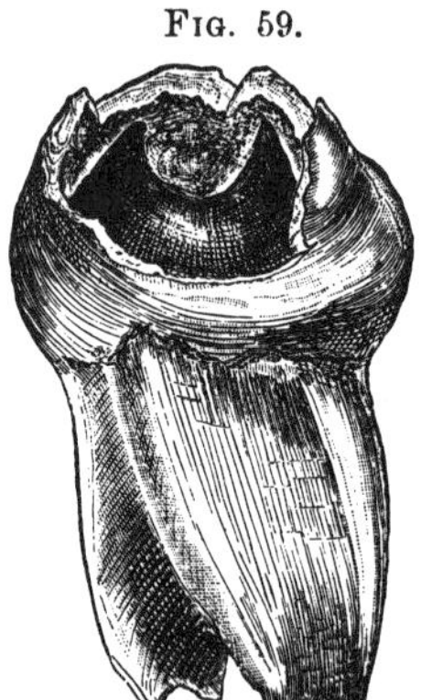

DECAY OF A MILK-MOLAR. The enamel-walls are broken off, while the dentine remains standing.

In other cases, again, the destructive process advances most rapidly along the line of the dentinal tubules toward the pulp. By this means a tube-shaped cavity is formed, as is often observed on the grinding-surface. These cases are usually designated as penetrating decay. But these terms, penetrating and undermining decay, must not mislead us, for there is no specific form of decay which shows a particular tendency to penetrate toward the pulp, nor is there one which especially avoids the pulp to spread laterally under the enamel. The causes and the entire process are identical; in both cases it depends only on the structure of the tooth, whether the decay presents itself as penetrating or undermining.

In poorly developed teeth, with many interglobular spaces, the destruction spreads rapidly on all sides under the enamel, following the course of the interglobular zone, whereas when the teeth are dense and completely dentinified the decay extends more rapidly in the direction of the dentinal tubules. It is barely possible that an infection with small cocci might cause the decay to spread laterally more rapidly than an infection with large cocci or bacilli, since the former could advance laterally through the fine branches of the tubules, whereas the latter would be obliged to keep more to the main track.

When the softened dentine is strongly saturated with liquids, as is the case in caries acuta, it has been designated as caries humida. The chronic form of dentine decay, in which the dentine is dry and brittle, is sometimes termed caries sicca.

c. Decay of the Cement.

Decay of the cement frequently occurs at the neck of the tooth. The layer of cement is, however, so thin here that the characteristic phenomena of cement-caries scarcely become apparent. Caries of the cement of the root occurs only when the latter is exposed, and is therefore comparatively rare.

The roots of molars which are laid bare by the recession of the gums and destruction of the periosteum show the greatest preference for decay.

Such roots are often covered with thick white or yellowish-white deposits, consisting of food particles, dead epithelium, mucus, and fungus masses, and not unfrequently present cases of typical decay of the cement.

The first symptom of cement-decay is an abnormal roughness or softness of the cement surface, which may be easily penetrated or scraped off with an excavator.

This phenomenon, which is also nothing but the softening of the cement, is followed by a loss of the surface-substance; thus a cavity is produced, or rather a depression, since it has little similarity with the cavities of the crown. Deep bulb-shaped cavities are hardly ever formed; they are for the most part shallow, widely extended excavations, without a distinct margin.

This is due to the fact that there are no circumscribed points of retention or foci of decay on the roots, from which alone the destruction could proceed. It therefore seldom happens that decay beginning at the root spreads from the cement to the dentine and destroys the latter to such an extent that the root-pulp is exposed.

A natural retention-center is formed at the point of bifurcation of the molar roots where it has been exposed by recession of the gums, and penetrating decay is consequently not seldom found here.

Discoloration has been erroneously regarded as the first stage of cement-decay also. Exposed roots almost invariably become more or less discolored in time, whether they are decayed or not, especially when they are not kept clean.

d. Decay of the Enamel-Cuticle.

It is impossible to follow the process of decay in the delicate membrane covering the crown of the tooth without the aid of the microscope. All we can see with the naked eye is a more or less pronounced discoloration surrounding the carious part of the membrane which has been detached by strong acids. Frequently a thickening and cloudiness are also detectable.

In pulpless and dead human teeth, even in artificial teeth carved from walrus-teeth, decay exhibits the same physical phenomena as in living teeth.

ACCOMPANYING PHENOMENA OF DENTAL DECAY.

As concomitant phenomena of dental decay I designate certain processes which manifest themselves either immediately or some time after the appearance of decay, and which, in my opinion, have been erroneously denominated as characteristics of it.

Those processes are: (1) transparency, (2) the pigmentation or discoloration of the decayed tissue.

"Coincident with the development of the opacity and the pigmental degeneration in the commencement of the carious affection of the dentine, an increased translucency is observed, frequently, in the portions adjacent to the boundary of the carious portion. With reflected light these portions have a horny appearance, similar to that found in senile roots, and with transmitted light they present hyaline bands and spots. The focus

Fig. 60.

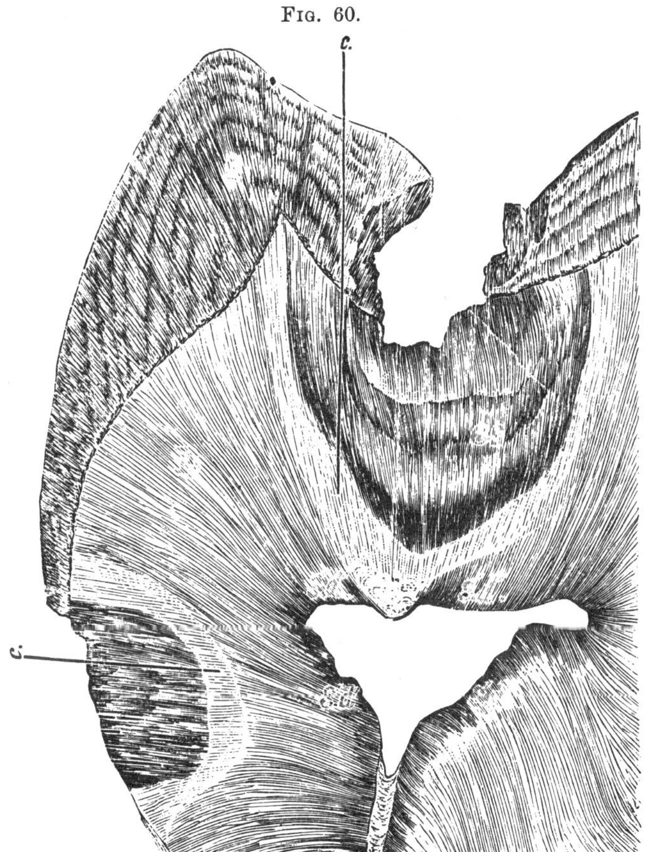

Portion of a Longitudinal Ground Section through the Crown of a Molar, Showing two cavities of decay, with the transparent zones at *c*. (After Gysi.)

(Herd) of the caries is surrounded by a diaphanous halo. The opaque, carious dentinal cone, therefore, is invested by a translucent zone, extending from the periphery toward the center; around a more spherical, carious portion of the dentine a crescentic diaphanous halo is sometimes met with (Fig. 60). The light portions, finally, vary exceedingly in respect of their outlines, according to the form in which the carious limits are extended, being radiated, kidney-shaped, etc." (Wedl.)

A true picture of transparency can be obtained only where softening and pigmentation of the dentine have not yet taken place; that is to say, where there is as yet no decay. The transparent portion here forms a cone whose apex points toward the

FIG. 61.

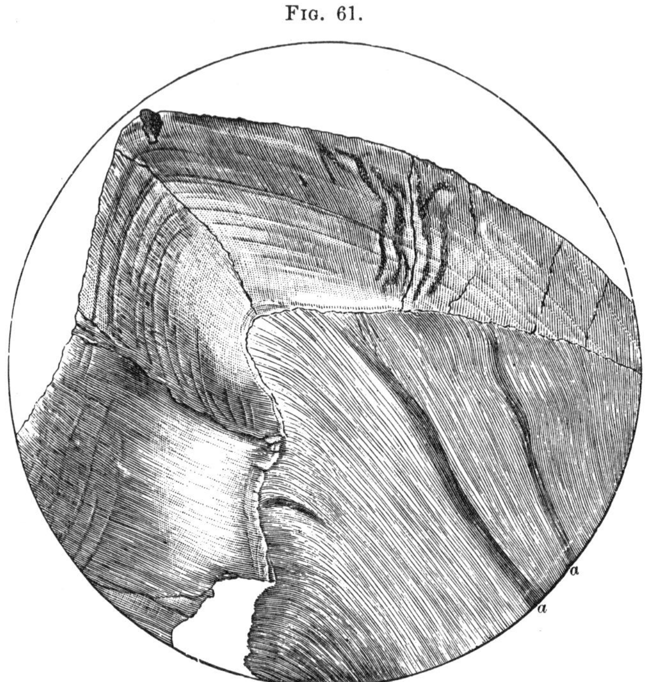

BEGINNING DECAY OF ENAMEL WITH TRANSPARENT CONE OF DENTINE.
Under weak power.

pulp and whose sides run parallel with the dentinal tubules. In most cases the transverse sections of these cones are, as far as my observations go, bounded by two opaque stripes (Fig. 61, *a*). Under the microscope, the dentinal tubules within these stripes are seen to be filled with irregular, angular granules or oblong particles.

I have not been able to discover analogous phenomena in

dead dentine. Through the kindness of the late Dr. Franz, I obtained no fewer than three hundred human teeth which had been worn in the mouth on plates. Nearly all of them showed different degrees of decay. I split about sixty which seemed specially suited for the purpose. One case only revealed a phenomenon resembling transparency, but even in this one case it was not possible to say that the change was not brought about while the tooth was still living. Again, the appearance in question is by no means peculiar to decay. We have seen that it does not accompany decay of dead teeth, whereas it is very common in sound teeth which have been worn off, also in teeth whose approximal surfaces have been slightly worn away by friction. It is found particularly in senile teeth, whose entire roots frequently become transparent, likewise in roots in the process of resorption, etc.; everywhere, in short, where the living dentinal fibers are slightly irritated. I have noticed a high degree of transparency in the teeth of old dogs which have been extensively worn away. It does not show the remotest similarity to decay, and, in fact, bears no direct relation to it, inasmuch as it is absent in dead teeth, and very frequently occurs in a marked degree and in typical forms in places where there is not a trace of decay, and where decay, on the whole, very seldom occurs. The same agents which produce decay may also occasion transparency of dentine, which explains the frequent simultaneous appearance of both phenomena.

The opacity of normal dentine is produced by the different coefficients of refraction of its component parts. If two substances, whether transparent or not, of different refractive power be mixed, an opaque substance will result, unless the one is soluble in the other. Thus water and oil are both transparent, but when mixed they are opaque. In a like manner the opaque foam is composed of two transparent substances, air and water. Furthermore, both glass and air are transparent, but when glass is pulverized, that is to say mixed with air, an opaque substance will result. The powdered glass can be made transparent again, when another substance having the same coefficient of refraction as glass is substituted for the air. Oil of cedar is such a body (approximately). This poured upon powdered glass restores its transparency. Now, dentine consists, on the one hand, of the basis-substance infiltrated with lime-salts, and on the other of the dentinal tubules, with their contents; and since both these constituents of dentine have different coefficients of refraction, an opaque tissue is formed. We may diminish the opacity—that is, increase the transparency—by filling the dentinal tubules with a substance which has the same coefficient of refraction as the basis-substance, or by transforming the basis-substance so as to make it resemble the contents of the tubules in respect to refraction.

In spite of the many attempts to account for the increased transparency of the dentine under certain conditions, its true cause has not yet been established with certainty. J. Tomes[107] and Magitot[108] explain transparency by the calcification of the dentinal fibrils. Both authors regard it as the result of a vital process—an attempt made by nature to impede the progress of the disease. Later, Tomes[109] seems to have doubted the correctness of his former views. C. Wedl[110] regards the transparency occurring in dental decay as identical with that appearing in the roots of senile teeth. He doubts the correctness of the calcification theory, without giving further expression to his own.

Leber and Rottenstein[58] ascribe transparency to a partial decalcification of the dentine.

Schlenker[72] seems to be of the same opinion.

It has also been attempted to explain the transparency of the dentine by the obliteration of the dentinal tubules brought about by the swelling of the basis-structure.

Since, however, the swelling or expansion of a porous body is not accompanied by obliteration of the pores, but, on the other hand, naturally implies a corresponding enlargement of them, an obliteration by swelling is a physical impossibility. According to Walkhoff,[111] "transparency has also been explained as the consequence of micrococci." I have found no such view expressed anywhere, either by Milles and Underwood or any other advocate of the chemico-parasitical theory of decay.

Walkhoff concludes from his experiments "that transparency must be regarded as a sclerotic action of the dentine-fibers, by which they form new basis-substance at their own expense. Its real nature is an increased and lasting physiological activity, which calls forth over-production of intercellular matter at the expense of the cells and primarily of their offshoots."

Black[112] disputes the view that transparency is to be looked upon as the expression of a vital process. He appears to regard it as the earliest stage of disintegration. According to the observations which I have made in reference to transparency, I am inclined to accept the vital theory. In my opinion we must choose here between two possibilities: either the basis-substance is decalcified and a form of transparency thus brought about, or the tubules are partially or completely filled with a substance which has a similar action upon light as the intertubular substance. *A decalcification, however, has most certainly not taken place in the transparency in question;* this is sufficiently proved by chemical analysis, while on the other hand many facts point to a vital process.

1. We know that the diameter of dentinal tubules in normal condition is much greater near the pulp than at the border of the enamel, and that it is much smaller in senile than in young teeth. These facts point to a gradual decrease of the diameter of the tubules after the dentine has already been formed. We also know that chronic excitations of any kind lead to "secondary" dentine formation on the inner surface of the dentine. May they not, then, also lead to an acceleration of the formation in the domain of the fibrils?

2. The microscopic examination of transparency shows as a matter of fact a decrease in the diameter of the dentinal tubules within the transparent zone. This at the same time signifies a diminution in the size of the fibrils.

3. The transparency is characteristic of living dentine.

4. Chemical analysis gives results which agree with this theory. According to my own determinations, dentine from the transparent part of a number of teeth (about twenty-five) gave, when dried at 102°–105° C., 71.9 per cent. ashes, while normal dentine from the same teeth gave 72.1 per cent. A second calculation, made by a chemist, yielded for transparent dentine 69.5 per cent., and for the normal dentine from the same teeth 68.0. We may conjecture from the rather small amount of ashes that

the dentine was not thoroughly dried before combustion; this latter determination is therefore not quite reliable, but at any rate shows that there is an increase rather than a decrease of lime-salts. The general conception, however, that this theory is compatible only with a high percentage of lime-salts is not quite correct. A formation of new dentine, whether it be at the periphery of the pulp or in the domain of the fibrils, does not occur without a preceding solidification of the outer layer of the odontoblasts or fibrils. If, therefore, a new formation of dentine takes place in the tubules at the expense of the dentinal fibrils, this occasions not only an increase of lime-salts, but also simultaneously an increase of the glue-giving basis-substance. We may therefore have a consolidation of the dentine, although analysis may not detect any marked increase in the percentage of lime-salts. In conclusion, this theory must not be confounded with the old calcification theory. The latter demands an impregnation of the fibrils with lime-salts only, the former a partial or total conversion of the fibrils into normal dentine.

2. Pigmentation of the Tissue in Dental Decay.

The pigmentation or discoloration usually attending decay of enamel or dentine is another secondary process which has erroneously been viewed as a stage of decay. Every degree of discoloration may be observed, from the normal color of the tissue to a yellowish, yellow, yellowish-brown, dark-brown, black. In the very first appearance of decay no discoloration is visible. This absence of discoloration is especially remarkable in secondary caries of enamel, the tissue being converted into a perfectly white powder.

Nor does rapid caries show any or but very little discoloration in the deeper parts, while chronic caries always exhibits a dark color, dark brown to black; in other words, *the intensity of the discoloration is in inverse proportion to the rapidity of the progress of the disease.* Besides, the discoloration of dentine does by no means occur in decay only. Wherever the dentine is laid bare, it may be more or less discolored in time. The black discoloration is especially common in worn-off teeth, and, indeed, not only in the case of smokers, but also of non-smokers, nor is it rare for the teeth of dogs to show a deep brown to black discoloration. Most authors concur in the view that the pigment arises from without, and is conditioned by causes which have nothing to do with the decay itself.

Watt explains it by the action of various mineral acids: muriatic acid conditions the white, nitric acid the yellow, sulphuric acid the brownish-black decay.

Clark [113] believes that the discoloration is called forth by the color-forming power of bacteria.

Black [112] explains the discoloration by the settling of coloring-matters into the partly decomposed tissue. These seem to be derived chiefly from the dark sulphurets formed in the mouth by the action of sulphuretted hydrogen upon such metallic elements as may be present. Others lay the blame on various foods and stimulants, coffee, tobacco, etc.

It is not to be denied that smoking may occasion a dark discoloration of dentine. It cannot, however, be the cause of pigmentation in dental caries, since the latter occurs in the cases of persons who do not smoke. Then, again, dentine is colored black also in the worn-off teeth of dogs; moreover, discoloration of dentine and coal-black deposits are very common in teeth of animals without decay.

In my judgment, the cause of discoloration in dental caries is exactly the same as that of the discoloration of any other organic substance which is decomposed by micro-organisms. This idea is presented at length in the chapter on chromogenic mouth-bacteria.

CHEMICAL CHANGES ATTENDING DECAY OF THE TEETH.

With very few exceptions, all investigators who have given any attention to the study of the phenomena of dental decay have been unanimous in the opinion that the softening of the dentine is caused by the extraction of the lime-salts.

The fact that we have to do with a genuine process of decalcification is so patent that I would have no excuse for presenting the experiments recorded below, if they were not of some value in showing the comparative degrees of decalcification in decayed dentine and in dentine artificially softened, as well as the comparative losses of the organic and inorganic constituents of the dentine.

A large number of analyses were made by myself, as well as by Dr. Jeserich, Prof. Liebreich, and others, in which decayed dentine was compared with dentine softened in a fermenting mixture of saliva and bread and in various acids. The results obtained showed the process to be identical in all cases. (See *Dental Cosmos*, 1883, p. 337.) In order to obtain results which would show at the same time the amount of loss suffered by the organic constituents of the dentine, I proceeded in the following manner:

I procured three perfectly fresh teeth which contained large quantities of carious dentine. These teeth were washed in a gentle stream of water to remove all remains of food, and the softened dentine removed *in one piece* with a spoon-shaped excavator. The joint volume of the pieces was then determined by an instrument specially constructed for the purpose, which gave the volume at once in cubic millimeters, and also by the ordinary picnometer. Then (from the same teeth) pieces of sound dentine were procured whose volume was determined in the same manner. The pieces were then dried for thirty hours at 105° C., and analyzed.

I give the result of one analysis:

187.2 cubic millimeters of sound dentine weighed	0.3600
" " " " carious " "	0.0821
Loss,	0.2779

The sound dentine gave on analysis 72.1 per cent. lime-salts . . . . =	0.2595
The carious dentine gave on analysis 26.3 per cent. lime-salts . . . . =	0.0192
Loss,	0.2403

The sound dentine contained 27.9 organic matter =	0.1004
" carious " " 73.7 " " =	0.0605
Loss,	0.0399

The carious dentine had accordingly lost on the whole seven-ninths of its original mass, the lime-salts had lost twelve-thirteenths, and the organic matter two-fifths.

In plain words, the carious dentine had suffered an almost complete decalcification, only one-thirteenth of the original amount of lime-salts being still present. The organic matter had suffered the comparatively small loss of two-fifths of its original amount. This loss is no doubt attributable, for the most part, to the direct action of the micro-organisms upon the more completely decalcified portions of the carious dentine.

The results of these experiments are too plain to require further explanation. They show an almost complete decalcification of the carious dentine, and a comparatively small reduction of the organic matter, also that the organic matter yields *last* to the destroying agents.

MICROSCOPICAL PHENOMENA OF DECAY.

1. Decay of the Enamel-Cuticle.

If we subject a piece of Nasmyth's membrane perforated by decay to a microscopic examination, we will find, in addition to its discoloration and clefts, an enormous number of round and oblong densely crowded bodies, which are easily recognized as bacteria, especially after staining (Plate, Fig. 6). They are sometimes so closely packed that the membrane itself is entirely lost to sight (Fig. 62). Wedl calls these corpuscles "the matrix of Leptothrix buccalis." They have, however, most probably no necessary genetic connection with thread-forming mouth-bacteria, but represent various kinds of bacteria, both monomorph and pleomorph. They exert the same destructive influence upon the enamel-cuticle as upon every organic substance; it loses its transparency, appears thickened and cleft in all directions, and

Fig. 62.

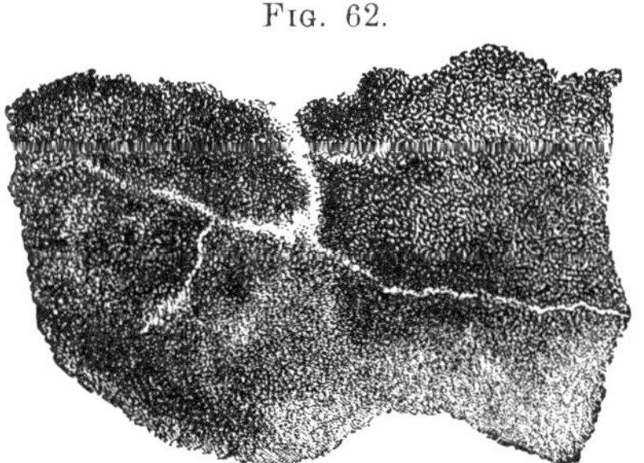

Small Piece of Enamel-Cuticle
Converted into a mass of bacteria by decay. 300 : 1.

particularly at the margin of the cavity ragged and in a state of dissolution. In the last stages of decay we see only a mass of bacteria (cocci, rods and threads), which is held together by the remnant of the membrane. The thickening of the membrane is for the most part, I think, due to the accumulations of bacteria. Sections of enamel in an early stage of caries, after being stained with fuchsine, clearly show that the membrane is loosened from the enamel on the decayed point, thickened and invaded by masses of bacteria. The membrane in this condition affords a matrix, that is, a point of retention, for bacteria, as well as for very minute particles of food, and thereby accelerates the progress of decay.

2. Decay of Enamel.

a. Preparation of Specimens.

The preparation of specimens of enamel suited for a study of the process of decay is very difficult. It is well known that it is impossible to decalcify enamel and to make sections of it with the microtome. We are restricted to the study of ground sections, and these necessarily give but an imperfect idea of the process, because the largest part of the decayed enamel is lost in grinding. Various methods have been proposed for the preparation of microscopically thin ground sections. Whichever method be applied, we first endeavor to split the tooth with a pair of splitting forceps in such a manner that the surface of cleavage passes approximately through the center of the cavity (which, of course, does not always succeed) and grind down each half on a rough corundum-wheel to the thickness of about 1 mm.; or the whole tooth is ground down from both sides, until the cavity is reached. By the latter process we obtain only one lamella, and consequently but one preparation, whereas the former yields two preparations. These lamellæ are then ground under water on a fine corundum-wheel as thin as possible without destroying too much of the diseased tissue. A smooth, firm cork is best suited for holding the piece against the wheel.

The method of A. Weil (p. 171) may also be applied to advantage, or we may follow the suggestion of Gysi:[114]

"Take a freshly-extracted tooth and grind it down with a coarse corundum-wheel to a pretty thin lamella, according as a transverse or a longitudinal section is desired. This lamella should then be ground on one side perfectly even on a fine stone, and then polished on the same side upon leather, coating with some fine polishing-powder until no rays are visible on this side anywhere. The lamella should then be cemented with the polished side down on a glass slide, such as is used for putting up microscopical preparations, with some thick Canada balsam, which is easily softened by heating, and then firmly pressing the lamella against the glass. Around the lamella are cemented some exceedingly thin pieces of covering-glasses, as used in microscopy.

"Practically it is best to cement on the other side of the glass a piece of cork, so that the slide can be easily managed during the further process of grinding. The lamella is then ground by hand on a fine and perfectly flat stone until all the thin covering-glasses are evenly touched. By this process the lamella is made of an equal thickness, with the covering-glasses cemented around it.

"The cover-glass pieces are then removed and the lamella ground still thinner; when thin enough, it generally detaches itself. All this grinding must be done with water on a water-stone. The final step is to polish it on this newly-ground side.

"The exceedingly thin plate procured in this manner should then be washed in alcohol, and every particle of polishing-powder brushed off with a fine camel's-hair brush. The ground section is now ready for mounting. For this purpose it is placed in absolute alcohol for five minutes or longer, by which every trace of water is removed. It is then transferred to oil of cloves to clear it; then placed on a clean glass slide, a drop of Canada balsam put on it, and covered with a thin cover-glass. The preparation is now finished and ready for examination under the microscope."

Charters White ("Elementary Microscopical Manipulation") recommends rubbing down the sections between two plates of ground glass, with the addition of some pumice-powder and water; a method which is said to give very good results.

Preparations of enamel are to be stained in the same manner as those of dentine. (See page 173.)

b. Appearances under the Microscope.

Microscopic examination of preparations of decayed enamel brings to light in many preparations nothing more than a depression (a loss of substance) with uneven margins (Fig. 63), a more or less pronounced pigmentation of the enamel in the vicinity of the depression, and a distinct appearance of the transverse striation of the enamel-prisms (Fig. 64).

Fig. 63.

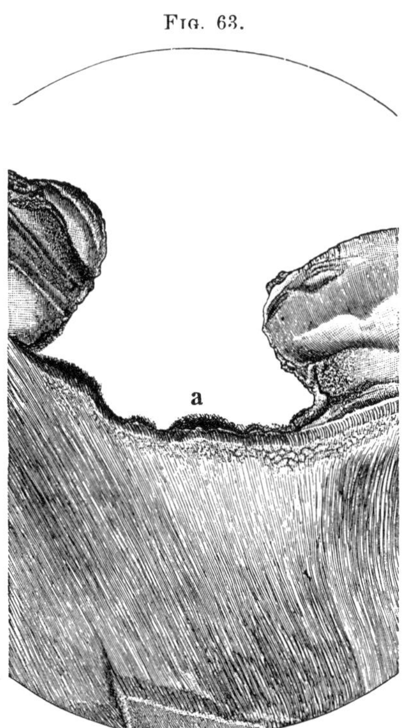

Underminining Enamel Decay.
a, Masses of bacteria lining the cavity. Circa 50 : 1.

Fig. 64.

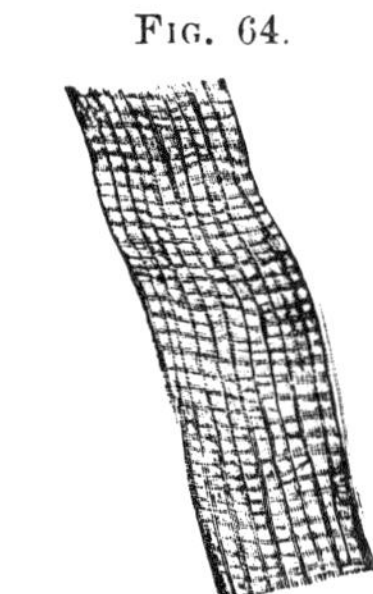

Pronounced Striation of the Prisms in Decay of Enamel.
250 : 1.

In other better prepared specimens the depression is seen to be filled with masses of micro-organisms which readily take on coloring-matter; the margin of the cavity is indented, the enamel cracked, the prisms falling to pieces. The spaces between the loosened prisms are, in these cases, often filled with the same fungal masses, whereas the latter never penetrate between the prisms of normal enamel. In grinding, the masses of bacteria, as well as the loosened prisms, are generally torn away.

After the enamel has once been perforated by decay, its further destruction proceeds principally from the inner surface. This statement may at first seem strange, but will be found on closer examination to be in accordance with the observed facts. The remains of food accumulating in every dental cavity do not, of course, attack the external, but the internal surface of the enamel. We will find, furthermore, in nearly all large cavities the decay extending from the dentine directly upon the inner surface of the enamel.

This latter form of decay, which we designate as secondary enamel-decay, is in many respects better suited for study than the primary, inasmuch as the diseased tissue is not torn away by mastication, etc., and not contaminated from without by foreign bodies.

The extent of the secondary decay of the enamel naturally corresponds to that of the dentine-decay; in large cavities on the grinding-surface of molars, almost the entire inner surface of the enamel may be found to be involved. Penetrating enamel-decay proceeding from within is rare. I have observed such cases usually in inferior molars, where decay proceeding from the grinding-surface perforates the enamel-wall from the inner side, breaking through the approximal wall of enamel to the outside. In secondary decay we find the enamel-surface coated with a white layer of softened enamel sometimes ½ mm. thick. If a small quantity of this be brought under the microscope in water, it is seen to be composed of enamel-prisms mixed with large masses of bacteria (Fig. 65). These prisms lie either singly or in groups; are 10–150μ long, and have sharp or rough extremities. The transverse striation is distinctly marked. In sections the margin appears indented, and the enamel-prisms

Fig. 65.

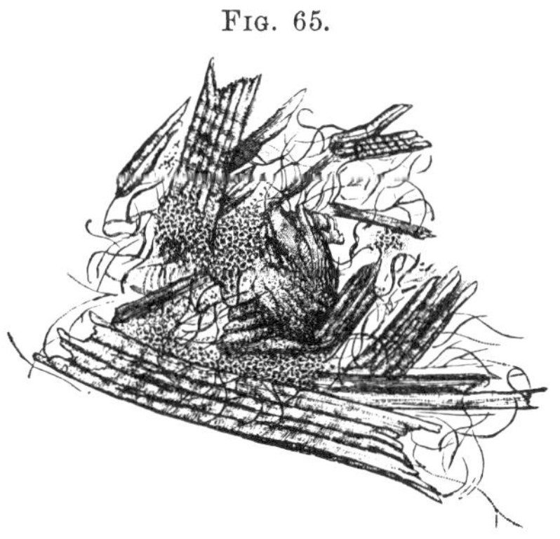

Disruption of the Prisms in Secondary Enamel-Decay. 400 : 1.

more or less dislocated. The whole looks as if the inter-prismatic substance were dissolved, *i.e.*, the connection between the prisms

FIG. 66.

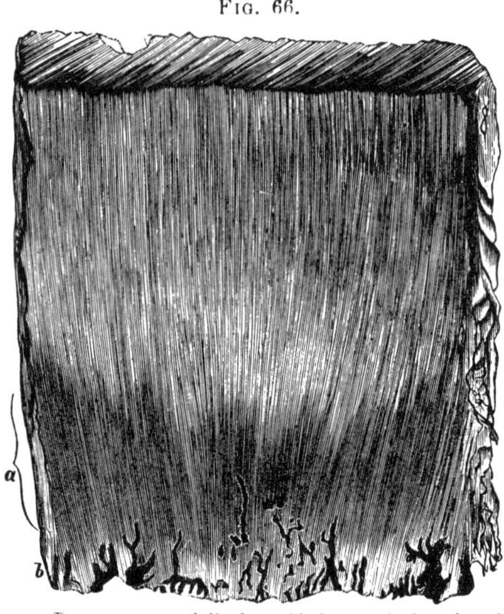

SECONDARY ENAMEL-DECAY. *a*, partially decalcified enamel which has slightly taken on the staining matter; *b*, zone of infected enamel showing masses of bacteria working their way into the decalcifying tissue. 70 : 1.

destroyed. Sections of enamel in secondary decay often show the bacteria forcing their way between the loosened prisms (Figs. 66, 67). About the same result is obtained where normal enamel is treated with diluted acids. The destruction of the enamel as it occurs in decay must be regarded as essentially a parasitico-chemical process. The loosening of the enamel-prisms is caused by acids concerning whose origin there can be no doubt; they arise in the mouth by fermentation of carbohydrates. The prisms thus loosened are sometimes mechanically removed; sometimes they remain on the spot, as in the case

FIG. 67.

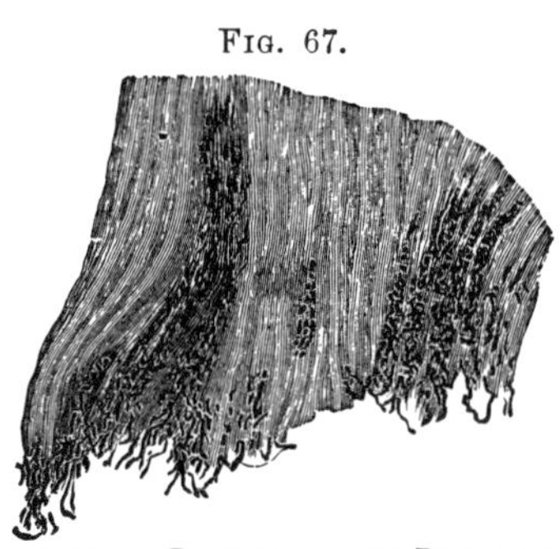

A SMALL PORTION OF THE BORDER of Fig. 66, showing the invasion of the diseased enamel by bacilli.

of secondary enamel-decay, until an opening is formed through which they escape. The bacteria directly participate in the process, inasmuch as they invade the broken-down enamel, perhaps drive the prisms farther apart, and destroy the remnant of organic matter. Micro-organisms do not exert a direct influence on normal enamel; their action upon the enamel in the first stage of decay is therefore indirect,—that is, they act by means of the acids which they produce. In the later stages of the process they exert also a direct action upon the diseased tissue.

3. Decay of Dentine.

a. Preparation of Specimens.

Various methods have been employed to prepare specimens of decayed dentine for microscopic examination. In the first place, ground sections of the decayed and the adjacent normal dentine have been made, in the different manners described for preparing sections of decayed enamel. Whoever has tried to grind softened dentine or any soft tissue will easily understand how difficult it is to obtain good specimens in this manner. Better sections might, perhaps, be prepared by previously hardening the decayed matter in absolute alcohol.

A method of grinding soft tissue, or a combination of soft and hard tissue, which v. Koch applied in the case of mollusks, has been employed by Weil[115] for grinding the soft tissues of the teeth. Weil first placed the tissue (2–5 mm. thick sections of the root or crown) into Müller's fluid, in order to fix the soft parts, which requires six to seven weeks. The objects were then thoroughly washed, and successively brought into a 30 per cent., 50 per cent., and finally 70 per cent. solution of alcohol to be hardened. They were then cut into smaller pieces by a fine bracket-saw, so as to facilitate the action of the coloring-matter in the subsequent staining process, and again placed for some time in a 70 per cent. solution of alcohol. He then stained them, extracted the water by means of alcohol, clearing them up in oil of cloves; the objects were then taken out of the oil, rinsed in pure xylol, and placed for at least twenty-four hours in a large quantity of chloroform; then they came for an equal length of time in a diluted solution of Canada balsam in chloroform, to which, after about twenty-four hours, was added as much hardened Canada balsam as would dissolve in it.

Weil now placed the teeth in a porcelain vessel, added enough of the solution to cover them, and then kept the solution over a water-bath at 60°–70° C.,—later at 80°–90° C. until the mass when cooled became as hard as glass; the teeth were then carefully taken out, the superfluous balsam removed, and the specimens were ready for grinding.

Sections of dentine are also frequently prepared as follows: Rather thick ground sections are made comprising both the normal and softened tissue; these are decalcified in diluted acid (chromic acid, etc.), and cut into microscopically thin sections by the microtome. Such preparations have the great disadvantage that we are not able to determine with certainty just where the decayed tissue stops and the artificially decalcified begins; nor can we tell exactly what changes of the dentine may have been caused by the artificial decalcification.

Having made and examined several thousand microscopic preparations of decayed dentine, I have found the following method to be the most recommendable, both on account of its extreme simplicity as on account of the excellence of the preparations which it yields and the few reagents to which it is necessary to subject the tissue.

Selecting a freshly-extracted decayed tooth, we wash out the cavity only sufficiently to remove the particles of food, and break away the margins of enamel so as to expose the softened dentine as much as possible. Then with a sharp instrument we dissect, so to speak, the decayed from the sound dentine, keeping hard upon the latter; by this means we may easily shell out nearly the whole of the softened dentine in one piece. Where the decay has approached near to the pulp, it is very easy to extend the cut quite to the pulp-chamber, by which means a thin layer of hard dentine will be contained in the mass removed.

The material thus gained is immediately cut on the freezing microtome. It is well to freeze the tissue in an aqueous solution of gum-arabic instead of in water. Such a solution has a higher freezing-point than water, and does not become so hard. By means of the freezing microtome several hundred very thin cuts may be prepared in a very few moments.

The objection has been raised to this method that it permits of securing sections of the softened dentine only, whereas we may wish to see what, if any, changes have taken place in the otherwise normal dentine just at or a little beyond the border of decalcification. I do not, however, attach much importance to this point, because a study of a few preparations soon teaches us that in the parts indicated but slight changes, or none at all, can be detected; besides, it is not difficult, with the help of the freezing microtome, from such pieces of dentine in which a *thin* layer of unsoftened dentine has been cut out along with the decayed, to make a few cuts containing both hard as well as decayed dentine, although the edge of the knife will be somewhat damaged by it. For the study of the phenomena of transparent dentine, a number of ground sections should be made from teeth in which the decay has made but little progress.

Unstained sections must be examined in water. But it is imperatively necessary to stain a large number of sections, especially in order to study the distribution of the bacteria in the tissue and the manner in which they demolish it.

b. Methods of Staining.

For the purpose of staining the tissue, picro-carmine or picro-lithio-carmine is, according to my experience, most suitable. The sections are placed in the concentrated solution for about fifteen minutes, then in a mixture of alcohol 70, water 29, muriatic acid 1, where they may remain from fifteen minutes to five hours, then for a short time into alcohol, to which have been added a few crystals of picric acid (till it turns slightly yellow). They are then cleared up in oil of cloves, and mounted in Canada balsam or glycerine. The dentinal fibrils and sheaths are colored red, the basis-substance pink, the bacteria light red, the decomposing parts yellow.

For staining the micro-organisms the basic aniline colors are best suited, fuchsine and gentian-violet being, according to my experience, preferable; methyl-violet, methylene-blue, and vesuvin not quite so good. The staining with fuchsine is carried out in the following manner: Enough of a concentrated alcoholic solution of fuchsine is added to water to turn it cherry-red. In this solution the sections are allowed to remain for three to five minutes, and are then placed (after Gram's method) for one to three minutes into a solution of iodine 1.0, iodide of potassium 2.0, distilled water 300.0. Then they are put into absolute alcohol, which must be renewed as soon as it becomes red. In the alcohol the color gradually disappears from the tissue, while the bacteria retain it. The sections must not be left in the alcohol too long, otherwise the bacteria will also give up a portion of their coloring-matter. Some experience is necessary in order to take out the cuts at the proper time. From the alcohol they are transferred to oil of cloves, then mounted in Canada balsam. By this method the parts infiltrated with bacteria, or the bacteria themselves, are colored red; everything else appears unstained.

I have obtained equally good, and, in fact, I have sometimes thought, better, results by simply treating the slightly overstained cuts with absolute alcohol, though the process is somewhat longer, it sometimes requiring an hour or more to decolorize the preparations, during which time the alcohol must be repeatedly changed. The preparations, when taken from the alcohol, must not show a diffuse staining, but rather a differential staining, some parts of the preparation appearing to the naked eye quite colorless and others bright red.

The other coloring-materials above mentioned are employed in the same way as fuchsine. Remarkably beautiful preparations may be obtained in a very few minutes by employing Günther's modification of Gram's method with gentian-violet.

The cuts are brought from absolute alcohol for one to two minutes in a deep violet solution of gentian-violet in aniline water, then removed on the point of a platinum wire, lightly touched to bibulous paper to remove the excess of coloring solution, placed for two minutes in the iodine-iodide of potassium solution, one-half minute in alcohol, ten seconds in 3 per cent. alcoholic solution of hydrochloric acid, then again one to five minutes in alcohol, then cleared in oil of cloves and mounted in Canada balsam.

I have not given much attention to the double staining of decayed dentine, but as far as my experience goes I have found that double-stained preparations, while they "show up" very well under low powers, are not as good for study as the single-stained.

Sections stained with gentian-violet may be after-stained by transferring them from the last alcohol bath to a solution of vesuvin one minute or picro-carmine one to three minutes, after which they must be returned to the alcohol, then to oil of cloves, etc.

A very good double stain may often be obtained if the sections colored with fuchsine are placed in a vesuvin solution for one to five minutes, then rinsed in water, put into alcohol for a few moments, then cleared up in oil of cloves and mounted in Canada balsam. The bacteria appear red, the dentine appears yellowish-brown. Double coloration does not, however, always succeed, and requires some practice to obtain good results.

Ground sections are to be stained in the same way as the cuts.

c. Appearances under the Microscope.

Preparations colored with fuchsine, when examined under very low power or even with the naked eye, show that the bacteria are not equally distributed throughout the mass of softened dentine. Sections parallel to the dentinal tubules (longitudinal sections) generally reveal on the outer margin corresponding to the external layer of dentine a deep-red coloration, which gradually diminishes toward the inner margin. Large tracts of decayed tissue, especially at the extremities of the specimen, often remain entirely uncolored. This necessitates the conclusion that the softening (decalcification) of the dentine extends further than the invasion of the micro-organisms. The appearance of comparatively large non-infected portions at the extremities or sides of the specimen may be explained by the accompanying diagram (Fig. 68).

FIG. 68.

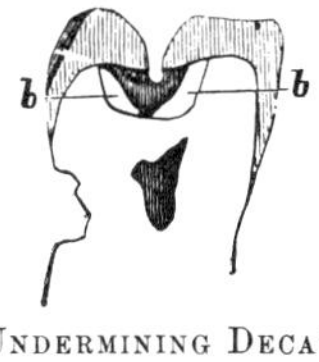

UNDERMINING DECAY.
b, zone of softened non-infected dentine.

This is intended to represent a case of undermining decay on the grinding-surface of a molar; the enamel has been broken through, and the softening (decalcification) has extended in all directions in the dentine with about equal rapidity. The micro-organisms, on the other hand, travel more readily in the direction of the dentinal tubules than at right angles to them, since in the latter direction they can advance only through the tortuous and narrow road of the fine branches of the tubuli. Consequently, while the micro-organisms almost or quite keep up with

FIG. 69.

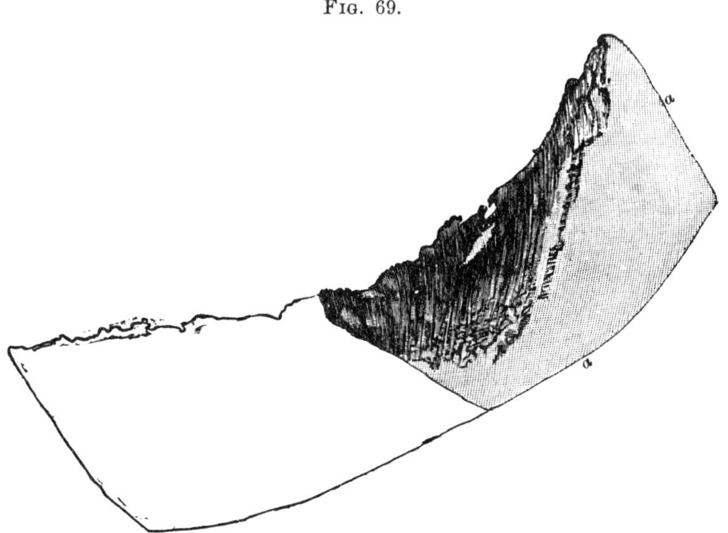

A CUT FROM A LARGE PIECE OF DECAYED DENTINE, left half only in outline. Shows at *a* an unusually large non-infected zone of decayed dentine. 20 : 1.

the softening in the direction toward the pulp, they fall considerably behind in the lateral directions, so that the invasion, particularly in the lateral direction, is usually much less extensive than the softening.

Fig. 69 represents the appearance under a low power of a preparation of decayed dentine in my possession.

Cases where there are many large interglobular spaces may form an exception to the rule. In such cases, the bacteria, following the course of the interglobular spaces, can advance very rapidly in both directions underneath the enamel (Fig. 70), though strangely enough, as first pointed out by Mummery, the interglobular spaces are often peculiarly free from infection.

The presence of these non-infected areas in decaying dentine, which I announced in 1883, was at first contradicted by some authors. Now, however, it is universally acknowledged. Among others, Watson writes, "I quite agree with Dr. Miller that there are areas of softened, non-infected dentine which contain no organisms." In fact, they are so easily detected that I am at a loss to understand how any investigator could have missed seeing them at once.

Under a somewhat higher power (forty to sixty diameters) we

FIG. 70.

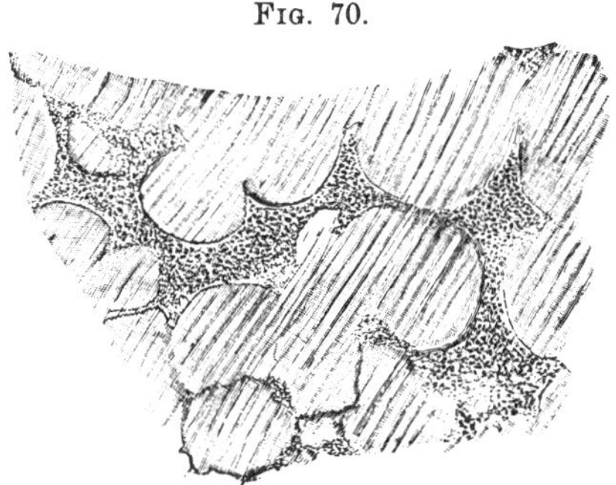

INTERGLOBULAR SPACES FILLED WITH MICROCOCCI. About 400 : 1.

may more easily follow the invasion. Occasionally we find that a majority of the tubules are infiltrated to the same depth; usually, however, the parasites penetrate the different tubules to very different depths. We also occasionally find that all or nearly all the tubules are filled with bacteria at the surface, while in the deeper parts only a few are infiltrated.

The advancing hordes of bacteria consequently present a very irregular, zigzag front toward the pulp. Laterally, however, the line separating the infected from the non-infected portions of the decaying dentine often appears quite regular and sharply defined (Fig. 71). These peculiarities are readily accounted for by the structure of the invaded tissue.

I have found in one case only the very remarkable mode of advance represented in Fig. 72. Here the invaders are seen

FIG. 71.

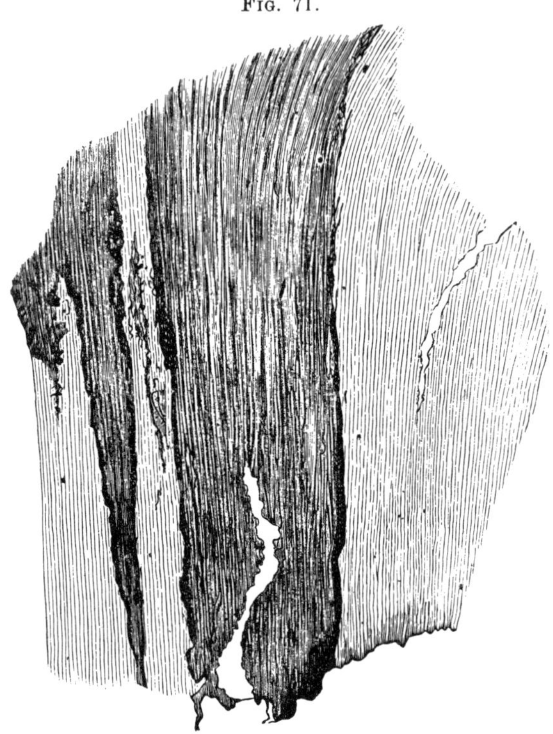

DECAYED DENTINE, showing that laterally the boundary between the infected and non-infected parts may be very regular. Circa 40 : 1.

FIG. 72.

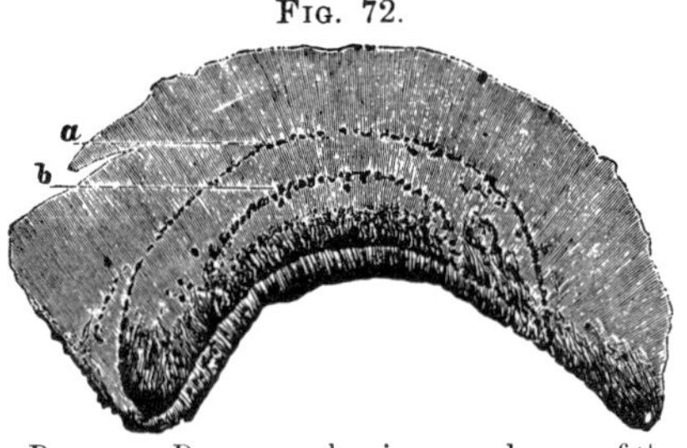

DECAYED DENTINE, showing an advance of the bacteria in three columns. Circa 15 : 1.

to advance in a manner which I can only liken to an army of men marching through a hostile country. Far in advance we

PLATE I.

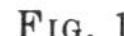

Fig. 1.

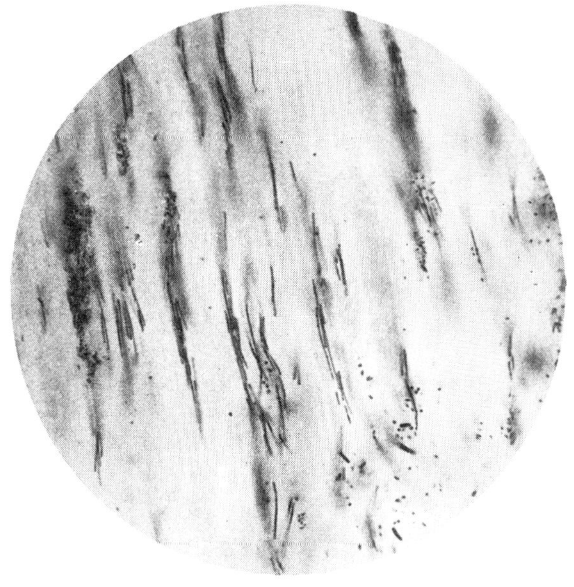

Longitudinal section of decayed dentine, showing infection with micrococci, bacilli and threads (mixed infection). 500 : 1.

Fig. 2.

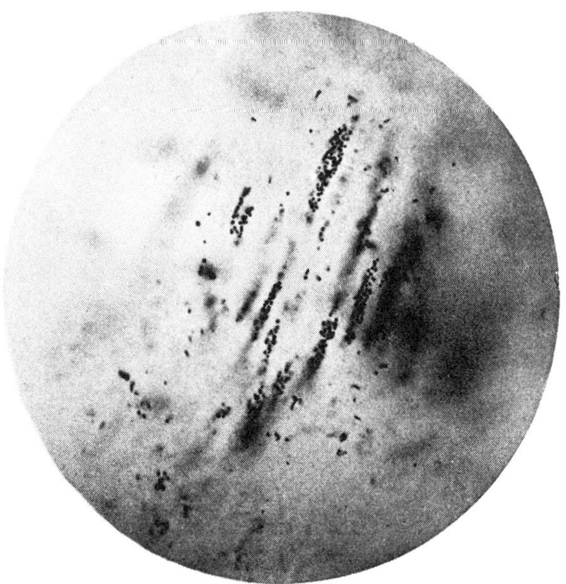

Longitudinal section of decayed dentine, showing infection with micrococci. 500 : 1.

see a very distinct line of pickets. This is followed by an interval which in the language of bacteria might be put down at several furlongs, since it is about one thousand times the length of an average-sized bacillus. Then comes the vanguard, and finally, after another interval, the main body of the invading hordes. I was not able to find any cause for this peculiar disposition of the forces.

A question which has often been mooted now arises: Can the bacteria penetrate into normal dentine? This question must be answered in the affirmative. Since the average diameter of the dentinal tubules is greater than that of the bacteria found in the mouth, it is but reasonable to conclude, *a priori*, that bacteria may under certain circumstances make their way into the tubules of apparently intact tissue. Under high power we also often observe that a small number of bacteria, outposts, as it were, have penetrated into the normal dentine without, however, producing any visible changes.

Fig. 73.

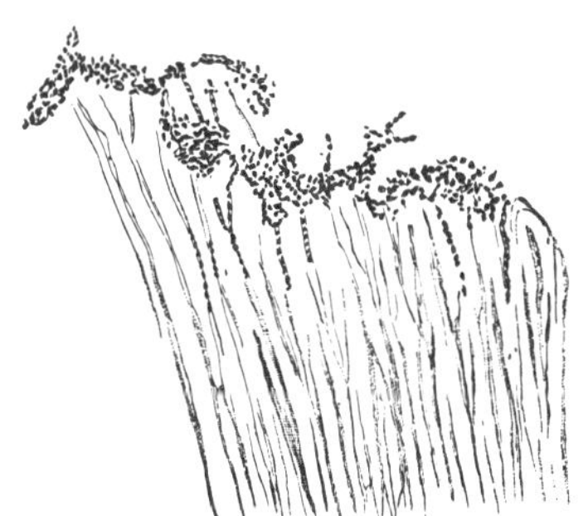

Micrococci penetrating the Canals of Solid Dentine, in a partially absorbed and abscessed but not decayed root. 700 : 1.

Fig. 74.

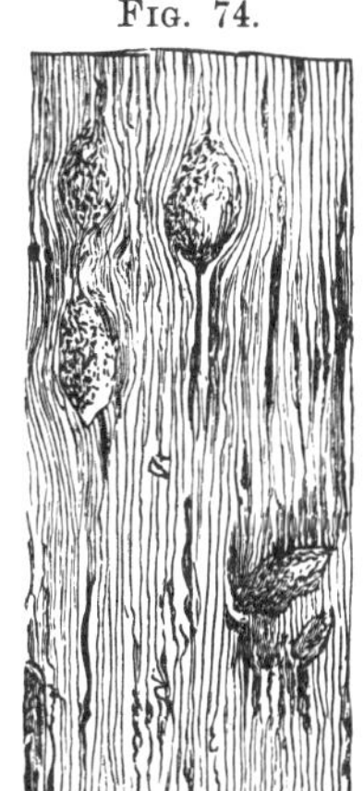

Longitudinal Section of Decayed Dentine, showing caverns, or foci of liquefaction, filled with bacteria. 150 : 1.

We notice also in partly resorbed, abscessed roots, particularly of milk-teeth (Fig. 73), that bacteria work themselves into the open ends of exposed tubules for a short distance. The great mass of bacteria, however, in decay of the dentine does not even penetrate up to the normal dentine, much less into it. From this it is evident that the proposition which I established in

1882 [116] is correct in every respect: "The action of acids always precedes the invasion of bacteria."

As is best seen in a longitudinal section under low power, numerous rounded or oval masses of from ten to one hundred micro-millimeters long and from five to fifty broad often appear in the domain of the infected dentine (Fig. 74). The masses consist of closely packed cells of bacteria, and correspond to the more or less ample enlargement of one or more dentinal tubules, by which the neighboring tubules are crowded together or bent out of their course. If these masses attain larger dimensions, the course of some of the tubules, together with the intervening basis-substance, is interrupted for a certain distance, thus forming a space or cavern in the dentine. These caverns being formed by the dissolving of the basis-substance by peptonizing bacteria, may be properly designated as liquefaction-foci.

Fig. 75.

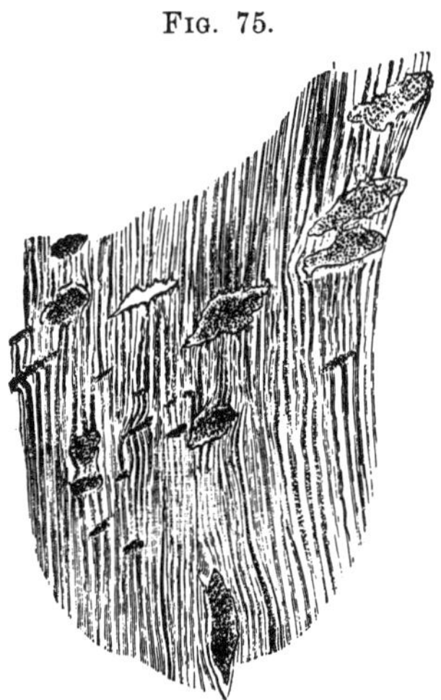

Decayed Dentine with Oblique Liquefaction-Foci. Circa 400 : 1.

Fig. 76.

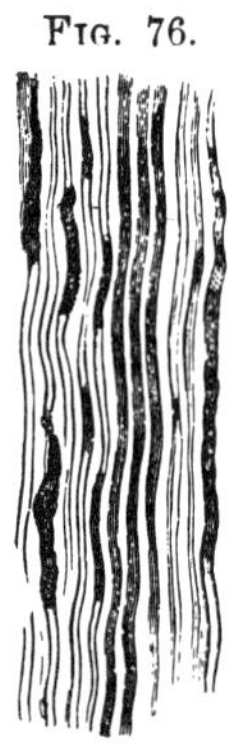

Uniform Enlargement of the Tubules in Decaying Dentine.

Such foci do not always have the form represented in Fig. 74; they may be tapering, triangular, crevice-shaped, etc. The crevice-shaped spaces frequently lie obliquely to the dentinal tubules, presenting the characteristic appearance shown in Fig. 75.

In some specimens all the tubules are enlarged to nearly the same extent (Fig. 76), occasionally to three or four times their normal size. This enlargement is caused partly by the dislodgment of the neighboring tubules, partly by the loss of the intertubular substance. Lastly, the destruction of the intervening substance causes a confluence of two or more adjacent tubules, producing long caverns running parallel to them. By the formation of caverns and by the fusion of adjacent caverns the dentine is broken up, becomes porous, and is gradually destroyed. The tubules are often attacked in groups, while others lying between these groups may be wholly free from infection. In other cases, however, every single canal is stuffed full of bacteria.

In Fig. 77 I have endeavored to reproduce an appearance very commonly met with in decaying dentine. This specimen

FIG. 77.

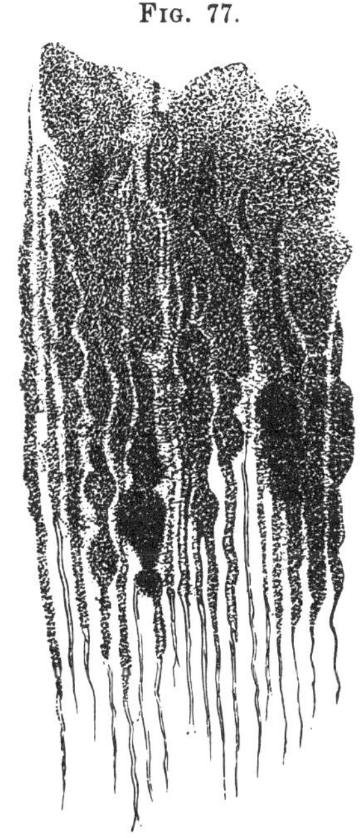

DECAYED DENTINE SHOWING TOTAL LIQUEFACTION OF THE BASIS-SUBSTANCE BY BACTERIA. 400 : 1.

FIG. 78.

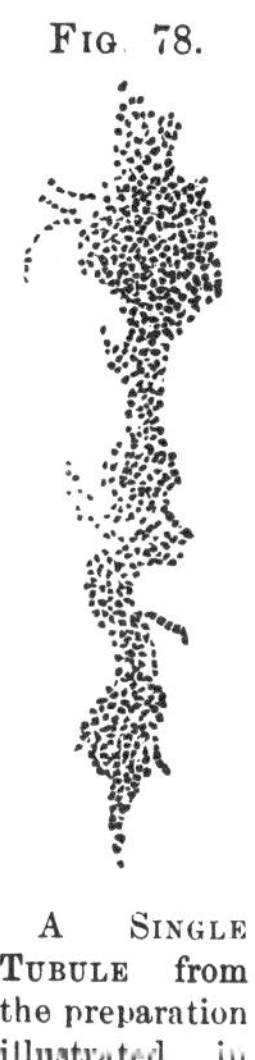

A SINGLE TUBULE from the preparation illustrated in Fig. 77.

clearly shows that the enlargement of the tubules always found in decayed dentine is due to the infection, and that a gradual fusion of the basis-substance may take place, beginning with the separate tubules, until nothing remains but a mass of bacteria held together by the remnant of the dentine. Fig. 78 shows a tubule from the same specimen under high power.

In rare cases the action of the bacteria is mostly restricted to the surface, and the dentine is gradually dissolved from the surface downward, without the formation of caverns within the dentine. I term this form of dissolution of dentine progressive superficial dentine dissolution, in contradistinction to that form represented in Figs. 74–78, which may be designated as parenchymatous dentine dissolution.

Not one of the morphological changes of dentine mentioned takes place without a previous invasion of bacteria.

FIG. 79.

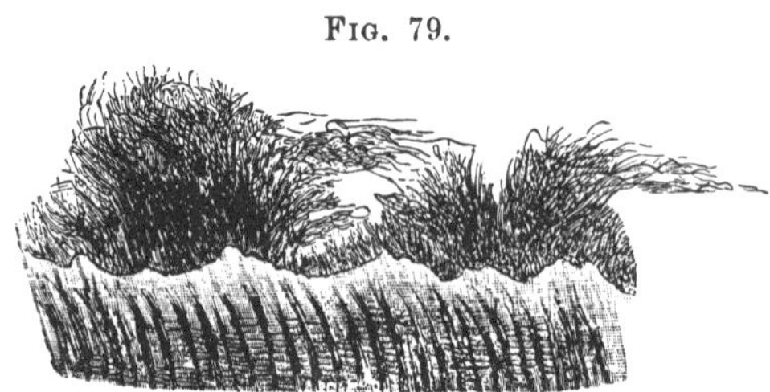

FRINGE OF LEPTOTHRIX THREADS on the border of a section of decayed dentine. 400 : 1.

In well-stained specimens the individual cells of the bacteria are clearly visible under a power of 400–500 diameters; although for a thorough study of the specimens oil immersion lenses and Abbe's condenser are desirable. With their assistance we see that the external margin of the specimen consists of broken-down dental tissue intermixed with enormous masses of micrococci, bacilli, and leptothrix threads. The latter often appear as fringes on the border of the specimen (Fig. 79), but are not found along the entire margin, while in some they are altogether lacking. In many cases, no doubt, they are torn away in preparing the specimens. It is seldom that they penetrate the dentinal tubules, unless the dissolution is already far advanced, and even then they are to be found mostly in the external layers. Tubules containing long, tortuous threads (Fig. 80) are therefore comparatively rare.

FIG. 80.

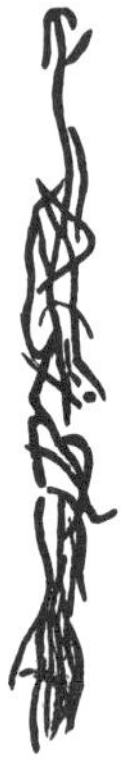

SINGLE TUBULE FILLED WITH THREAD FORMS. 1100 : 1.

If we examine a somewhat deeper zone, we usually find the tubules filled with micrococci and rods only, the former decidedly preponderating. These two forms of bacteria generally occur in separate tubules; thus we often see a tubule

PLATE II.

FIG. 1.

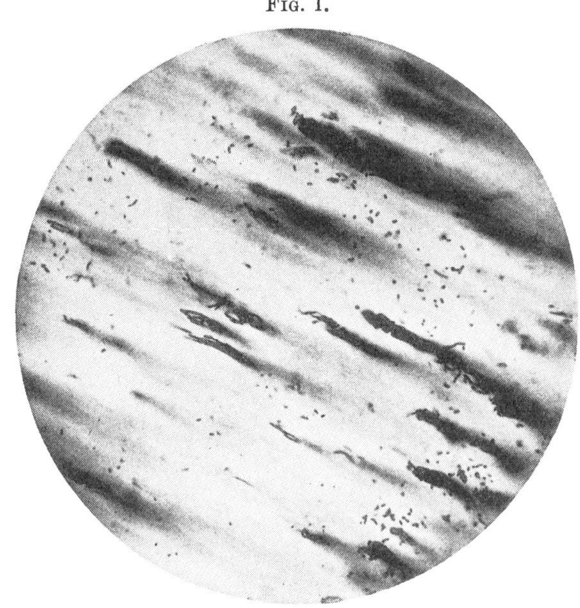

Diagonal section of decayed dentine. Infection with micrococci, bacilli and screw-forms. 500 : 1.

FIG. 2.

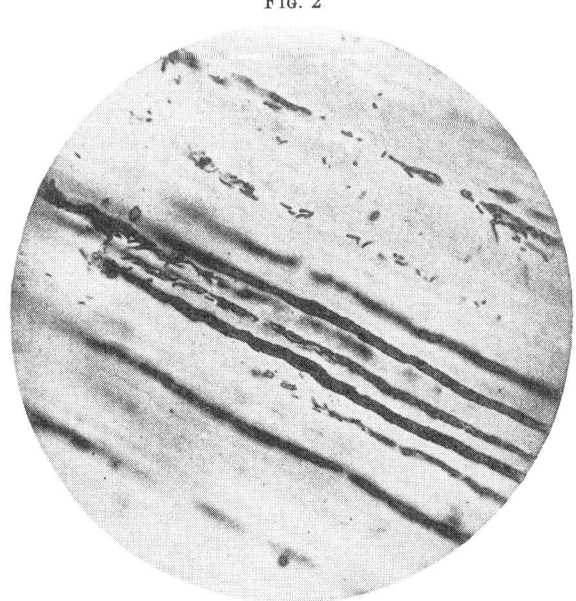

Longitudinal section of dentine artificially decayed. Infection with bacilli. 500 : 1.

stocked only with micrococci (Fig. 81), the adjacent one only with rods (Fig. 82); there are, however, tubules packed with a mixture of both (Fig. 83), while it rarely happens that one extremity of a tubule is filled with rods, the other with cocci.

We have consequently in decay of the teeth to do with a so-called mix-infection (Fig. 84).

Fig 81.

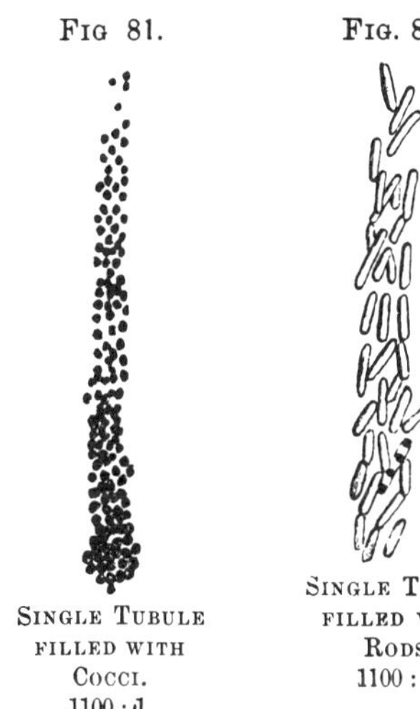

Single Tubule filled with Cocci. 1100 : 1.

Fig. 82.

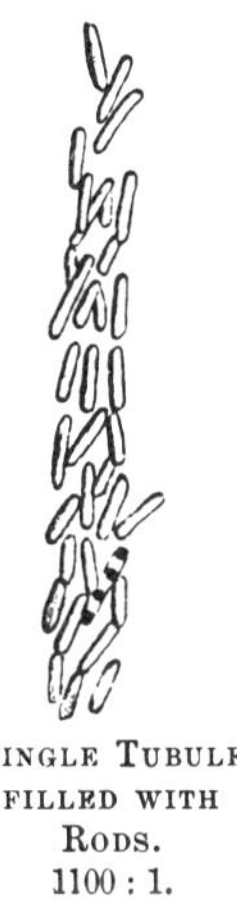

Single Tubule filled with Rods. 1100 : 1.

Fig. 83.

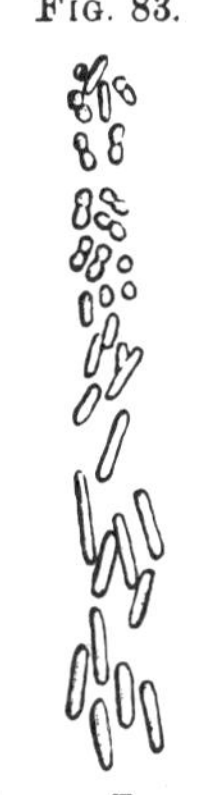

Single Tubule showing a Mixed Infection or Infection with a Pleomorphous Bacterium. 1100 : 1.

Fig. 84.

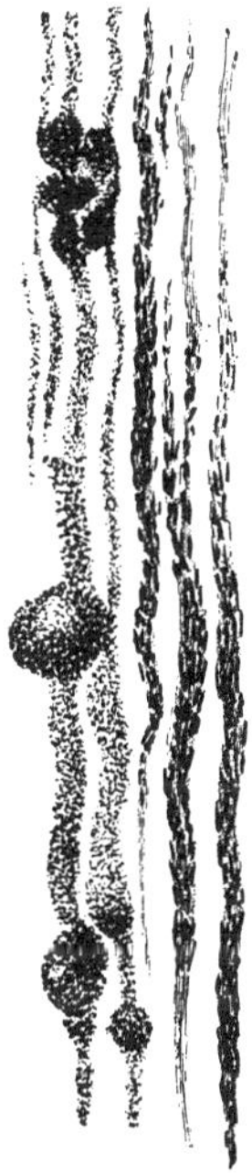

Decayed Dentine showing a Mix-infection with Cocci and Bacilli. 400 : 1.

It is true that we often meet with specimens which appear to contain cocci alone (whether of one or of different varieties the microscopic examination does not tell). On the other hand, I have in my possession a few preparations which exhibit a pure bacillus infection, particularly in circumscribed portions.

This, however, must not lead us to believe that there is a bacillus-decay and a micrococcus-decay which are distinguished by characteristic phenomena; decay caused by the different bacteria reveals no such distinctions, consequently I do not consider it as proved that caries chronica, acuta, acutissima, etc., are caused each by its own specific bacterium.

In general that species of bacterium which possesses the

highest ferment activity (in other words, acid-forming power) and the highest peptonizing power (*i.e.*, dissolving power for albuminous substances) and is able to flourish with a limited supply of air will, *cæteris paribus*, cause a more rapid destruction of the tooth-substance than another having these qualities in a minor degree. A mouth-bacterium which in respect to these properties excels all others in such a degree as would be necessary to explain the difference between caries acuta and caries chronica will most probably never be discovered. The rapid advance of acute caries is to be explained rather by the resistlessness of the tooth's structure and the favorable conditions for fermentation obtaining in the mouth.

Successfully stained cuts of decayed dentine furnish preparations which to the eye of the bacteriologist and pathologist are not only of exceeding great beauty, but also demonstrate with such clearness the intense action of micro-organisms upon dentine that no doubting Thomas can look at them and then have the hardihood to deny their significance. In Fig. 85 I have endeavored to reproduce the microscopic appearance of a specimen in my possession (and of which I presented duplicates to Dr. Cunningham, of Cambridge, England, and to Dr. Allan, of New York). If the reader can imagine the basis-substance in this preparation stained yellowish-brown and the micro-organisms red, and further take into account that by slightly lowering or raising the tube of the microscope or by moving the preparation one constantly brings new and different pictures into focus, and, lastly, that the most skilled draughtsman and xylographer come very short of nature, he may then form some idea of the beauty of this specimen. The dentine is completely riddled by the masses of bacilli and threads.

A section cutting the tubules at right angles shows under a power of three hundred diameters that the tubules filled with micro-organisms are distended from one to four times their normal diameter, and that often two or more of the enlarged tubules are converted into one by the liquefaction of the membranes and the intervening substance (Fig. 86). This melting together of the tubules increases as we near the outer border of the specimen (corresponding to the surface of the cavity) until it is no longer possible to distinguish the separate tubules; we then see only irregular masses of bacteria, of different sizes, which are more or less contaminated by the detritus (débris) of the decomposing dentine. These impure masses are what Abbott

FIG. 85.

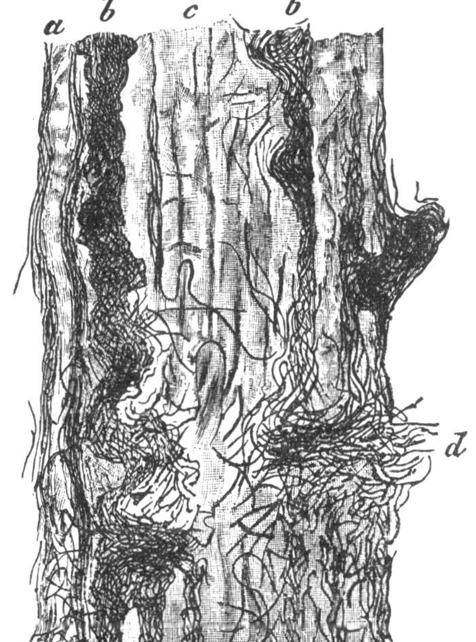

LONGITUDINAL SECTION OF DECAYED DENTINE SHOWING INFECTION WITH ROD- AND THREAD-FORMS. *a*, tubule distended, but walls still comparatively intact; *b*, *d*, tubular walls broken through and the dentine in a state of complete dissolution; *c*, tubules out of focus. Circa 500 : 1.

calls "embryonic elements." Since they are not homogeneous, they take up the coloring-matter unequally at different points, and therefore occasionally present figures that may bear a certain faint resemblance to cells.

Fig. 87 represents an appearance frequently observed in cross-sections. A number of adjacent tubules are enlarged to such an extent that their walls finally touch or even flatten one another. In such cases they form five- to six-sided prisms. The question arises: What has become of the intertubular substance?

A slight compression of the intervening substance may doubtless be caused by the pressure from within the tubules, but its total compression, as shown in Fig. 87, is altogether inconceivable. Now, since the micro-organisms cannot penetrate into the intertubular substance through the intact dentinal sheath, the above occurrence can be explained only by the hypothesis that

FIG. 86.

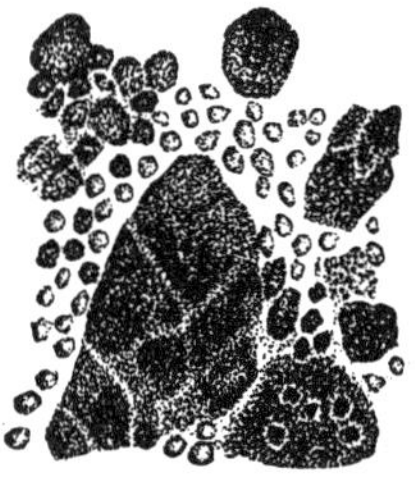

CROSS-SECTION OF DECAYED DENTINE.
Showing the distention of the tubuli and formation of liquefaction-foci.
400 : 1.

FIG. 87.

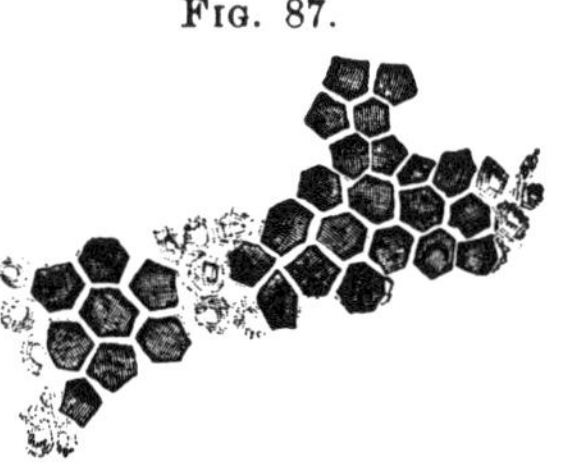

CROSS-SECTION OF DECAYED DENTINE.
The tubules through reciprocal pressure have assumed the shape of 5–6 sided prisms.

they form a pepsine-like diffusible ferment, which dissolves the intervening substance, while Neumann's sheath remains intact. I am not, however, at all sure that I have hit upon the right explanation of this phenomenon.

In the deeper zones of decayed dentine the bacteria lie exclusively in the tubules and their ramifications, and a direct invasion of bacteria into the intertubular substance only exceptionally takes place; the dissolution of the latter progresses from the surface or from the lumen of the tubules.

At the neck of the tooth the external layer of dentine is either devoid of tubules, or they are so narrow that the entrance of the bacteria is greatly impeded. Caries at the neck of the tooth consequently presents phenomena which differ somewhat from those of other parts. This applies especially to chronic dry caries at the neck of the tooth, which leads to intense pigmentation. Under the microscope the external margin of a longitudinal section exhibits a layer consisting of masses of bacteria from which numerous leptothrix threads radiate. Below it the dentine appears interspersed with many triangular fissures, with their bases toward the border and their longer diameter parallel to the tubules (Fig. 88).

The fissures are almost always filled with micro-organisms, especially with cocci. I suspect that they are not formed by

FIG. 88.

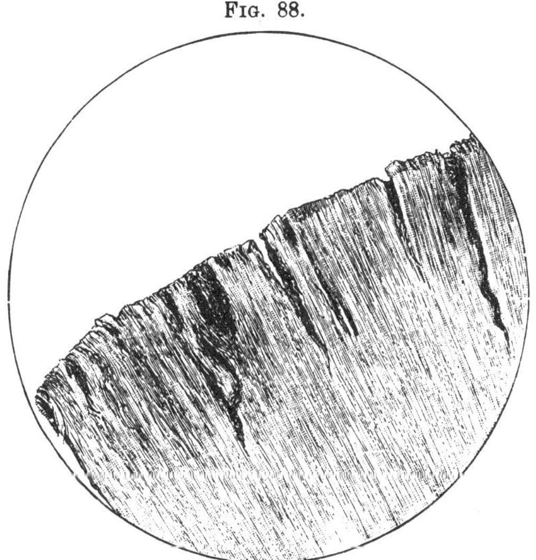

APPEARANCE OF DECAY AT THE NECK OF THE TOOTH.
The fissures are filled with bacteria. Circa 50 : 1.

bacteria, but by the contraction of the external layer of dentine, and that masses of bacteria, as well as very small food-particles, enter them afterward. Each fissure thus affords a point of retention or a caries-center from which the infection of the dentine proceeds.

Specimens stained with picrocarmine frequently exhibit peculiar appearances, which cannot always be easily explained. Longitudinal sections under three hundred diameters show on the margin a reddish fringe of leptothrix threads, mingled with micrococci, and below this a yellow layer about one-fourth of a millimeter wide. Besides, the parts in a state of disintegration are generally of a yellowish color. In the parts that are only softened, but not infected, as well as in the masses of bacteria, the red color prevails. Now and then scattered, greatly enlarged tubules are seen to be filled with shining, yellow, homogeneous contents, and only under a very high power does its granular character become evident.

Cross-sections also often present a very peculiar appearance. They reveal more or less numerous, scattered, greatly enlarged tubules, filled with red-colored micrococci, and about as many scattered, enlarged tubules of strongly refractive, homogeneous yellowish contents (Plate III, Fig. 5). I am not able to state why these various tubules are so differently affected by coloring matter; it occurs in artificial as well as in natural decay.

Fuchsine specimens also occasionally exhibit tubules of deep red, apparently homogeneous contents. In such cases it may be shown that the specimens have been over-stained, which makes it impossible to distinguish the closely-crowded cocci.

We now come to a series of phenomena which have been widely discussed, but not yet definitely explained. They are (1) the thickening of Neumann's sheaths; (2) the breaking up of the dentinal fibrils into rods (pipe-stems); (3) the occurrence of granular, not vegetable, elements in the tubules.

FIG. 89.

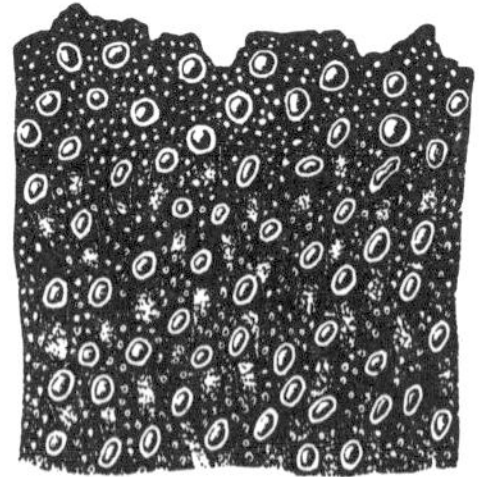

THICKENING OF THE DENTAL SHEATH.
(Neumann's sheath.)
(After Wedl.)

THICKENING OF NEUMANN'S SHEATH.

According to some authors, a thickening of the walls of the dentinal tubules (Fig. 89), that is, of Neumann's sheaths, is an invariable accompaniment of decay. According to Neumann, this thickening proceeds until the lumen of the tubules is totally obliterated, while Tomes assumes only partial obliteration. He compares a dentinal tubule with its thickened walls to the stem of a tobacco-pipe.

Leber and Rottenstein, on the other hand, found not a contraction, but a distention of the tubules with thickened sheaths. They examined several teeth made of the ivory of the hippopotamus, as well as three human teeth, worn on a plate, which had become carious in the mouth, and discovered that the microscopic changes of the dentine described above occur in such teeth also. In all cases the tubules were more or less, sometimes very extensively, dilated by a substance generally stained red by carmine. The specimens from the ivory teeth particularly presented these changes in a very high degree.

Opinions vary greatly concerning the cause of this thickening. Tomes[117] considers that "the diseased condition has, perhaps, undone the work of development and thrown light on the question how this was effected; it might almost be said to have restored the outline of the formative cells: the tissue is to a certain extent broken up into its histological elements. Under the microscope the section looks as though it might have been built up of multitudes of tobacco-pipe stems, united by an intervening substance. Such is the condition when disorganization has advanced up to a certain point; at a later period short lengths of the walls of the tubes (dentinal sheaths, Zahnscheiden of Neumann) are found isolated; and finally the whole tissue breaks down into minute granular particles which are, by degrees, washed away in the saliva."

Leber and Rottenstein[58] do not seem to be satisfied with their own attempts to explain the thickening of Neumann's sheaths; still it seemed to them most probable "that the thickening of the walls of the dilated tubules is brought about mechanically by the compression of the surrounding substance." In their judgment, the thickening cannot be caused by acids.

I have examined numerous specimens of natural and artificial decay stained with picrocarmine, fuchsine, hæmotoxylin, etc., and indorse the view of Leber and Rottenstein, that a contraction of the lumen of the dentinal tubules is seen only in cases where it existed before the softening commenced. Further, that the thickening of the dentinal sheath is not a vital process, since it may be clearly observed in specimens of artificial decay.

This phenomenon might perhaps be explained, in part at least, by the pressure of the fungal masses in the tubules, by which a compression of the walls is caused. This supposition receives support from the fact that a thickening of the dentine may also be observed around the larger masses of bacteria in decayed dentine. When examined under the microscope, the dentine bordering such masses may often be seen to differ from the surrounding tissue by its higher refractive power.

By the action of acids upon carious dentine I have succeeded in producing appearances greatly similar to, if not identical with, the thickening described above. The resisting dentinal sheaths (tubules), especially such as are filled with bacteria, are loosened from the basis-substance and then more or less bent at the

FIG. 90.

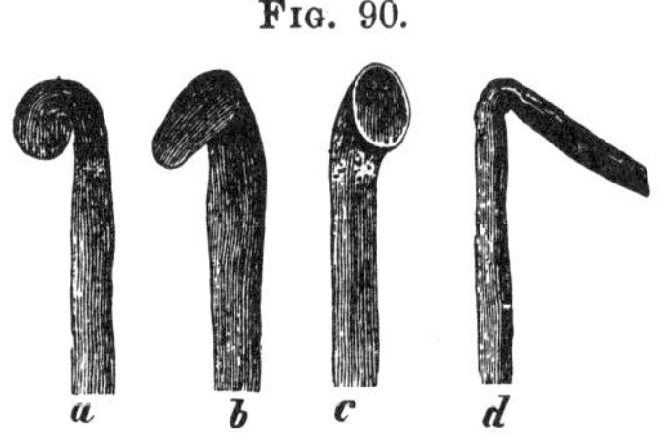

APPEARANCE OF DENTINAL SHEATHS produced by the action of strong acid on decayed dentine. 1100 : 1.

FIG. 91.

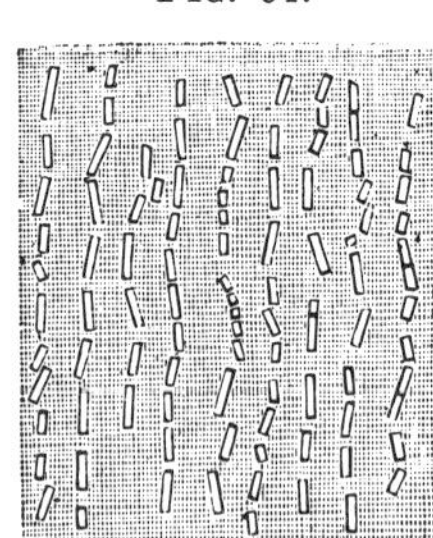

ROD-SHAPED, NON-VEGETABLE ELEMENTS in decayed dentine.

loosened extremities (Fig. 90, *a*, *b*), or flattened out (Fig. 90, *c*), or, lastly, torn from their beds altogether (Fig. 90, *d*). On the whole, however, it will be seen that I am not able to throw much light upon this question, and must leave it for further investigation to settle.

The appearance of rod-shaped elements or fragments in the tubuli of decayed dentine was first noticed by J. Tomes, and is no rare phenomenon either in natural or artificial decay. Fig. 91, taken from a specimen of artificial caries, gives a fair idea of it. J. Tomes[118] endeavored to explain this phenomenon by the consolidation of the dentinal fibrils, while Wedl[91] regards this view as not proved. Later Tomes[117] writes, "These rods may be portions of consolidated fibrils, or they may be bits of the sheaths of Neumann, or they may be mere casts of the enlarged tubules."

The fact, however, that these rods disappear often completely as soon as they are brought into contact with dilute sulphuric acid appears to me to render the view that they are bits of the dentinal sheaths untenable. The rods are easily isolated by crushing a section of dentine containing them in a drop of water on an object-glass. If the specimen be now covered with a cover-glass and dilute sulphuric acid allowed to flow through it from the margin in the usual manner, we may clearly observe, under a high power (1000 to 1500), how the pieces suddenly dissolve, leaving behind a hardly visible granular detritus, and in

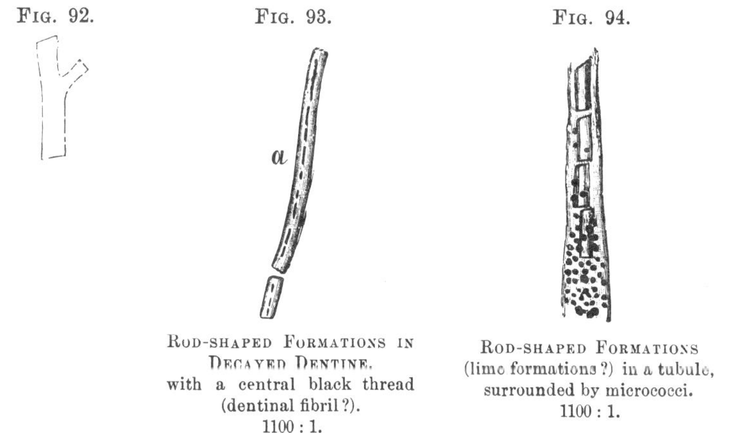

FIG. 92. FIG. 93. FIG. 94.

ROD-SHAPED FORMATIONS IN DECAYED DENTINE, with a central black thread (dentinal fibril?). 1100 : 1.

ROD-SHAPED FORMATIONS (lime formations?) in a tubule, surrounded by micrococci. 1100 : 1.

some cases disappearing altogether. In one case I plainly saw the form represented in Fig. 92 appear at the instant when the acid came in contact with a larger fragment.

I do not regard it as improbable that the products in question are lime formations; to me, however, they look more like cylindrical casts of the dentinal tubules than calcified fibrils. And indeed these pieces, when greatly magnified, are sometimes seen to contain filaments which may be regarded as the remains of dentinal fibrils (Fig. 93). The tubular structure may sometimes be directly ascertained under high power. I have never found micro-organisms in these rod-like products, but have repeatedly seen them mixed together with cocci, in much enlarged tubules

(Fig. 94). This would seem to justify the hypothesis that after the formation of these lime-casts an invasion of the micro-organisms and an enlargement of the tubules takes place, loosening the casts from the walls of the tubules. At any rate, we have here not a vital but a chemical process, since the fragments in question are very common in artificial decay. The fact that I have never noticed the characteristic crystals of sulphate of lime, after treating the separate rods with sulphuric acid, appears at first to tell

FIG. 95.

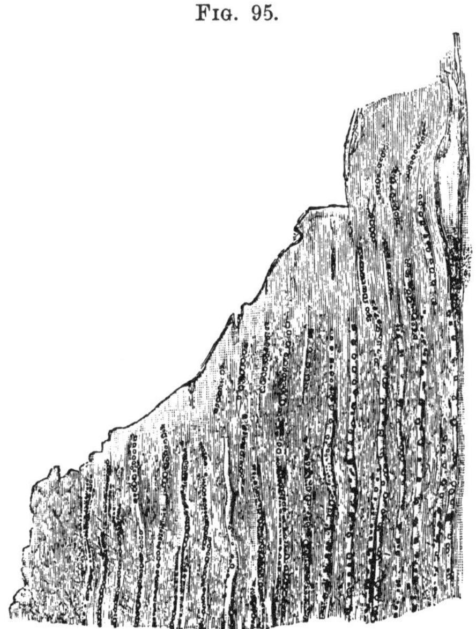

ROWS OF SHINING GRANULES IN THE TUBULES, in decay of a tooth worn on a plate.

against the hypothesis that these elements consist of lime-salts; the quantity of lime in one fragment may, however, be too small to give the crystal test.

The rods do not dissolve in organic acids; they even become more distinct after treatment with lactic and acetic acids. Three tests with alcohol and chloroform had no effect.

The occurrence of rows of shining, irregular grains in the tubules (Fig. 95) is frequently observed in the beginning of caries. Sometimes this deposit is made in a zone just in front of the advancing caries, so that many have regarded it as an attempt on the part of the living pulp to retard the progress of the disease. But we can easily prove that such is not the case, since the process occurs in living as well as in dead teeth. In accordance with the above view, Tomes, Magitot, and others took these granules for lime-granules; Wedl, Black, and others regard them as fat. By crushing the above-mentioned casts (page 191), grains are also produced in the tubules which bear considerable resemblance to those which occur naturally) Fig. 96).

FIG. 96.

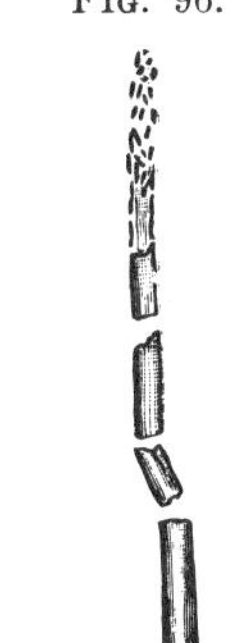

ROD-SHAPED FORMATIONS IN DECAYED DENTINE breaking up into granules. 1100 : 1.

I regard it therefore as not improbable that the granular bodies have the same origin as the rod-shaped (pipe-stems).

4. DECAY OF CEMENT.

Decay of cement is confined chiefly to a very thin layer at the

FIG. 97.

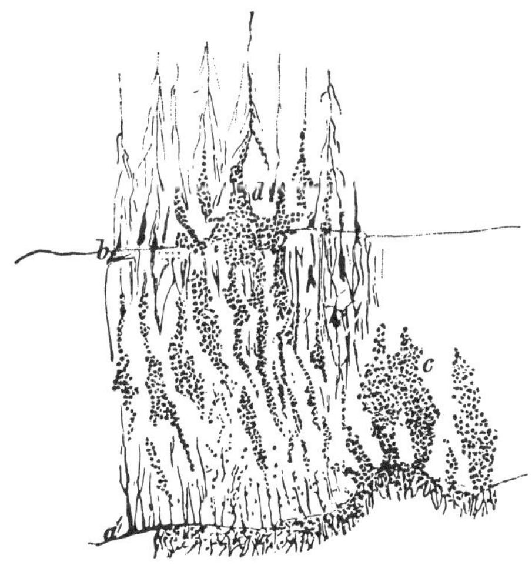

APPEARANCE OF DECAY IN CEMENT WITH PRONOUNCED DEVELOPMENT OF THE CEMENT-CANALS. *a*, surface of cement covered with various bacterium-forms; *b*, border of the dentine; *c*, enlargement of the cement-canals and formation of liquefaction-foci; *d*, spreading of the decay into the dentine. 1100 : 1.

neck of the tooth. The decalcification and dissolution of the cement proceeds either from the surface inward, in the form of a progressive superficial dissolution of the cement, or the cavities of the cement become infiltrated with bacteria, giving rise to a parenchymatous dissolution, accompanied by phenomena very similar to those of dentine-decay. Its similarity to the latter is especially striking in places where Sharpey's fibers are well developed. Immediately following decalcification these fibers, or rather canals, are infiltrated and enlarged by bacteria which gradually liquefy the intervening tissue (Fig. 97). In this way the tissue is rarefied, and finally totally destroyed. I possess several specimens in which this form of cement-caries has been artificially produced.

FIG. 98.

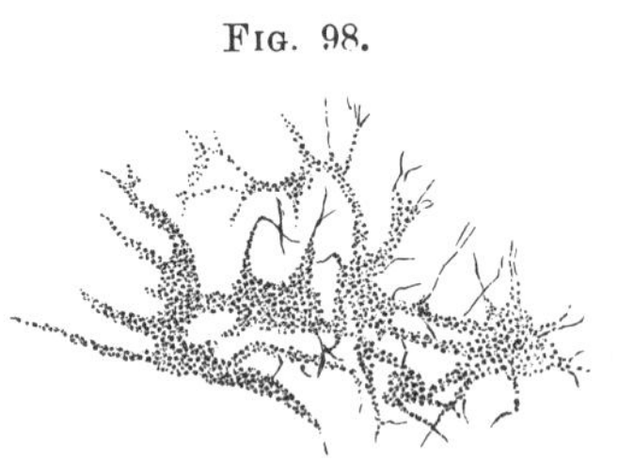

DECAY OF CEMENT.
Enlargement of the lacunæ and gradual liquefaction of the basis-substance by bacteria. 800 : 1.

When cement-corpuscles are present, they or their offshoots (as far as I have had opportunity to examine such cases) are infiltrated with bacteria and swollen (Fig. 98). I was not able to determine any such inflammatory reaction on the part of the cement as occurs, say in bone or cartilage.

DECAY OF TEETH WORN ON PLATES.

Some authors state that decay of human teeth, worn as artificial teeth, just as decay of natural teeth devoid of living pulps, is exactly identical with and shows all the phenomena of decay of living teeth. Other eminent authors, on the other hand, describe appearances (transparency, thickening of Neumann's sheath, etc.) which, they claim, occur in living teeth only. My observations lead me to believe that all the phenomena of decay, with the exception of transparency, which, strictly speaking, cannot be regarded as a phenomenon of decay, occur in dead as well as in living teeth. In fact, I have reproduced all artificially.

ARTIFICIAL DECAY.

The attempt to procure artificial decay has been made by many investigators. Magitot made extensive experiments in order to determine the action on the teeth of various acids and salts, as well as of fermenting albuminous substances and carbohydrates. The fermentative substances especially showed a pronounced action in the course of two years; when a tooth was so protected that the agent touched it at one point only, nothing but the exposed place was softened and destroyed. In this way a cavity was produced which could in no wise be distinguished from a natural cavity of decay. Magitot ascribed this action to the acids arising in the fermenting mixtures, overlooking the further work of the bacteria; he also neglected, unfortunately, to determine by microscopical examination whether the tissue showed phenomena identical with natural decay.

Similar experiments were afterward made by a number of investigators, among others by Milles and Underwood. The latter[119] constructed a large incubator, in which a mixture of milk, bread, meat, saliva, and carious teeth was kept for six months at blood temperature. No changes resembling caries occurred, and this is easily conceivable from their own statements: "The putridity of the baths was, however, so offensive that it was with some relief that we decided to abandon this particular experiment. . . . My health and appetite suffered from constant exposure to all these putrid smells."

Milles and Underwood say nothing about the reaction in these baths, but this "putridity" leads us to conclude that it most probably was alkaline. It cannot have been acid, since we are told that the dentine was "not a bit softened." Now I think that we are all pretty well agreed that there can be no caries without acid; hence the failure in the above experiment.

In a second experiment the same authors subjected fragments of teeth to the action of a mixture of saliva and bread for three months.

It is not stated whether they renewed the mixture in this time. It would be a serious mistake not to have done so, because many bacteria are very sensitive to the action of their own products, and would be devitalized long before the close of the experiment. (See page 14.) Besides, a thick felt of yeast-fungi formed on the surface of the flasks, which probably also materially interfered with the course of the experiment. In this experiment they obtained softening, but no discoloration. A microscopical examination does not appear to have been made.

They came finally to the conclusion that artificial decay is an impossibility, because the bacteria of decay lose their specific power when cultivated out of the mouth.

Nevertheless, I affirm that a destruction of the tooth-substance may be brought about artificially which the most practiced microscopist will not be able to distinguish from real decay as it occurs in the human mouth. In fact, not one of the many microscopists who have made the attempt has been able to determine which of a given number of preparations were artificial and which natural.

The chief object of my experiments was to produce the microscopic appearances of decay of the teeth, since it had already been proved by Magitot beyond doubt that by various means *macro*scopical appearances may be produced which are identical with those found in decay.

I cut up a number of teeth which were perfectly sound, but of different density, into pieces of different size, and placed them in a mixture of saliva and bread. This mixture was kept for three months at a temperature of 37° C., and during the course of the experiment repeatedly renewed. At the end of this time I showed a number of these pieces to a well-known dentist of thirty-three years' standing, and asked him if these were not peculiar cases of decay. He replied by saying that he saw such cases every day in his practice. In many pieces the dentine was softened through and through, in all to a considerable depth. When the softening had penetrated through the dentine to the inner surface of the enamel, the latter was found covered with a layer of white powder exactly as it is found in natural decay. Cracks and fissures in the enamel had an opaque, whitish appearance, and in many cases could be easily penetrated by a sharp instrument. At the neck of the tooth the dentine was likewise much softened, though not to so great a degree as on the crown. The border of the enamel was rough, and so brittle that in many places an instrument could be inserted between the enamel and the dentine. On the grinding-surface, in such cases where the structure of the tooth was imperfect and full of fissures or depressions, the whole tissue had been converted into a soft mass such as is often found on the surface of third molars.

In two cases, apparently on account of a defect of structure, the cusps of the teeth had been attacked. On those points where the acid had penetrated through the enamel, its action upon the dentine could be followed in all directions; where the enamel was hard and thick, without cracks or other defects, it had not even lost its natural polish.

All of the phenomena observed in cases of so-called white decay were present in these cases of artificial decay. If the mixture was allowed to stand until the reaction became alkaline, or if the pieces were exposed to the air or to the action of different articles of food, such as coffee, tea, tobacco, fruit, etc., all possible shades of color were produced just as they are found in the mouth.

These experiments show, among other things, to what an extent the resistance which the tooth opposes to the destroying factors depends upon the structure; further, it furnishes an answer to the question why all teeth under the same conditions do not become decayed in the same degree. A tooth of sound structure, protected by sound enamel, will resist the action of an acid many years, whereas a soft, imperfectly developed tooth under the same conditions would show decay in the course of a few weeks.

Sections of these pieces showed all the microscopic changes which have been described as characteristic of decay of dentine. (See Figs. 99 to 101.) The canaliculi were filled with bacteria, and at many points were much distended; the thickening of Neumann's sheaths and the swelling of the fibrils could also be well observed. A well-known dentist and histologist, to whom I showed one of the preparations, at once called my attention to the varicose swelling of the fibrils and to the distended canaliculi, not knowing that he had an artificial preparation before him. Up to the present, not one who has made the attempt has been able to distinguish a specimen of artificial from one of natural decay at its side.

When Atkinson[120] says, "There is not one of these cases that cannot be discovered in an instant as to which is natural and which artificial," and bases this declaration on the ground that "in every one that was artificial the micro-organisms followed the line of the tubules without striking into the consolidated intertubular substance," he makes a double mistake which I

FIG. 99.

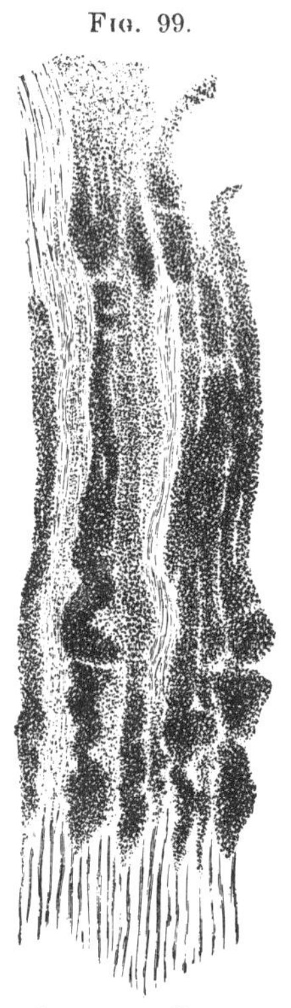

ARTIFICIAL DECAY.
Tubules infiltrated with cocci, distended and in parts running together through the liquefaction of the intertubular substance. Circa 400 : 1. Compare Fig. 77.

FIG. 100

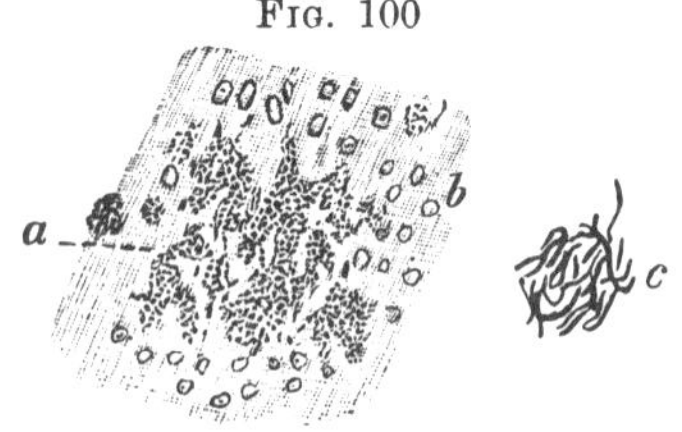

ARTIFICIAL DECAY.
a, tubules distended and melted together; *b*, normal tubules: *c*, tubule under high power (1100 : 1). Cross-section.

FIG. 101.

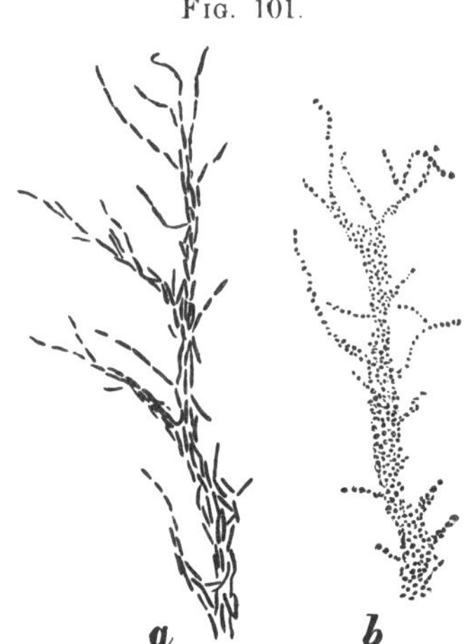

TWO TUBULES FROM ARTIFICIAL DECAY.
a, filled with rods; *b*, with cocci. **Only those branches lying in one plane are represented. 1100 : 1.**

think he will correct himself when he shall have acquired a thorough knowledge of the appearances of natural and artificial decay under the microscope.

One does not require to examine a very large number of preparations in order to discover that both in artificial as well as in natural decay the micro-organisms in the deeper parts of the decaying tissue are confined strictly to the tubules, whereas those nearer the surface, although they do not *strike into* the basis-substance, yet they gradually liquefy it, and thus produce caverns or microscopic holes in it which they immediately fill up.

My experiments have been repeated and their results confirmed by Foerster. Since 1884 I myself have repeated the experiments a number of times, and have somewhat changed the conditions by adding meat to the mixture and changing it every second or third day. Not unfrequently the course of the experiment is interfered with by the appearance of yeast-fungi, particularly of Saccharomyces mycoderma, in the mixture. This fungus appears as a white, thick, dry, felty skin upon the surface of the mixture, and uses up the acid. In the course of a few days putrefaction sets in and the mixture shows an alkaline reaction, by which the course of the experiment is interfered with. If no such disturbance occurs, the pieces will be so far decalcified in a week that they may be easily taken up with a needle; after five weeks sections may be prepared, and by making sections each successive week one will be enabled to observe how the micro-organisms in the course of time penetrate deeper and deeper into the tissue and gradually bring about its destruction.

I do not look upon discoloration as an essential phenomenon of decay, and do not therefore trouble myself about the color of the dentine in artificial decay. It has appeared to me that where nitrogenous substances were present the discoloration appeared sooner than if only carbohydrates were used. A decalcified tooth placed in a mixture of saliva and meat will become discolored in a few days or weeks.

CARIES OF ANIMAL TEETH.

It is commonly believed that dental caries either does not occur at all in animals, or at best so seldom that the few cases which may have been observed are to be regarded as striking exceptions. And indeed we must grant that the teeth of animals, compared to those of modern civilized races, are relatively seldom attacked by caries. But if we compare the teeth of certain kinds of animals with those of uncivilized human races which subsist principally on meat, we arrive at quite different conclusions. The animals referred to are such as live on the same food as civilized human beings, especially dogs and other domesticated animals that feed on substances which form acids by fermentation.

All writers on this subject are, I believe, unanimous in the opinion that decay is exceedingly rare in the case of carnivora.

Bland Sutton, who has occupied himself with this study for many years, found only a small number of decayed teeth in carnivora, and these almost invariably in animals living in captivity for some length of time.

I have obtained information confirming these observations from the directors of various zoölogical institutes and veterinary colleges.

On the other hand, according to my experience, every considerable collection of dogs' skulls will be found to contain one or more decayed teeth, nor is decay of very rare occurrence in horses and apes.

In two hundred and ninety-five dogs' skulls, mostly of bull- and lapdogs, I found eighteen cases of decay; in six, two teeth were decayed; in each of the remaining twelve, one. In two other cases probably incipient decay (I could not decide with certainty whether the teeth were really decayed or not); these two are therefore not included in the above number. In all these cases it was invariably the first upper molar that was decayed, which is explained by the fact that this tooth possesses deep retaining-points for food-particles on the grinding-surface. The fourth bicuspid also frequently showed signs of decay, but no cavity. Decay occurs in these skulls in the proportion of 6 : 100, which signifies much higher percentage than has been found in Esquimaux and various Indian tribes. I succeeded in obtaining material from the dry, decayed tooth of a dog, which being soaked for a few hours in water, and then cut on the freezing microtome and stained with fuchsine, yielded very fair microscopic specimens. Through these specimens I was enabled to establish the interesting fact that decay of dog teeth is accompanied by exactly the same phenomena as that of human teeth

(Fig. 102). Here also, as far as my observations reach, micrococci are the chief destructive agents. In twenty wild dogs, forty foxes, and forty jackals I discovered no decay. Among forty-four apes I found one having a molar tooth with a large cavity extending to the pulp, and two molar teeth with small cavities on the grinding-surface. Of a small number of porcupines' skulls examined, one had a molar completely broken down by decay, nothing being left but the thin walls.

FIG. 102.

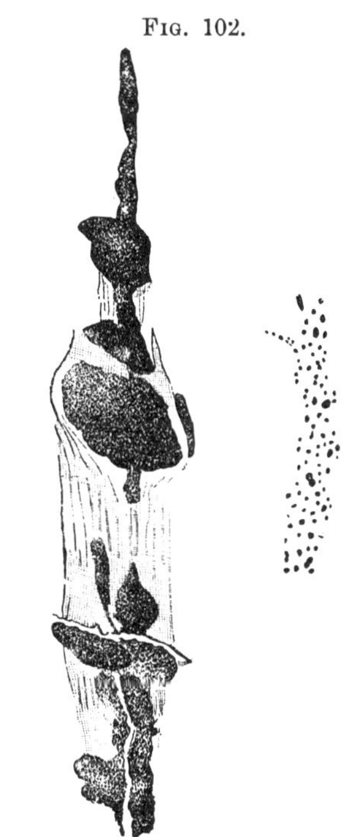

GROUP OF TUBULES FROM DENTINE OF THE DECAYED TOOTH OF A DOG. 400 : 1. In the side figure, piece of a tubule in the beginning of the infection. 1100 : 1.

In horses, decayed teeth are frequently found. In the pathological collection of the Berlin veterinary school there are two skulls in which nearly all the molars show pronounced decay on the grinding-surface. Other skulls also had decayed teeth. Out of about forty normal skulls in the collection of the agricultural school I found but one tooth which I could with certainty pronounce as decayed. But it is exceedingly difficult to recognize decay in old, dry teeth of horses unless it be already far advanced. Dr. Galbreath mentions three badly decayed teeth which he saw in the collection of Prof. Dr. Günther, of Hanover.

The microscopical examination of decayed dentine from the horse also showed the phenomena characteristic of human caries, —invasions of bacteria, enlargement of the tubules, etc. (Fig. 103).

I have found the searching for decay in dry teeth of sheep skulls no easy matter. The many folds, islands, and spaces which are filled with remnants of food, and always intensely discolored, render it still more difficult to perceive small cavities here than in horses' teeth.*

FIG. 103.

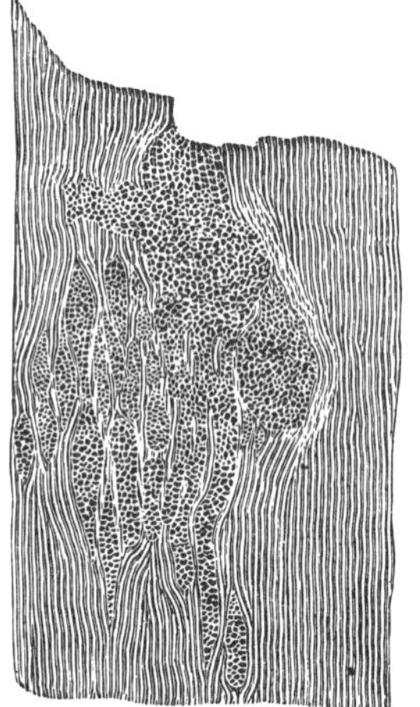

DECAYED DENTINE FROM A HORSE'S TOOTH, showing the destruction of the tissue by bacteria. 800 : 1.

I have examined a few pig skulls and found but one small point of decay. Since pigs eat much fermentable food, we should expect decay more frequently, in spite of the alkalinity of their saliva, if the teeth were not so compact, and particularly if the animals were not slaughtered at so early an age (two to three years).

The conditions which explain the comparatively rare appearance of decay in animal teeth are, in my opinion:

1. The firm structure of animal teeth.
2. The nature of their food (but little fermentable).
3. The alkalinity of their saliva.
4. The comparatively short time during which the teeth are exposed to the causes that produce decay.

SPOTANEOUS HEALING OF DENTAL DECAY.

The process of decay, if not retarded by the proper treatment, usually results in the complete destruction of the crown. Cases, however, occur (comparatively seldom) which strangely deviate from the usual course, in that the destructive process ceases spontaneously, and the already softened dentine becomes hard again. This process is most frequently observed in the permanent first molars, but it also occurs in milk-teeth. Some years ago I examined the mouths of a boy and girl (twins, three years old)

*In more than one hundred skulls I could not establish with certainty the presence of any trace of decay. I was, on the other hand, astonished at the frequency of exostoses and destructive processes on the roots of sheep teeth.

whose teeth were in a very bad condition. All the front and several molar teeth were so much decayed that I entertained but little hope of saving them.

I made temporary fillings in a number of the teeth, and directed the little patients to be sent back again in two months. At the end of this time they punctually returned, but as the decay had apparently made no progress in the unfilled cavities, nothing further was done. All of these unfilled cavities, eight in the front teeth and three in the molars, healed completely, the dentine became hard and smooth, and no further loss of substance occurred.

The healed dentine retains the color of the carious dentine, is almost as hard as the normal, and according to the determinations of Dr. Cohn, of Berlin, contains a much greater percentage of lime than decayed dentine. Microscopic examinations of healed dentine have not, as far as I know, been made. In two cases of healed decay I prepared some sections, but was not able to note anything characteristic. The invasion of the bacteria in the cases examined had been superficial, a fusion of the basis-substance had not taken place, and the dilatation of the tubules was confined to the external layer. Results obtained from the examination of only two cases are, however, naturally not to be relied upon too implicitly.

Opinions concerning the cause of this healing vary. According to some authors, it is to be explained by a renewed deposit of lime-salts in the softened dentine. Such a deposit could of course occur only in places not yet invaded by bacteria. Others maintain that no vital process of any kind, as a redeposition of lime-salts, can take place in the completely developed dentine. They regard the healing as being due merely to the dehydration (drying) of the dentine. As is well known, the decayed dentine of extracted teeth becomes somewhat hard. Further experiments are necessary to determine which of these views is correct.

If we accept the dehydration theory, we shall find it very difficult, I am afraid, to explain how the dentine, continually bathed with liquid as it is, can at all dry out in the human mouth, particularly how it can dry out in one tooth and not in others which may be decayed in the same mouth. We shall, furthermore, in case the experiments of Cohn should be confirmed, be unable to account for the smooth, shining surface and the increased percentage of lime-salts in the repaired dentine. If we, on the other hand, accept the recalcification theory, we have to choose between two possibilities,—(1) the possibility of a recalcification of the dentine; more or less complete restoration of the lime-salts of the decayed dentine through the medium of the pulp (a virtual restitutio ad integrum), which would not be in accordance with the conception of Hoppe-Seyler (page 149); (2) the possibility that new dentine may be formed at the expense of the fibrils in the manner described under transparency of the dentine. Without pronouncing my adherence to the vitalistic theory, I think I may say that I am not quite satisfied with the dehydration theory. We have here another subject for experiment.

CHAPTER VIII

ETIOLOGY OF DENTAL DECAY.

HAVING acquainted ourselves with the physiological properties of the chemical and organic ferments occurring in the oral cavity, as well as with the nature of the fermentations excited by them, and having furthermore examined the chemical and microscopical changes of the dentine characteristic of decay, and shown the possibility of producing decay artificially, we now come to the question: What is the cause of dental decay?

Dental decay is a chemico-parasitical process consisting of two distinctly marked stages: decalcification, or softening of the tissue, and dissolution of the softened residue. In the case of enamel, however, the second stage is practically wanting, the decalcification of the enamel practically signifying its total destruction.

After having discussed the processes of fermentation in the mouth, it is not difficult to determine the source of the acids which effect the decalcification. They are derived chiefly from particles of amylaceous and saccharine substances which lodge in the retaining-centers and there undergo fermentation. The presence of an acid reaction in cavities of decay and in caries-centers may be easily determined by the simple test with blue litmus-paper. The test should not be made at the surface, but in the deeper layers, after the remains of food and outer layers of carious dentine have been removed. I examined two hundred and thirty cases in regard to this question, and found the reaction acid in two hundred and twenty-five, neutral in four, and alkaline in one case. The latter five cases may be explained by the predominance of albuminous substances (meat, gangrenous pulp-tissue, etc.) in the cavity at the time of examination.

Inasmuch as the fermentation of carbohydrates gives rise to the production chiefly of lactic acid, and since lactic acid even in dilute form speedily acts upon tooth-tissue (decalcifies it), there can be little doubt that the acid reaction and the decalcification of the dentine are produced in a great part by this acid. The accuracy of the supposition may be easily proved by the Ewald test. If we place a large piece of decayed dentine in a test tube containing the solution given on page 106, and allow the tube to stand in the dark for some time, a yellowish zone like a halo will be formed about the piece, indicating the presence of lactic acid with tolerable certainty, since we know that the other substances which give this test (page 107) are not formed except in very minute quantities.

The acids formed in the mouth by fermentation of starch are quite as injurious to the teeth as those formed from sugar. The assertion that starch is not injurious to the teeth rests upon no experimental basis. On the other hand, it has been irrefutably established by experiment that saliva containing starch at blood temperature shows an acid reaction as soon and develops as much acid in a given space of time as saliva containing sugar.

If we divide a quantity of saliva into a number of equal portions, and add to each an equal quantity of different carbohydrates (sugar, bread, potato, starch, etc.), we shall find that those containing bread and potato not only show an acid reaction sooner, but even develop more acid in a given time than the portions to which sugar has been added. Starch-paste and sugar, as far as my observations go, react about equally strong.

Some very interesting experiments were performed by Ellenberger and Hofmeister,[121] which show that under certain circumstances starch-paste, too, is more rapidly transformed into lactic acid than sugar. An alkalinized pancreas-extract containing grape-sugar kept at a specified temperature did not develop an acid reaction till after forty-eight hours or more, whereas on the addition of starch-paste an acid reaction appeared in twenty-four hours. " Sugar in statu nascendi seems to be transformed into lactic acid more quickly than in its ordinary state. In all experiments on digestion with starch-paste, lactic acid is rapidly developed."

In all cases the starch is first transformed into grape-sugar by the ptyaline of the saliva or of the pancreatic juiçe, and is then split into lactic acid by the lactic acid ferment of various bacteria. Now, it is well known that many chemical bodies possess other affinities at the moment of their formation than at other times. According to the experiments referred to, this appears to be the case with sugar. For other reasons, also, I consider starch and amylaceous substances more detrimental to the teeth than sugar, particularly as sugar, being readily soluble, is soon carried away or so diluted with the saliva as to be rendered harmless, whereas amylaceous matter adheres to the teeth for a greater length of time and consequently manifests a more continued action than sugar.

Hesse's[122] observations in respect to caries of bakers' teeth lend support to this opinion. He writes, "In the Dental Institute of this city [Leipzig] I have had the opportunity of seeing a great number of patients among the industrial and working classes, and have been particularly surprised at the bad condition of the teeth of our bakers. They are affected by caries to such a degree that I have been able in many cases, since my acquaintance with this phenomenon, to determine the calling of a patient by the condition of his teeth. There can be little doubt that we have here to do with a disease which stands in causal connection with the calling, and the theory of caries recently propounded by Miller gives a satisfactory explanation of it. A few confectioners' children are the only individuals I have seen who could bear comparison with bakers, although their teeth were not in quite so bad a condition. Probably the millers may be able to compete with the bakers, and it would be desirable to be enlightened on this point."

Busch, on the contrary, is of the opinion that "baker caries" is due rather to the inhalation of sugar-dust than to that of flour-dust.

Different sugars manifest but little difference in their capability of being split up into acids. Those kinds belonging to the grape-sugar group—grape-sugar (dextrose), fruit-sugar (levulose), lactose (galactose), and maltose—are directly fermentable and decompose according to the equation: $C_6H_{12}O_6 = 2C_3H_6O_3$. Cane-sugar (saccharose) and milk-sugar become fermentable only after hydratization.

$$\underset{\text{Cane-sugar.}}{C_{12}H_{22}O_{11}} + H_2O = \underset{\text{Dextrose.}}{C_6H_{12}O_6} + \underset{\text{Levulose.}}{C_6H_{12}O_6}. \quad C_6H_{12}O_6 = \underset{\text{Lactic acid.}}{2C_3H_6O_3}$$

There seems to be no considerable difference of time in respect to the beginning of the fermentation of the grape-sugar and cane-sugar groups: the one is apparently about as detrimental to the teeth as the other.

Fermentable albuminous substances mixed with saliva develop but small quantities of acid, which soon disappear. They are not injurious to the teeth, even though retained for some length of time; they may even retard the progress of decay by neutralizing the acid through their alkaline products. The most diverging opinions prevail in regard to the participation of different substances in fermentations arising in the mouth, none of which rest on solid foundations. Above all, the conception that albuminous substances (meat) putrefying in the mouth produce acids is totally erroneous.

The facts mentioned on pages 27 and 115 cannot leave us in doubt on this point. It seemed to me desirable, however, to refute the above views experimentally, and at the same time to establish the relative significance of different carbohydrates as acidifiers. For this purpose I made over two hundred experiments with human saliva, and also a few with the saliva of dogs and rabbits. 4.0 c.cm. of fresh saliva were mixed with 0.5 g. of the food to be tested, and the reaction as well as the quantity of free acid determined after the lapse of a certain time.

The results obtained are given in the following table. The "acid unit" signifies that quantity of acid which is necessary to neutralize 0.1 c.cm. of a 0.5 per cent. solution of caustic potash.

Material.	Duration of experiment.	Acid formed in acid units.
Bread (dry)	12 and 30 hours	22 and 72
Starch	" " "	20 " 42
Cane-sugar	" " "	17 " 37
Grape-sugar	" " "	19 " 40
Potato (boiled)	" " "	24 " 75
Corn (in milk)	" " "	24 " 77

Material.	Duration of experiment.	Acid formed in acid units.
Bread (1.0 g.) . .	12 and 30 hours	35 and 110
Sugar (2.0 g.) . .	" " "	20 " 41
Rice . . .	" " "	25 " 72
Macaroni . . .	" " "	20 " 76
Meat . . .	" " "	0 " —3*
Meat (raw) . .	" " "	— " —5
Fish . . .	" " "	0 " —5
Eggs . . .	" " "	0 " —
Cheese . . .	" " "	0 " (?)
Spinach (in water) .	" " "	0 " 0
Potato (raw) . .	" " "	0 " 0
Salad (raw) . .	" " "	0 " 0
Fat	" " "	— " (?)

In but one series of experiments with dog saliva I obtained the following figures (reaction strongly alkaline at the beginning of the test):

Material.	Duration of experiment.	Reaction.
Starch . .	$4\frac{1}{2}$, 12, 20, and 35 hours.	always alkaline.
Meat (cooked)	" " " " " "	" "
Meat (raw) .	" " " " " "	alkaline, putrid smell.
Sugar . .	" " " " " "	"
Bread . .	" " " " " "	acid after 20 hours.
Potato . .	" " " " " "	" " 12 "

For rabbits' saliva.

Material.	Duration of experiment.	Reaction.
Grass	$4\frac{1}{2}$ to 12 hours.	alkaline.
Turnips . . .	$4\frac{1}{2}$ " 35 "	up to thirty

hours alkaline, then an acid reaction set in, but not so strong as when the turnips were crushed in water.

The fresh saliva of both animals showed a strong alkaline reaction.

The few experiments made for the purpose of comparing the acidifying power of raw and cooked food seem to indicate that

* The sign — denotes an alkaline reaction.

raw vegetable food is less fermentable than cooked. Should further researches prove that this is indeed the case, the cooking of food would have to be reckoned among those customs of civilization which have a detrimental influence upon the teeth.

It is well enough known that acids, brought into the mouth as medicines or with the foods, may have a deleterious action on the teeth. An excess of sour fruit, grapes, lemons, etc., and the continued use of acids or acid compounds doubtless has a decalcifying action on the teeth, attacking first not the concealed but the exposed parts.

Schlenker[72] calls attention to certain substances which, coming into contact with the teeth, either as food or as medicine, are generally injurious, some to such an extent that their decalcifying action becomes visible to the naked eye in the short space of five minutes. I do not attribute too great an importance to the influence of such substances, nor do I underrate them, since a slight injury of the enamel or dentine caused by such agents may give rise to decay at points which otherwise would have escaped.

An acid reaction of the saliva is equally detrimental. This is said to occur in rheumatism, gout, gastro-enteritis, diabetes mellitus, dyspepsia, and various disorders of the alimentary tract, in fevers (typhus, intermittent fever, etc.), in diseases of the lungs, etc., and during pregnancy. According to some authors, the mucus also, under certain circumstances, has an acid reaction, and the attempt has been made thereby to explain pathological phenomena, particularly at the neck of the tooth (wedge-shaped defect, neck decay). Our knowledge of the properties of mucus is unfortunately too limited to determine accurately the part it plays in decay of the teeth. (See page 42.)

With less reason, it appears to me, Tomes, Black, and others ascribe a destructive (probably meaning a decalcifying) action on the neck of the tooth to the "acid secretion" of the irritated gums. No conclusive facts have been adduced for this supposition. On the other hand, it is well known that decay very seldom occurs in cases of pyorrhœa alveolaris, in which the gums are in a state of irritation for months together. Whenever decay does accompany inflamed gums, we invariably find pockets or spaces which, by retaining food-particles, serve as centers of fermentation and consequent decay.

According to Coleman,[123] the acid reaction of decayed dentine is caused by the formation of an acid phosphate of lime, arising from the disintegration of the lime-salts.

Bridgman[124] explains the acidification by an electrolytic decomposition of the buccal juices.

The second stage of caries, the dissolution of the softened dentine, is caused by bacteria. We have seen that many mouth-bacteria have the faculty of dissolving coagulated albumen or albuminous substances, of peptonizing or converting them into a soluble modification. We have also seen that the basis-substance of dentine consists of an albuminous substance. The explanation of the second stage of decay is therefore very easy, the more so, since the liquefaction of the softened dentine by bacteria is directly detectable under the microscope and may be easily accomplished experimentally. The dissolution of dental cartilage (in fact, decay in general) has been designated as putrefaction, on the whole an ill-chosen term, inasmuch as the characteristics of putrefaction (alkaline reaction and bad odor) are entirely wanting in a cavity of real decay. The decaying dentine shows an acid reaction and emits a sour smell.* This stage of caries, therefore, is a digestive process. The dental cartilage is dissolved by the bacterium-ferment, as albumen by the pepsine of the gastric juice.

We must rid ourselves of the impression, which the application of the very unscientific and unprofessional name of bugs to bacteria has no doubt tended to spread, that the parasites of the human mouth make holes in the dentine by boring into it as a worm bores into wood or by gnawing at it as a dog gnaws at a bone. Bacteria have no apparatus for boring, nor do they have mouths or any provision for breaking off small portions of solid substances which they then swallow whole or take directly up at any point of their periphery after the manner of an amœba. They nourish themselves alone by substances in a state

* Of course the odor of a gangrenous pulp or of suppurating gums, etc., must not be confounded with that of the dentine.

of solution, and if we present them solid substances they themselves must liquefy them before they can make any use of them for their own nourishment.

Upon this power of bacteria to liquefy substances of an albuminous nature depends the destruction of the softened dentine, —in other words, the second stage of dental decay.

The objection has been raised against the chemico-parasitical theory of caries, that the reaction of the saliva in any mouth is no criterion for the extent of decay in that mouth. When the reaction of the saliva is alkaline, decay has been found to be extensive; and, on the other hand, cases have been reported where an acid reaction of the saliva was not accompanied by a corresponding amount of decay. None but a very superficial investigator, however, would draw conclusions from a simple examination of saliva.

The rapidity with which the process of destruction of the teeth in any mouth advances is evidently directly proportional to the intensity of the fermentations going on in the retention-centers, and inversely proportional to the density of the tooth-substance. Now, both of these factors are virtually independent of the reaction which the saliva may show on escaping from the ducts. A prolonged strong acid reaction of the saliva would indeed render the fluids of the mouth less adapted to the development of bacteria, and in so far as the acid could penetrate the centers of fermentation tend to decrease the intensity of such fermentation. Such a decrease would, however, be compensated for by the action of the acid itself.

The case becomes very different when we turn our attention to the free surfaces of the teeth. A prolonged acid reaction of the saliva would of necessity manifest its disastrous influences upon these surfaces sooner or later, according as the teeth are soft or dense in structure. Consequently, if anyone can show me a case in which an acid condition of the saliva has persisted for some months (not one in which the saliva chanced to react acid just at the moment of examination, or one in which the acid reaction was caused by bad litmus-paper, or by handling the paper with sweaty fingers, etc.), I shall have no difficulty in pointing out places at which its action is plainly manifest.

The total absence of decay in a closed root-canal which has for years been harboring a putrid pulp and innumerable bacteria is a still less warrantable objection to the above-mentioned theory. It evinces an entire ignorance of the vital conditions and fermentative action of bacteria. For, in the first place, the bacteria in a closed root-canal either perish, or, what happens more rarely, become inactive as soon as the nutriment in the pulp is consumed,—*i.e.*, in a few days. In the second place, even though they could really vegetate for years in a root-canal, we should still have no reason to expect decay, because the carbohydrates, essential to the formation of acids, are wanting. The reaction of a putrid pulp is invariably alkaline.

Leber and Rottenstein[58] discovered after boring into two incisors, which had a peculiar blue color without exhibiting a trace of decay externally, that the entire interior of the teeth was brown, completely softened up to the enamel, and that even the root was hollow. Such very exceptional cases "must not be identified with common caries." They are of such rare occurrence that no satisfactory explanation of them has yet been offered, and every one who reads the report of them can only shrug his shoulders and wait for the day when he may have an opportunity to examine such a case personally, an opportunity which but rarely comes even once in a lifetime.

The view that during the disintegration of the pulp the acid necessary for the softening of the dentine was formed, is untenable, first, because the reaction of putrid pulps is always alkaline; secondly, because even in case an acid reaction should take place, under peculiar circumstances, all bacteria of the pulp would be destroyed long before even a fraction of the quantity of acid requisite to decalcification would be formed. We cannot ascribe this occurrence to a process of nitrification, such as occurs in the soil, since this demands free access of air.

In support of the inflammation theory, a difference has been assumed between decay of living and dead teeth. It has been asserted that the softened layer of dentine is much thinner, dryer, and blacker in dead than in living teeth. Every practitioner has surely seen phenomena which seem to agree with this assertion, but a satisfactory explanation may be found without much trouble. The alkaline products of the putrefying pulp and of the inflamed suppurating or disintegrating gums neutralize the acids formed in the dental cavity by fermentation. The process of decalcification ceases, partially at least, whereas the dissolution of the already softened dentine proceeds. The decalcified layer of dentine must gradually become thinner under such circumstances. If a just extracted carious tooth be kept in a putrefying albuminous solution for some length of time, the softening of the dentine completely ceases, while the dentine which has already been softened gradually disappears.

THE MICRO-ORGANISMS OF DENTAL DECAY.

Our knowledge of the micro-organisms most directly concerned in the destruction of the substance of the tooth is as yet very deficient. We have been able to establish the fact that all micro-organisms of the human mouth which possess the power of exciting an acid fermentation of foods may and do take part in producing the first stage of caries; also, that all possessing a peptonizing or digestive action upon albuminous substances may take part in the second stage; and, finally, that those possessing both properties at the same time may take part in the production of both stages. But whether there is any one bacterium which may *always* be found in decayed dentine, and which might therefore be entitled to the name of *the* bacterium of tooth-decay, or whether there are various kinds which occur with considerable constancy, we are not able to say.

During my experiments upon the bacteria of decay in the year 1883, I isolated four different kinds of bacteria from decaying dentine. These I described in the *Independent Practitioner* for July, 1884.

I have frequently met with them in more recent investigations, and they have also been observed by others. I do not consider the experiments I then made sufficiently extensive or conclusive to be incorporated here, and experiments now in progress, with new methods and larger material, are not yet concluded, it being necessary to examine at least fifty to one hundred different teeth in order to arrive at satisfactory results.

The researches recently made by Vignal and Galippe,[125] and reported in *L'Odontologie*, although not yet concluded, appear to be deserving of more notice.

The investigators named have examined eighteen decayed teeth, in all which they found four different kinds of bacteria; a fifth kind they met with eight times, and a sixth five times.

1. The first kind met with is a short, thick bacillus, not forming chains. It has a length of 1.5μ, and is almost as thick as it is long. In puncture-cultures, in gelatine, it grows tolerably rapidly, forming a white trail, and begins to liquefy the gelatine at the end of the third or fourth day, turning it white and opaque. In plate-cultures it forms small, slightly prominent colonies, which having attained a diameter of two to three millimeters spread out in the liquefied gelatine.

2. The second kind is a bacillus 3.0μ long and about one-half as thick, slightly constricted in the middle. Its cultures are similar to those of the preceding, except that its colonies spread out more upon the surface of the gelatine before liquefying it.

3. The third kind is a bacillus quite similar to the preceding, showing, however, no constriction. It is square at the ends, and forms quite long chains, particularly in liquid media. It does not liquefy the gelatine, but slightly softens it.

4. The fourth kind is a very small, thin bacillus, almost as thick as long, so that it might at first be mistaken for a coccus. It forms a white trail in the gelatine, which it speedily turns yellow and then liquefies.

5. The fifth kind, found but eight times, is a bacillus with rounded ends, which forms at first a white trail in the gelatine and then liquefies and clouds it.

6. The sixth micro-organism, found but five times, is a very large coccus. It was found only in advanced stages of decay, where the canaliculi were already considerably dilated, it being too large to enter the sound tubuli.

It forms trails in the gelatine, which it does not liquefy, and to which it lends a whitish aspect.

In a memoir, soon to be published, Galippe and Vignal promise to present in detail the characters of the cultures above mentioned.

PREDISPOSING CAUSES OF DENTAL CARIES.

In contradistinction to the exciting causes of caries, we characterize as *predisposing* such conditions of individual or of all teeth which divest them of their normal power of resisting exciting causes, or by which they offer them especial points of attack.

Predisposing conditions are only found in the teeth themselves, in their development, position, etc., while, on the other hand, all external agencies are to be considered as exciting causes. It is therefore not logical to regard gout, *e.g.*, as a predisposing cause, because it is accompanied by an acid reaction of the saliva. The action of an acid on the teeth will always be the same, whether it is secreted by the mucus or salivary glands, or formed in the mouth by fermentation, or introduced from without; it is invariably an exciting, not a predisposing cause.

1. The structure of the teeth plays the most important part as a predisposing cause of dental caries. Poorly developed, soft, porous teeth, with many large interglobular spaces, are highly predisposed to caries. As a lump of table-salt dissolves more rapidly in water, on account of its porosity, than an equally large piece of rock-salt, porous dentine is more rapidly decalcified than well-developed, firm dentine, because the acid may the more readily penetrate the tissue, and because less acid is required to decalcify a porous than a hard tooth. It may easily be proved by experiment that poorly developed dentine is much more rapidly attacked by acids than sound dentine. (See page 196.) Not only does the decalcification, but also the destruction of the cartilage, advance more rapidly in the former case, because the micro-organisms, in many cases at least, enter the interglobular spaces and more readily pervade and destroy the entire softened tissue.

2. As a second predisposing factor I designate abnormally deep fissures or blind holes (foramina cœca) in molars and superior lateral incisors, especially in cases where the enamel also is poorly developed. By their continual retention of food-particles, such points directly induce caries, and offer but little resistance to it in consequence of the absence of an intact protecting cover of enamel.

3. In the third place, fissures or cracks in the enamel are regarded as a predisposing cause. I have not, however, been able to convince myself that decay frequently starts from these enamel-cracks, often found in senile teeth. They are usually too narrow to permit the entrance of food-particles, and consequently do not serve as points of retention.

4. In the fourth place, teeth are predisposed to decay by a crowded, irregular position. An instructive example is furnished in cases where the first bicuspid stands inside of the arch, so as to form a triangle with the second bicuspid and the cuspid; or the second bicuspid forms a triangle with the first bicuspid and first molar. It is impossible to keep the space between these three teeth clean, and fermentation and acid formation continually occur there and attack the teeth. Not only in such cases, but wherever a crowded position of the teeth favors the retention of food-particles, or renders their removal difficult, a predisposition to caries prevails. The form of a tooth is not without influence; teeth with convex approximal surfaces touching each other at one point only (Fig. 104) are, *cæteris paribus*, less subject

FIG. 104. FIG. 105.

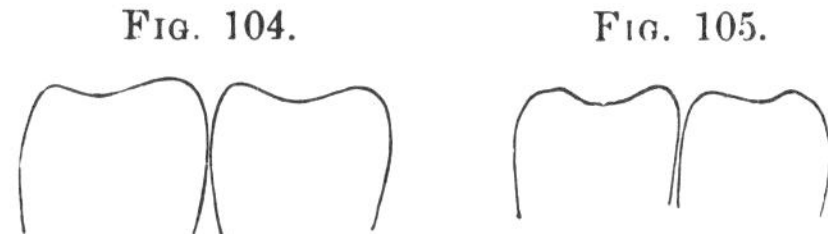

to caries than teeth with flat or slightly concave surfaces (Fig. 105), because the latter cannot be kept so clean, either spontaneously (by the tongue, etc.) or with the brush.

5. A recession or loosening of the gums from the neck of the tooth not only lays bare the dentine, but also permits the entrance of food-particles between the necks of the teeth or into the pockets formed by the loosening of the gums, by which means a further predisposing cause for caries is furnished.

6. Many consider pregnancy as a predisposing cause. It is not to be denied that during pregnancy women are particularly subject to caries. The reason for this is, however, probably to be sought in the fact that the patients generally neglect the care of the mouth during that time, and that the buccal secretions

assume an acid reaction; these are both exciting causes of decay. Pregnancy itself can only be regarded as a predisposing cause in so far as it effects a loosening of the gums or a change in the structure of the teeth by a withdrawal of the lime-salts to build up the fœtal skeleton. Whether such an extraction takes place has not been definitely ascertained.

7. Many believe that a predisposition to caries may be inherited. It cannot be denied that badly developed, irregular teeth may be and are inherited, and in so far inheritance may be considered as a predisposing cause of caries.

8. Wedl, Tomes, and others mention as predisposing causes various general diseases, as rheumatism, gout, diabetes, gastroenteritis, dyspepsia, cancer of the stomach, scrofula, rachitis, and tuberculosis. These diseases may indeed furnish the exciting causes of caries by imparting an acid reaction to the buccal juices, but how they can predispose the teeth themselves to caries is not readily apparent, unless they render them more easy of access to the exciting causes by concomitant gum-diseases as described under 5.

I doubt whether climatic or geological conditions have much to do with the origin of caries. Esquimaux, Lapps, Icelanders, Arabs in Nubia, Patagonians, etc., have the best teeth in spite of unfavorable climatic conditions.

INFLUENCE OF CIVILIZATION ON DECAY.

That decay of the teeth is not a disease peculiar to civilization is proved by the manifold observations which have been made on the skulls of ancient and modern uncivilized races in Europe and America. A visit to any anatomical or anthropological museum and an examination of a large number of race-skulls will convince every one of the correctness of this assertion. Such examinations have been made by Broca, Magitot,[126] Mummery,[127] Barrett,[128] myself,[129] and many others, and invariably led to the same conclusion, that decay has occurred in all races, civilized as well as uncivilized, and at all times.

Races subsisting solely on meat (Greenlanders, etc.) come near forming an exception to the rule, yet they appear to be not absolutely exempt from decay. (See page 221.)

That the frequency of decay is greater in civilized races than among savages has also been established by numerous observations. Mummery's interesting communications are especially worthy of mention. He found decay among the old Britons of the dolichocephalous type in 2.94 per cent., among the brachycephalous Britons in 21.87 per cent., among the Anglo-Saxons in 15.78 per cent., among the Romano-Britons in 28.67 per cent., and among the ancient Egyptians in 41.66 per cent.

There is no doubt that a deterioration of the teeth accompanies the progress of civilization. The reasons for this are many. The mode of life of most uncivilized races not only conditions a sound, well-developed body, but the osseous system, of course including the teeth, shows the same vigorous development, and above all a compact structure. An individual whose youth is spent in the open air, unrestricted in his bodily freedom, is likely to possess a body better developed in all its parts than one who has been brought up in a modern school-room.

The quality of the food also exerts an influence on the teeth not to be underrated. They form no exception to the rule that an unused member will be less perfectly developed than one constantly used.

The pressure brought to bear upon the teeth by mastication causes a more lively circulation in the periosteum and in the pulp, thereby inducing an increased deposit of lime-salts or a more complete calcification. Practical experience also teaches that children brought up on soft food (broths, paps, etc.) generally have bad teeth. If a race of human beings or of animals were to make no use of their teeth for several generations, we should expect to find a gradual deterioration of the dental structure. It is, to say the least, highly probable that the soft quality of many of our foods, as compared to those of uncivilized races, conditions a soft, porous dental substance, as well as an imperfect development of the jaw-bone, and a concomitant crowded position of the teeth.

Then again, the chemical composition of the food is of great influence upon the origin and extension of caries. Whoever grants the truth of our proposition,—no caries without acid,—and recognizes the fermentative processes in the mouth as the chief source of the decalcifying acids, and has verified our table (pages 208, 209), will hardly deny the correctness of this statement.

A person living on such foods only as undergo no acid fermentation in the mouth (meat, raw vegetables, roots, etc.) will, I am convinced, be but comparatively little afflicted with caries. If this supposition were well founded, a comparison of the frequency of caries among races subsisting on meat alone with that of races who consume vegetable or mixed foods would yield higher figures for the latter. Caries should also then be more frequent in phytophagous animals than in carnivora.

That such investigations are connected with enormous difficulties is apparent. It is extremely difficult or altogether impossible to eliminate other simultaneously present, especially predisposing causes. In the second place, the statements of certain authors concerning the food of savage tribes do not always agree, and furthermore suitable material for these examinations is extremely scarce in most anatomical collections.

Very interesting and valuable figures have been gathered by Mummery, which are meant to establish the relation of caries to the healthy or unhealthy manner of life of a given race.

These figures, with a few changes which concern the nourishment of the races specified, and with the addition of those which I have deduced from various anatomical and anthropological collections, are presented in the following table:

Ancient Races.	No. of Skulls.	Caries.	Percentage of Caries.	Food.
Ancient Britons (dolichocephalous.)	68	2	2.94	Meat (beef, wild boar).
Ancient Britons (brachycephalous.)	32	7	21.87	Mixed food (meat, fish, oats, wheat, beans, roots, etc.).
Ancient Britons (exploration of Greenwell.)	59	24	40 68	
Ancient Britons (mixed.)	44	9	20.45	
Romano-Britons	143	41	28 67	
Anglo-Saxons	76	12	15.78	
Ancient Egyptians	36	15	41.66	

MODERN RACES.	No. of Skulls.	Caries.	Percentage of Caries.	Food.
Esquimaux	81	2	2.46	Meat and fish.
North Americans . . . (coasters.)	63	2	3.17	Meat and fish, probably not quite exclusively.
North Americans . . . (interior.)	22	2	9.09	Mostly meat, some vegetables.
South Americans . . .	26	7	27.00	Principally meat.
Feejee Islanders . . .	38	2	5.26	Human flesh and mixed food.
Polynesians	79	8	10.12	Mixed food.
Sandwich Islanders . .	21	3	14.28	" "
New Zealanders . . .	66	2	3.30	Human flesh, pork, fish, roots.
Australians	132	27	20.45	Mixed food.
Tasmanians	33	9	27.27	" "
Chinese	50	21	40.20	" " mostly vegetable
East Indians (north) . .	152	9	5.92	" "
East Indians (south) . .	71	10	14.84	" "
Africans (east)	32	8	25.00	" "
Kaffirs	49	7	14.28	" "
Africans (west)	236	66	27.96	" "
Lapps	22	1 (?)	4.54 (?)	Meat or fish, milk, cheese.

The Gauchos, a cattle-breeding tribe, inhabiting the pampas of La Plata, and subsisting on meat, are said to be free from caries, while a related tribe in Chili, that subsists on bread, beans, meat, etc., showed 19.3 per cent. of caries. Again, those Gauchos who live in cities, and who eat mixed food and much sugar, also suffer much from decay of the teeth.

A hasty examination of several skulls led Black[130] to the supposition that those races which consume much sour fruit are less afflicted with caries than those living on meat and grain. But when we remember how the teeth are destroyed by a grape cure, we can only regard the result of Black's investigation as accidental, particularly as it was but a "hasty" one.

In one point, however, all examinations coincide. All authors call attention to the fact that the Esquimaux, certain meat-eating tribes of North American Indians, Icelanders, and, as far as I have observed, Lapps also, are almost entirely exempt from caries.

The immunity of these races cannot, it seems to me, be explained by the favorable hygienic mode of life, climatic influences, etc., alone. They often suffer from famines; various diseases are frequent, especially among the Lapps, and the latter, as well as the Esquimaux, are becoming extinct. That the númber of inhabitants of Iceland has remained stationary for the last few centuries is said to be due to "volcanic eruptions, frequent epidemics, unhealthy mode of life, famines, etc."

I think therefore every one will agree with me that the conditions prevailing in the countries named are not to be regarded as conducive to a perfect development of the human body.

Those factors which contribute to restrict the occurrence of decay of the teeth are, in my opinion, (1) a mode of life favorable to the development of the whole body, (2) the use of food which is sufficiently hard to afford the teeth the exercise necessary for their vigorous development, (3) the use of food which does not undergo an acid fermentation in the mouth.

CHAPTER IX.

PROPHYLAXIS OF DENTAL DECAY.

To every one at all acquainted with the nature of that condition of the teeth denominated as decay, caries, etc., and with the causes by which it is produced, it must be apparent that there are four ways by which we may counteract or limit the ravages of this disease. We may endeavor (1) by hygienic measures to secure the best possible development of the teeth; (2) by repeated, thorough, systematic cleansing of the oral cavity and the teeth, to so far reduce the amount of fermentable substances as to materially diminish the production of acid, as well as to rob the bacteria of the organic matter necessary to their rapid development; (3) by prohibiting or limiting the consumption of such foods or luxuries which readily undergo acid fermentation to remove the chief source of the ferment-products injurious to the teeth; (4) by the proper and intelligent use of antiseptics to destroy the bacteria, or at least to limit their number and activity.

That a great influence is exerted upon the process of fermentation in the human mouth by the mechanical cleansing mentioned under 2 may be easily proved by the following experiment: Take 10.0 c.cm. saliva from the mouth in the morning before cleansing it, add 0.5 gr. starch, and place the mixture in the incubator. Then cleanse the mouth and teeth most thoroughly with the brush, toothpick, floss silk, etc., after which take 10.0 c.cm. again (easily obtained by chewing a quill toothpick or in the manner described on page 40), add 0.5 gr. starch as before, and place also in the incubator. The first mixture not only shows signs of fermentation sooner than the second, but also forms much more acid in a given time. That different kinds of foods and luxuries play vastly different rôles in the fermentations of the human mouth must be apparent to every one from the table given on pages 208, 209.

The substances which give rise to fermentation in the mouth accompanied by the development of acid, belong almost without exception to the group of the carbohydrates. The general opinion that putrefying meat gives rise to products which attack the teeth is, I repeat it, entirely unfounded and erroneous. The products of a putrefying mixture of saliva and meat (whether cooked or raw) are always alkaline, and when meat has remained for some time between the teeth it may even act as a preventive to decay in so far as it tends to neutralize the acids produced by the fermentations of carbohydrates. The latter, however, are, as a rule, unless the albuminous substances preponderate to a great degree, more than sufficient to satisfy the basic products of the albuminous fermentation (putrefaction), so that in case of mixed diet the reaction will still be acid, not so strongly, however, as in purely amylaceous diet.

Most authors give sugar the chief place among those foods which exert an injurious action upon the teeth—again a conception which is not quite right. It is true that the constant breathing in of sugar-dust exerts a very destructive effect upon the front teeth in particular, known as sugar-decay (Zuckercaries). In general, however, the chief rôle in the production of decay is performed by bread, potatoes, etc., not only because they produce more acid, but because they, on account of their insolubility, may remain for a long time sticking to or between the teeth, whereas the readily soluble sugar is soon diluted or carried away. In my opinion, sugar can equal bread in its destructive action upon the teeth only when it is consumed as an ingredient of sticky, insoluble substances.

Naturally, we cannot think of making the attempt to banish the carbohydrates from the list of the foods and luxuries of civilized races; but we may accomplish a great deal for the teeth if we prevent the constant and unnecessary consumption of sweets, etc., indulged in by many young and not a few adult persons.

The Use of Antiseptics in the Prophylactic Treatment of Decay.

When at the beginning of the present decade, through the most exact methods of bacteriological investigation now in use, the true (parasitic) cause of one disease after another was brought to light, we had many reasons to hope that the helpless position of medicine in the presence of the severest infectious diseases was soon to be changed. As yet, however, our expectations have not been realized. With the exception of the still somewhat doubtful triumphs of Pasteur over anthrax and hydrophobia, very little advantage whatever has resulted to therapeutics from the eminent bacteriological discoveries of the last ten years. Consumption, cholera, typhus, diphtheria, syphilis, have not become less terrible through the discovery of the specific micro-organisms of these disorders.

Diseases which come under the treatment of the dentist form no exception to this statement. The fact that decay of the teeth is of parasitic origin having been once established, the thought suggests itself that we ought to be able by means of properly chosen antiseptic materials not only to arrest decay, but to prevent its appearance. This is, indeed, the avowed object of the very many antiseptic mouth-washes now in the market. As a matter of fact, however, there is no evidence that anything whatever has as yet been accomplished in the prophylactic treatment of the teeth through the use of antiseptic mouth-washes, and it is evident that anyone who would discover some means by which the often fatal ravages caused by decay of the teeth might be held in check would thereby confer a great boon on humanity.

It would, however, be going too far if we were to adopt the views of those who have expressed the opinion that by proper care of the teeth and constant use of antiseptic washes from childhood on, decay would be entirely banished from the human mouth.

This view is too optimistic for various reasons: chiefly because there are places in every denture which will remain completely untouched even by the most thorough application of the antiseptic, or the antiseptic will reach them in so diluted a condition that it possesses little or no action. If a very thorough mechanical cleansing has not preceded the antiseptic, its action upon the centers of decay will be equal to little more than zero.

A great difficulty lies further, in the fact that nearly all materials which possess antiseptic action are either contraindicated altogether in the mouth, or that they may be used only in very dilute solutions, either because they are injurious to the general health, or locally to the mucous membrane or to the teeth themselves. Finally, many otherwise useful antiseptics are excluded because of their bad taste and smell.

For these reasons the preparation of a mouth-wash which possesses an antiseptic action of any importance is accompanied by the greatest difficulties.

Determinations of the antiseptic power of different materials have been made in great number. Some of them which refer especially to those materials which are made use of in the human mouth may find place here.

Koch[131] found for anthrax bacilli the following numbers:

	Evident retardation of the development	Complete prevention of the development
	was produced by a concentration of	
Sublimate	1 : 1000000	1 : 300000
Thymol	1 : 80000	——
Oil of turpentine	1 : 75000	——
Oil of peppermint	1 : 33000	——
Chromic acid	1 : 10000	1 : 5000
Oil of cloves	1 : 5000	——
Iodine	1 : 5000	——
Salicylic acid	1 : 3300	1 : 1500
Oil of eucalyptus	1 : 2500	——
Hydrochloric acid	1 : 2500	1 : 1700
Camphor	1 : 2500	——
Benzoic acid	1 : 2000	——
Permanganate of potash	1 : 1400	——
Carbolic acid	1 : 1250	1 : 850
Boric acid	1 : 1250	1 : 800
Chinin	1 : 830	1 : 625
Benzoate of sodium	1 : 200	——
Alcohol	1 : 100	1 : 25
Table-salt	1 : 64	——

According to Miquel, the development of bacteria in bouillon is prevented by the following antiseptics in the given concentration:

Mercurous oxide	1 : 40000	Carbolic acid	1 : 313
Peroxide of hydrogen	1 : 20000	Permanganate of potash	1 : 286
Bichloride of mercury	1 : 14300	Arsenious acid	1 : 270
Nitrate of silver	1 : 12500	Boric acid	1 : 130
Iodine	1 : 4000	Borax	1 : 14
Salicylic acid	1 : 1000	Alcohol	1 : 10.5
Mineral acids	1 : 500 to 1 : 333		

In the *Deutsche medicinische Wochenschrift* for 1884 I gave in the form of a table the results of a series of experiments which I undertook for the purpose of determining the action of a number of antiseptics upon the bacteria of the human mouth. This table, to which a number of materials have recently been added, follows here:

Antiseptics.	Development of Bacteria prevented by
Bichloride of mercury	1 : 100000
Nitrate of silver	1 : 50000
Peroxide of hydrogen	1 : 8000
Iodine	1 : 6000
Iodoform	1 : 5000
Naphthaline	1 : 4000
Salicylic acid	1 : 2000
Benzoic acid	1 : 1500
Permanganate of potash	1 : 1000
Oil of eucalyptus	1 : 600
Carbolic acid	1 : 500
Hydrochloric acid	1 : 500
Biborate of sodium	1 : 350
Arsenious acid	1 : 250
Chloride of zinc	1 : 250
Lactic acid	1 : 125
Carbonate of sodium	1 : 100
Listerine	1 : 20
Absolute alcohol	1 : 10
Chlorate of potash	1 : 8

It is evident that it would not do to tax the value of these materials for therapeutic purposes exactly according to the above numbers. Whoever, for example, would consider bichloride of mercury, particularly for dental purposes, two hundred times as active as carbolic acid would make a great mistake, since the former can as a rule be applied only in dilute solutions, whereas the latter may usually be made use of in concentrated form.

In connection with the antiseptic materials used in the human mouth, the question of their adaptability demands particular consideration; and in regard to this point I have examined a number of the materials used in the treatment of the human mouth in the same form and concentration as they may be made use of in the form of a mouth-wash. Usually in rinsing the mouth the solution remains from a few seconds to at most a minute in connection with the mucous membrane and the teeth; and we need accordingly for the purpose of sterilizing the oral cavity a material which in the adapted concentration is able to devitalize bacteria inside of a minute. How far this is accomplished by the means at our command may be seen from the following table:

Antiseptic.	Concentration.	Time necessary for devitalization.
*Salicylic acid	1 : 100	¼ minute
*Benzoic acid	1 : 100	¼ "
Listerine	——	¼ to ½ minute.
Salicylic acid	1 : 200	½ "
Bichloride of mercury	1 : 2500	½ to ¾ "
Benzoic acid	1 : 200	1 to 2 minutes
Borobenzoic acid	1 : 175	1 to 2 "
Thymol	1 : 1500	2 to 4 "
Bichloride of mercury	1 : 5000	2 to 5 "
Peroxide of hydrogen	10 per cent.	10 to 15 "
Carbolic acid	1 : 100	10 to 15 "
Oil of peppermint in agreeable strength	——	5 to 10 "
Permanganate of potash	1 : 4000	more than 15 minutes
Boric acid	1 : 50	" " 15 "
Oil of wintergreen	——	" " 15 "
Tincture of cinchona	1 : 18	" " 15 "
Lime-water	——	no action.

The above experiments were made in the following manner:

A determined quantity of a pure culture of a ferment bacterium of the mouth is brought into 0.5 c.cm. of the antiseptic to be tested, and then in determined intervals single drops of this mixture are brought into test tubes containing 5 c.cm. of a nutritive solution. If a development of bacteria does not take place in any tube or tubes, it may be taken as an indication that the bacteria were devitalized in the corresponding time.

* Salicylic and benzoic acids may be applied in this concentration only on the brush.

Control experiments were naturally made at the same time. A number of tests which I made with a coccus found in a case of mycosis tonsillaris benigna led to the same result.

It appears from the above experiments that only few of these substances are serviceable for the purpose of cleansing the mouth. The bichloride of mercury is the most active, not only because it has the highest antiseptic power, but because its action continues for a longer time. Even after the solution has been removed from the mouth, traces remaining retain their antiseptic action, even when they have been diluted from one to two hundred times by the fluids of the mouth. None of the other materials possess this property in so high a degree. Furthermore, sublimate appears to penetrate particles of food, deposits, etc., more rapidly than the other materials given. I have satisfied myself by many experiments that it is possible, after a complete mechanical cleansing of the mouth, to obtain by means of sublimate (1–2500) an almost perfect sterilization of the mouth. Unfortunately, the application of the bichloride of mercury is limited, on account of its very poisonous properties.

As for salicylic acid, many are of the opinion that it attacks the teeth (decalcifies them), and that it consequently should never be used in the mouth. On the other hand, others deny this action. I myself have seen it used for years without any evil consequences, and do not fear to use it now and then in the strength of 1–200 or 1–300.

In all diseases of the human mouth in which antiseptics are indicated, particularly in acute infectious diseases, salicylic acid may be used for a short time without any danger to the teeth. For continual use perhaps the milder, though somewhat weaker, benzoic acid in the concentration of 1–200 is preferable, unless it should turn out that this also may have an injurious effect upon the teeth.

Listerine has proved to be a very useful and active antiseptic. This is a preparation of Lambert & Co., in St. Louis, consisting of oil of eucalyptus, borobenzoic acid, wintergreen oil, etc.; it owes its antiseptic property probably more to the borobenzoic acid than to the oil of eucalyptus. It is to be applied on the brush in cleansing the teeth, or slightly diluted as a mouth-wash.

For cleansing root-canals, cavities, etc., the more powerful antiseptics are of course preferable.

Wintergreen oil and similar aromatic substances, which usually form an important constituent of mouth-washes, have as far as I have examined them, in an adaptable concentration, very little antiseptic action, unless the oil of peppermint is an exception. This possesses considerable antiseptic action, and is consequently as a constituent of mouth-washes to be preferred to the other ethereal oils. According to Black,[132] however, oil of cassia, oil of cinnamon, and oil of cloves have a much higher antiseptic action than the oil of peppermint. The results obtained by Black, in so far as they refer to the oil of cloves and oil of peppermint, are in direct contradiction to those obtained by Koch, who found that the oil of peppermint has an action nearly seven times as strong as that of the oil of cloves. This difference is no doubt to be accounted for in the difference of the bacteria experimented upon.

If we compare the two tables last given, we find some apparent contradictions. For example, listerine, which is, according to one table, forty times weaker than a 10 per cent. solution of the peroxide of hydrogen, devitalizes bacteria much more quickly than the latter. I am able to explain this remarkable difference only on the supposition that the rapidity with which an antiseptic acts need by no means be proportional to its strength. We must furthermore distinguish clearly between those substances which only *prevent development*, as indicated in the first three tables, and those which devitalize, as indicated in the last table. It is possible that an agent may prevent the development of bacteria in very dilute solutions, and yet not devitalize them even in more concentrated condition.

In the third place, it may be readily conceived that a highly diffusible substance may penetrate the cell-membrane more quickly and therefore act more rapidly than a less diffusible one, even though the latter may retard or prevent development in a much more dilute condition.

Recently I have tested salol, aseptine, and the acetate of aluminium in a similar manner. Salol is a very agreeable antiseptic, but in my experiments it showed very little action.

Aseptine compared with thymol, sublimate, carbolic acid, etc., is a very weak antiseptic, but it has the advantage that it may be applied in concentrated solutions. Acetate of aluminium is an old medicament still adhered to by many physicians; it combines considerable antiseptic power with a strong astringent action. The strongest solution which may be used in the human mouth had in some cases a marked action, but on the whole not strong enough to encourage me in its use.

I finally made a series of experiments with various mixtures, my aim being to combine a number of antiseptics in such a manner as to produce the greatest possible antiseptic action with the least possible action upon the mucous membrane and the teeth, etc.

My experiments were made on the following mixtures:

(1)	Water	50.00	(4)	Water	50.00
	Alcohol	5.00		Alcohol	5.00
	Tinct. eucalypt.	0.75		Tinct. eucalypt.	0.75
	Benzoic acid	0.15		Benzoic acid	0.15
	Thymol	0.0125		Thymol	0.0125
				Bichloride of mercury	0.025
(2)	Listerine	25.5			
	Water	25.0	(5)	Water	25.00
				Aseptin	25.00
(3)	Aseptin	25.00		Salol	5.00
	Water	25.00		Alcohol	5.00
	Alcohol	5.00		Acetate of aluminium	1.50
	Tinct. eucalypt.	0.75		Benzoic acid	0.15
	Benzoic acid	0.15		Thymol	0.0125
	Thymol	0.0125		Tinct. eucalypt.	0.75

These mixtures are not mouth-washes, but they might serve as bases for mouth-washes, as indicated below.

The alcohol was added only as a solvent, not because of its antiseptic powers.

As a mouth-wash, we need above all a solution which acts *quickly*, and which does not simply prevent the development of micro-organisms while it is acting, but which devitalizes them.

There are agents which, even in very dilute form, if applied constantly have a powerful antiseptic action, inasmuch as they prevent the development of such micro-organisms as may be present without, however, devitalizing them; such agents are of no more value as antiseptics in the treatment of the oral cavity than an equal amount of distilled water. It is seldom that any-one in rinsing his mouth will retain the wash longer than one minute, and an antiseptic mouth-wash, to be efficient, should be able to devitalize the micro-organisms with which it comes in contact within this short time.

Solution No. 4 accomplishes this for nearly, if not for all, micro-organisms in the vegetative form. A solution which devitalizes spores in one minute is out of the question, and, in fact, is not at all necessary, since the conditions which lead to the formation of spores do not exist in the mouth, where we find almost exclusively the vegetative forms.

This solution (No. 4) has a decided action in one-fourth to one-half of a minute; in one minute the sterilization is nearly or quite complete.

Next to this came the solutions Nos. 5, 3, and 1, in close order; the addition of aseptin and acetate of aluminium, both of which, but particularly the former, are antiseptics of considerable strength, did not produce the hoped-for increase in the action of the solution. The addition of salol had, as I anticipated, no effect whatever. These solutions produced a decided diminution in the number of colonies in half a minute; a complete sterilization usually required two minutes, sometimes even longer.

Nearly as strong as these solutions was a 50 per cent. solution of listerine, which also has the advantage of a very agreeable taste and odor.

Now, it very often happens that the centers of decay about the teeth are filled with particles of food, and we do not in such cases have liquids to sterilize, but solid substances impregnated with micro-organisms; what effect can we produce upon these by the action of the solutions given above?

To determine this question, a second series of experiments was made in the following manner:

Small porous bodies (bread, meat, paper, etc.), of as nearly the same size as possible, were saturated with bouillon containing certain micro-organisms, or with stale saliva, then subjected to the action of the antiseptic solutions during a specified length of time, after which they were brought into culture-gelatine and the number of colonies which developed determined. The stronger the antiseptic and the longer the time of exposure, the less will be the number of colonies which develop in the culture tube. As control, the experiment was repeated, using sterilized water instead of an antiseptic solution.

To avoid transferring too much of the antiseptic to the culture tube, each piece was placed for an instant on sterilized blotting-paper, to remove the excess of liquid. I give the results of one of these experiments below. In this solution No. 4 was made use of, and *small* pieces of bread charged with bacteria subjected to the action of the solution 20, 35, 55, 70, 90, and 120 seconds respectively. The control tube developed 4500 colonies:

Tube	1 (20 seconds action)	developed	420	colonies.
"	2 (35 " ")	"	46	"
"	3 (55 " ")	"	250	"
"	4 (70 " ")	"	13	"
"	5 (90 " ")	"	1	colony.
"	6 (120 " ")	remained sterile.		

It may appear strange that tube 3 should develop more colonies than tube 2, but such irregularities often occur, owing to the fact that it is not possible to obtain pieces of bread or meat of *exactly* the same size and consistency. The result of the experiment is, however, very clear. When large compact pieces were used (as large as a pea, for example), such as may sometimes be found in cavities of decay, it required as much as ten to fifteen minutes to effect a complete sterilization. The lesson is plain. Even such a powerful wash as the one under consideration will accomplish but little in sterilizing the human mouth when the centers of decay are stuffed full of food. This is also the reason why excessive smoking, notwithstanding the fact that tobacco-smoke is a powerful antiseptic, does not insure the teeth against decay; the smoke passes over the surface, but does not penetrate to the point of action. It follows that the use of the mouth-wash should always be preceded by the thorough use of the brush or toothpick, removing at least all larger particles of food and opening the spaces between the teeth, so that the wash may penetrate to the vulnerable point. If this is conscientiously done, I think that we have in solution No. 4, and, in a less degree, in the other solutions specified, a powerful means of preventing the excessive ravages of decay. The solutions 1 and 4 may be made use of in the following form:

No. 1.	Thymol	0.25 grams.
	Benzoic acid	3.00 "
	Tincture of eucalyptus . . .	15.00 "
	Alcohol	100.00 "
	Oil of wintergreen	25 drops
	(or oil of peppermint	20 ")

In use, enough of this mixture is added to a mouthful of water to produce a decided cloudiness.

The wash, no doubt, may be rendered softer and more palatable by the addition of glycerine, tincture of catechu, or something of the kind. Perhaps some one who is interested in mouth-washes will kindly undertake the task.

No. 4 is prepared in the same way, with the addition of 0.8 bichloride of mercury:

Acid. thymic.	0.25
Acid. benzoic.	3.00
Hydrarg. bichlorid.	0.80
Tinct. eucalypt.	15.00
Alcohol absolut.	100.00
Ol. gaultheriæ	gtt. xxv.

One naturally hesitates to prescribe a mouth-wash which contains bichloride of mercury, but I think a more thorough consideration of the question will show that it is not so reprehensible an act as may at first appear.

The strength in which the bichloride is used in the mouth is about $\frac{1}{2000}$. Let us suppose that the patient swallows of the solution two grams daily (as a matter of fact, one need not swallow any at all); it would require one hundred days to have swallowed 0.1 gram of the salt, which is the maximum dose for one day. In this matter, however, reasoning is of little value;

nowhere is the saying in medicine, experience is of greater value than reasoning, truer than in questions dealing with the physiological action of the salts of mercury. I, myself, have made extensive use of the above formula without a trace of any physiological or toxicological action, and if a sufficient number of members of the profession would make a trial of this solution upon themselves, and report the results, a great deal would be done toward solving the question of the advisability of recommending the wash in practice.

The taste of the bichloride is exceedingly disagreeable, even in dilute solutions; it may to a certain extent be disguised by the use of rose-water in place of aqua destillata as a solvent, as suggested by Allan.

Unfortunately, our pharmacopœia is not yet so rich that the physician or dentist can restrict himself to the use of good-tasting medicaments.

I have been informed by some who have used the bichloride as a mouth-wash that whereas it has most excellent effect in all suppurative diseases of the gums, it discolors the teeth. This of course would be a serious disadvantage if it should prove to be true. All the discoloration I have ever observed could be readily removed with brush and powder.

On the whole, however, the fear of a possible toxic effect from the bichloride, which, in consideration of the fact that certain individuals are extremely sensitive to the action of this drug, we shall scarcely be able to escape from, will probably prevent its ever being extensively introduced except for occasional use in acute infectious and putrid conditions of the mouth. I personally have never prescribed it for prolonged use, except for a few friends who were in a position to control its action. From such the only complaint I have heard has been of its bad taste.

Witzel is enthusiastic in his praise of sublimate in the treatment of putrid and septic conditions of the mouth. "A few drops of a 2 per cent. ethereal solution of sublimate in a glass of water suffice to remove for a short time the most offensive smell from the mouth." "Syringing the alveoli with sublimate 1–1000 followed by the injection of six to eight drops of a 2 per cent. solution into the septic parts . . . . as most sovereign medicament in case of septic alveolitis." In septic wounds following extractions, syringing with sublimate 1–1000 twice a day was continued for eight days with most beneficial results, etc.

In the last few years a large number of different materials have been recommended as disinfectants for the mouth. The most of them, however, have been as yet too little tested to enable us to give an estimation of their value.

Von Kaczorowski [133] recommends iodine-chloride of sodium solution (Natrium chloratum 1 per cent., Tr. Iodi 0.5 per cent.), one-half to a whole teaspoonful every quarter to half hour.

Truman praises hydronaphthol, which he finds as efficient as it is harmless.

Black [132] recommends a mixture of carbolic acid 1, oil of wintergreen 2, oil of sassafras 3. Others recommend iodol, sozoiodol, betanaphthol, sanitas oil, etc.

Witzel [134] recommends his so-called 20 per cent. solution of sublimate, for root-treatments, which, however, is said to discolor the teeth. Personally I use a 1 to 5 per cent. solution for the same purpose, and a ½ to 1 per cent. solution for syringing abscesses or suppurating wounds after extraction, and for the latter purposes in particular find it decidedly superior to either 2 per cent. carbolic acid or 5 per cent. peroxide of hydrogen.

Busch [135] has obtained most beneficial results from the use of peroxide of hydrogen, particularly in putrid and septic conditions of the gums, and is of the opinion that no other antiseptic at present in use is to be compared with this. He adds a sufficient quantity of the so-called 10 per cent. solution to water to produce about a 2 to 3 per cent. solution for rinsing the mouth.

Harlan has also enriched the dental materia medica with a considerable number of new antiseptics.

I lay no particular value on tooth-powder as a means of cleaning the teeth. It is true that the external surfaces, particularly of the front teeth, may be kept whiter by the use of tooth-powder, but the centers of decay are more liable to become stopped up than to be cleansed by tooth-powder, particularly when they contain insoluble constituents.

Somewhat more recommendable I find the tooth-soaps, in so

far as they dissolve fatty substances without attacking the teeth, and, furthermore, possibly make the penetration of the bristles of the tooth-brush into the center of decay somewhat more easy. They should be made of neutral soap, and have a neutral or slight alkaline reaction. Under all conditions, however, the chief thing is the thorough mechanical cleansing of the teeth.

THE ANTISEPTIC ACTION OF FILLING-MATERIALS.

It will scarcely be questioned by anyone acquainted with the nature of those diseases of the teeth which we treat by filling, that in a great many cases, if not in all, the probability of success would be greatly heightened if the filling-material could be made to exert a permanent antiseptic action upon the walls and margin of the cavity. This is more particularly true of all cases where, for some reason or other, carious dentine is left in the cavity at the time of filling; and such cases constantly occur in every dental practice. There are, I hope, very few practitioners in dentistry who place so high an estimate upon their own skill and thoroughness, or so far overlook the imperfection in the structure of the dentine, as to imagine that they excavate every cavity perfectly. Many even *prefer* leaving a thin layer of softened dentine in the cavity to removing it, if the pulp would thereby be exposed. Others, no doubt, for very humane reasons, sometimes excavate less thoroughly than they otherwise would do, in order to spare their patient the excessive pain accompanying the operation, or because the patient cannot or will not bear the pain. Most of us, for the sake of our backs, toward the end of a hard day's work, now and then decide that a difficult cavity is ready to fill when a careful examination of it might still reveal soft points. It is not necessary, however, to enumerate other cases in which the preparation of the cavity is not quite faultless; most readers will no doubt be able to suggest many more.

Now, it may appear remarkable that, while so much attention has of late years been bestowed upon the antiseptic treatment of root-canals and the employment of antiseptic materials for filling them, very little attention has been given to the subject of the antiseptic materials for filling cavities of decay; iodoform cement being, as far as I know, the only material which was introduced with this object in view. That it does not accomplish its object will, I think, be apparent from the experiments recorded below.

METHODS.—I.

Various methods may be employed for determining the antiseptic action of filling-materials. The two which I have made use of are exceedingly simple, and at the same time very instructive. In applying the first of these methods we proceed as follows: A tube of ordinary nutritive gelatine is infected with a bacterium from the oral cavity, which grows rapidly at room temperature without liquefying the gelatine. The gelatine is then melted, slightly shaken, so as to distribute the fungi equally throughout the solution, and poured upon a horizontal sterilized glass plate, upon which we drop pieces of the filling-material or other substances whose antiseptic action we wish to determine. As soon as the gelatine becomes stiff we place the plate in a damp chamber. A plate prepared in this way, without the addition of any material having an antiseptic action, will become cloudy and opaque in the course of twenty-four to forty-eight hours, through the development of innumerable colonies of bacteria. If, however, the pieces of filling-materials which we have dropped upon the plate possess an antiseptic action, the development of the fungi in their neighborhood will be retarded or altogether prevented, and each piece will appear surrounded by an area of transparent gelatine whose size will depend upon the activity of the antiseptic employed. Most of the filling-materials in use were tested by this method in respect to the antiseptic action, with the result that the only one which possesses such action and retains it for an indefinite time after it has been inserted is copper amalgam.* Not only freshly-mixed fillings, but pieces of old, half-worn-out fillings, taken from teeth extracted in the polyclinic of the Dental Institute, and even pieces of *dentine* from teeth which had been filled with copper amalgam, in-

* Regarding an unexpected antiseptic action of certain preparations of gold which might appear to furnish an exception to this rule, see the experiments described below.

variably manifested a retarding or preventing action upon the growth of bacteria. (Fig. 106.)

These results accord exactly with those which I obtained by entirely different methods in 1884 (*Independent Practitioner*, June), and which have been called in question by Bogue and others.

Of course it must not be inferred from these remarks that a little piece of copper amalgam dropped into a liter of bouillon will keep it from spoiling. Nor would an experiment of this nature be a just test of the antiseptic action of a material used in filling.

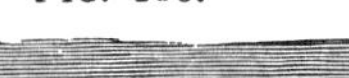

Fig. 106.

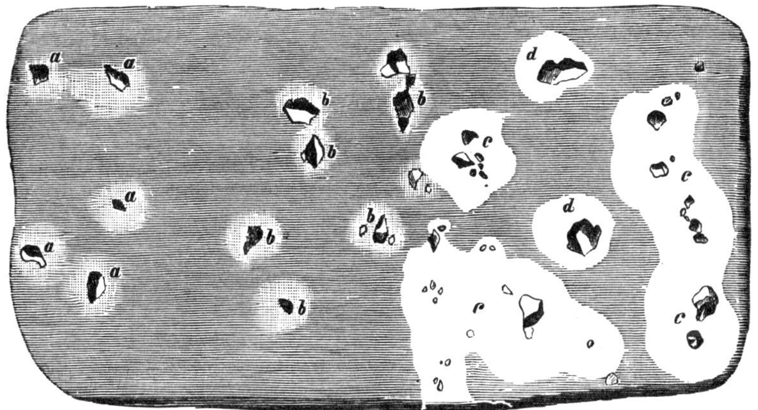

An inoculated gelatine plate containing: *a*, pieces of oxyphosphate cement one day old; *b*, pieces of gold amalgam one day old; *c*, pieces of an old copper amalgam filling, age unknown; *d*, pieces of stained dentine from a tooth which had been filled many years previously with copper amalgam.

If the filling prevents the progress of decay in softened dentine under it or in immediate contact with it, and if it retards the progress of fermentation in fine spaces (leakages) between it and the marginal wall, then it is doing a great deal toward preventing the recurrence of caries, which another filling not possessing antiseptic properties would not do.

That so much is accomplished by copper amalgam, I am, I believe, justified in concluding from the experiments enumerated above, and more particularly from those made under the second method and described below. It is a view, moreover, pretty generally accepted by all operators who have had opportunity of observing the action of copper amalgam fillings, that they do possess a preserving action upon tooth-substance. I, along with most others, formerly accounted for this action upon the supposition that copper amalgam does not shrink while setting. I meet almost daily with amalgam fillings, not containing copper, which admit of the point of an excavator being inserted between the filling and the margin of the cavity, whereas copper amalgam fillings appear to hug the walls of the cavity perfectly.

FIG. 107.

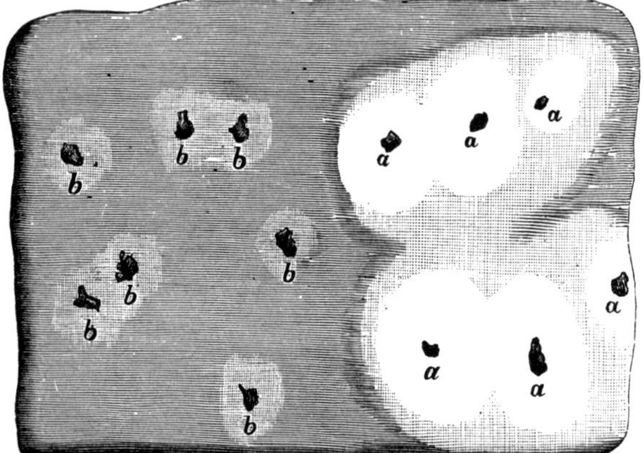

AN INOCULATED GELATINE PLATE containing pieces of freshly-mixed cement. *a*, oxychloride; *b*, oxyphosphate. A very marked hindrance in the development of the bacteria is noted around the pieces of oxychloride: around the pieces of oxyphosphate it is scarcely perceptible. Plate twenty-four hours old.

Elliott,* however, found by a very extended series of experiments that copper amalgams do contract, and some of them to a surprising degree. Elliott's results are corroborated by the evidence of J. Boyd Wallis,† who claims that the slight contraction is a distinct advantage in the case of soft and sensitive teeth, because of the more speedy formation of the oxide or sulphide, which, being absorbed by the surrounding dentine, protects it from further progress of decay. "Pulps dying under copper amalgam

* Transactions of the Odontological Society of Great Britain, December, 1888.

† *Dental Record*, February, 1889.

fillings do not so readily decompose, owing to their becoming charged with antiseptic cupric salts."

Other materials experimented with by the first method were gold amalgam, oxychloride of zinc (agate cement), oxyphosphate of zinc (Caulk's cement), gutta-percha, gold, tin, and tin-gold.

Gold amalgam, freshly mixed, caused a slight retardation in the development of bacteria ; old pieces had no effect. Oxychloride of zinc, fresh, had a very marked action. (See Fig. 107.) Pieces which had lain twenty-four hours in saliva and bread lost their antiseptic power. Oxyphosphate of zinc, fresh, had a slight, in-

Fig. 108.

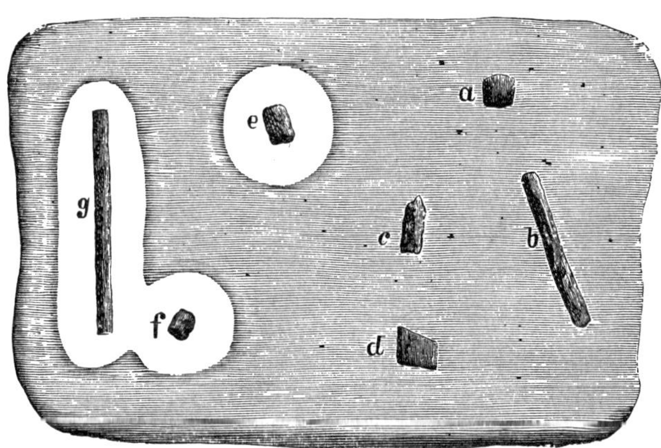

Inoculated gelatine plate containing Pack's pellets and Abbey's foil No. 4, folded to make strips of No. 32. *a*, *b*, *c*, *d*, annealed ; *e*, *f*, *g*, unannealed. The latter have retarded the growth of the bacteria in their neighborhood, as is shown by the gelatine remaining clear. Plate twenty-four hours old.

constant action (Fig. 107), sometimes none at all. After twenty-four hours' exposure in a mixture of saliva and bread, it showed no action whatever ; gutta-percha and tin proved completely inactive.

The results obtained with gold were very peculiar and perplexing. Some preparations of gold manifest a decided restraining effect upon the development of bacteria, so that if a pellet is dropped upon the plate it will after twenty-four to forty-eight hours appear surrounded by a perfectly round circle of transparent gelatine, separated from the clouded gelatine by a sharp border. Within this zone the bacteria develop very slowly, so that the cloudiness appears much later than on other parts of the plate. The antiseptic action of Pack's pellets was particularly marked. Plugs of the unannealed pellets made in holes bored in wood showed considerable action, even after they had lain for forty-eight to seventy-two hours in a mixture of saliva and bread. Also Abbey's soft foil and quarter-century foil showed similar action, but in a somewhat less degree. Other preparations showed varied effects; some were almost or quite indifferent. *The antiseptic action was completely destroyed by annealing the gold beforehand* (Fig. 108). Some preparations of sponge gold and platinum gold acted in a similar manner, and even old gold fillings now and then showed considerable antiseptic action.

I shall not attempt to give any explanation for these facts now. Different explanations suggest themselves, none, however, with which I have been quite satisfied. Nor will I at present endeavor to answer the question whether the action is strong enough to be entitled to any consideration as a saving property of unannealed gold. I am inclined to think that it would be rather venturesome to assert that it is.

Tin-gold was less active than gold alone.

I applied this method of testing the antiseptic property of filling-materials to a few other substances; among them to iodoform, which did not have the slightest action in checking the growth of the micro-organisms tested.

II.

In order to make a direct test of the action of fillings upon carious dentine or upon the micro-organisms contained in it, we proceed as follows: A number of freshly-extracted teeth which are extensively decayed, not, however, so as to expose the pulp, are cleansed of the remains of food, and only partially excavated, so as to leave a thick layer of carious dentine in each cavity.

The cavities are then filled with various substances whose antiseptic action we wish to test, and the teeth placed in a mixture of saliva and bread and kept for three days at a temperature of 30° C. to 40° C. At the end of this time they are taken out, washed in pure water, placed for a moment in sublimate

1–1000, then in a larger quantity of sterilized water to remove the sublimate, after which they are dried with sterilized bibulous paper. We then take the teeth by the root or roots, rest the side of the crown upon a small anvil, and strike a sharp blow upon it with a hammer. The filling flies out, exposing the untouched surface of carious dentine. We now with a sterilized spoon-shaped excavator remove a small piece of the carious dentine and place it upon a previously prepared plate of sterile nutritive agar-agar. The plate is then put away in a moist

FIG. 109.

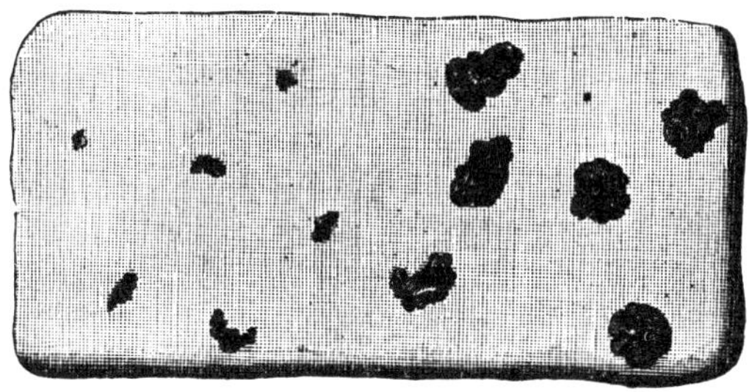

A STERILE AGAR-AGAR PLATE, containing in the left half pieces of dentine from a cavity which had been filled with copper amalgam, in the right half pieces from a cavity which had been filled with gold amalgam. The former have remained sterile, whereas an extensive growth of bacteria has taken place around the latter. Plate three days old.

chamber at or near the temperature of the human body. If now the bacteria in the carious dentine have been killed by the action of the filling-material, or if the dentine has been so acted upon by the material as itself to become antiseptic, no growth will develop around it; otherwise we will find in the course of forty-eight to sixty hours that the piece of dentine becomes surrounded by a growth of varying extent.

In examining the plates, a low power of the microscope should be used in cases where a growth is not visible to the naked eye. Furthermore, a slight cloudiness or precipitate which sometimes forms around pieces impregnated with copper salts must not be mistaken for micro-organisms; and lastly, a development of bud-fungi (yeast-fungi, Saccharomycetes), or mould-fungi (Hyphomycetes), which is very frequently observed, must not be mistaken for bacteria (Schizomycetes).

The following materials were examined by this method:

1. Copper amalgam (Lippoldt's). Fifteen teeth were treated as described, and the carious dentine examined by culture. In not a single case did a development of bacteria take place. They had either been devitalized or the dentine itself had become antiseptic. In two cases bud-fungi developed; in one case mould-fungi.

2. Gold amalgam, ten teeth. In all cases a development of bacteria took place around the dentine, to say nothing of bud- and mould-fungi (Fig. 109).

3. Oxyphosphate, eight teeth. Result same as with gold amalgam.

4. Oxychloride of zinc, eight teeth. In seven cases a growth of bacteria formed, though very much retarded when compared with the oxyphosphate or gold amalgam. In one case the piece remained sterile.

5. Iodoform powder mixed with phosphate cement, one tooth. Development of bacteria unchecked. In another case the floor of the cavity was covered with powdered iodoform and oxyphosphate filled over. Pieces of dentine taken from the cavity after three days and transferred to the culture plate were soon surrounded by a growth of bacteria and bud-fungi.

6. Powdered sulphate of copper incorporated with cement or with gutta-percha, or simply strewn upon the bottom of the cavity before filling, nine teeth. No trace of bacterial growth appeared in any case.

From these results we are forced to the conclusion that copper amalgam fillings exert a marked antibacterial influence upon the walls of the cavities containing them, that oxychloride cements have an appreciable though markedly less effect, and that oxyphosphate and gold amalgam are wanting in any such action. We learn, furthermore, that by incorporating certain antiseptics into the mass of the filling or covering the bottom of the cavity before inserting the filling we may produce an effect analogous to that of copper amalgam.

Can any application of these results be made in practice? I think so, though I am certainly not in favor of being over-hasty in drawing conclusions.

Personally, I have always had much faith in the preservative properties of copper amalgam fillings, because I have had abundant opportunity to observe the splendid results obtained by its use even when very little care was taken in its insertion. The experiments which I have made have naturally served to strengthen my confidence in this material, in consequence of which I have been using it to some extent in my practice. At the cervical margin I often put a layer of copper amalgam, and then fill the rest of the cavity with some other material. In cases of complicated caries extending under the gum and very near the pulp, where phosphate fillings are utterly unreliable, and even combined with gutta-percha often very unsatisfactory, and where it is not considered wise to risk a permanent filling at once, I protect the neck of the tooth by copper amalgam, allowing a very thin layer to extend over the floor of the cavity in order to thoroughly sterilize the dentine and keep it sterile. I then fill the remaining part of the cavity with cement or gutta-percha, with the intention, in case all goes well, of replacing it in some months by a permanent material.

I am inclined to believe that the use of antiseptic materials may be accompanied by excellent results also for capping exposed pulps, particularly when they are not in a healthy condition, or contain germs of infection, as well as for covering the floor of the cavity in all cases where the pulp is protected by but a thin layer of dentine, which is very often more or less softened, or even infected with bacteria. For this purpose sulphate of copper, incorporated with gutta-percha or with some soft cement like oxysulphate, would, I am convinced, go far to effectually sterilize the thin layer of dentine covering the pulp, and thereby to prevent not only the decomposition of such softened dentine as may have been left over the pulp, but also the infection of the latter, which is very often the cause of pulp-troubles arising under fillings.

The sulphate of copper, however, seriously stains dead teeth in the course of three days, and would probably act with equal rapidity upon living teeth, so that its use would be on that account very much restricted, if not altogether contraindicated. Dr. Cunningham, of Cambridge, informs me, however, that he has been using the sulphate of copper in this manner for some time, without any discoloration resulting.

Various substances suggest themselves, which, being incorporated with cement or gutta-percha, might do good service as antiseptic dressings over diseased pulps or over softened dentine; first of all, naturally, the bichloride of mercury. Which of the many available antiseptics, however, is best adapted to the purpose must be determined by further experiments in the laboratory and in practice.

The practice of treating exposed pulps, whether healthy or diseased, to a bath of concentrated carbolic acid has been sharply criticised by various writers. There are nevertheless many practitioners in high standing who treat all exposures of the pulp in this manner, and claim to obtain better results than by any other method. I will not venture to say that this may not be so, because the ill effects of so severely cauterizing the pulp-tissue may be balanced by the good effects of thorough antiseptic treatment. If we, however, could attain the same object by the use of less irritating agents, our probability of success would be much greater.

Further experiments relating to this subject are now in progress, and will be reported in due time.

THE ACTION OF TOBACCO UPON THE TEETH.

Five grammes of old Virginia plug were boiled fifteen minutes in 50 c.cm. of water, the loss by evaporation being constantly replaced; the decoction was then filtered, and a portion added to an equal volume of saliva with sugar. This produced a mixture scarcely stronger than that which many veteran chewers carry around in their mouths all day, and in it the bacteria led only a miserable existence.

Much more remarkable, however, was the action of tobacco-smoke upon the micro-organisms of the mouth; the smoke from the first third or last quarter of a Colorado Claro cigar being found amply sufficient to sterilize 10 c.cm. of a beef-extract-sugar solution, previously richly infected with bacteria from decayed dentine.

The apparatus used for this experiment (Fig. 110) explains itself. A current of water passing through the part B in the direction of the ↘ produces a current of air through the part A, in the direction of the ↘, which draws the smoke from a lighted cigar through the solution. The rate at which the cigar smokes may be regulated at will by the cock of the hydrant. The results of my experiments, which I[136] published in 1884, have been completely confirmed by an extended series of experiments by Tassinari.[137]

FIG. 110.

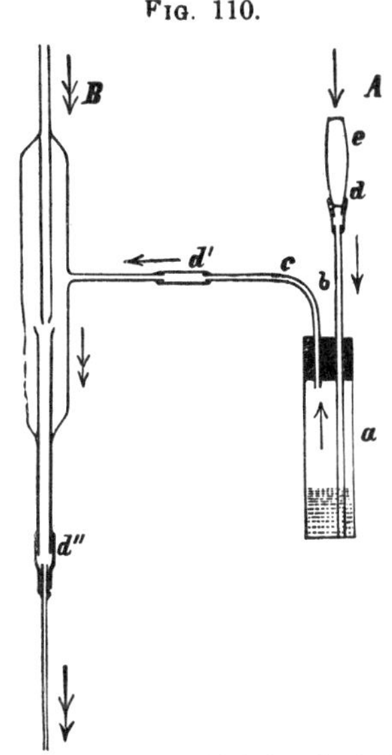

a, glass cylinder with infected solution; *b*, *c*, glass tubes; *d*, *d'*, *d''*, rubber tubing; *e*, cigar (Colorado Claro); *B*, water air-pump; *A*, current of water passing through *B* in the direction of the double arrow produces a partial vacuum in the bulb, and consequently a current of air in the direction of the arrow or through the cigar, which if lighted will smoke at a rate determined by the pressure under which the water is flowing.

In consideration of the strong antiseptic power of tobacco-smoke, we might be inclined to infer that tobacco-smokers should never suffer from decay of the teeth; it is evident, however, that there are many points in the dental arch, particularly when the teeth are not kept scrupulously clean, to which the smoke never penetrates.

THE STERILIZATION OF TEETH FOR THE PURPOSE OF IMPLANTATION.

It is well known that operations designated as replantation, in which a diseased tooth is extracted, cleansed, and returned to its alveolus again, and transplantation, in which a tooth taken from one individual is planted into the alveolus of another, which has been emptied by extraction, have now and then been performed by individual dentists for two and a half centuries.* Since some few years, a similar but more serious operation is being

* Dupont, Remède contre le mal des dents, 1633, recommended for toothache the extraction and replantation of the tooth.

performed, which consists in making an artificial alveolus at any point of the dental arch, which may have been toothless for an indefinite length of time, and consequently contains no alveolus, and often but little alveolar process, and then implanting the proper tooth in this artificial alveolus.

For this purpose teeth are often used concerning whose origin, whether from healthy or diseased individuals, nothing is known; and it becomes a question of great importance, for the patient as well as for the operator, whether or not infectious diseases may not be communicated in this way.

John Hunter[138] (1786), in whose time the operation of transplantation seems to have been extensively performed, describes seven cases in which it was followed by serious disturbances of an infectious nature. Hunter, who combatted the tendency then existing to ascribe all such disturbances to syphilitic inoculation, was forced to admit the transmission of syphilis in two out of the seven cases. He also readily admits the possibility of such inoculations through dental operations.

J. C. Lettsom[139] (1786) reports a number of cases which came under his notice, some of which he pronounced undoubted syphilis. He gives the following description of one case *resembling* syphilis: Eight weeks after the transplantation of two teeth the patient has a painful sensation between the roots, followed by ulceration through the gums and by soreness of the glands of the neck and throat. Within three or four days efflorescence of the skin appears, advancing to an eruption resembling syphilis. Inflammation and ulceration of the tonsils also occur, together with fever in the evening and profuse sweats in the morning. The teeth gradually loosen and almost fall out. Exophthalmia in one eye. Eight weeks later a similar attack came on. Both attacks were successfully treated with mercurials.

Of all cases of transplanting one in twenty have this disease, and one-fourth of these die.

In my judgment, the dentist who undertakes the above operation without having previously convinced himself that the tooth to be implanted is in a perfectly aseptic condition, or most certainly contains no specific germs, commits a serious wrong.

But how can we thoroughly sterilize a tooth? We must, in

the first place, reconcile ourselves to the fact that a complete sterilization of a suspected tooth with the conservation of the periosteum is absolutely out of the question. It is not alone necessary to sterilize the surface of the tooth, but the whole substance of the tooth; and since under certain circumstances the cement-lacunæ, as well as the dentinal tubules, may contain bacteria, it is not to be supposed for a moment that we can reach and kill them in these portions without injuring the pericementum. The transplantation or implantation of a tooth with living pericementum is therefore practicable only in such cases where the tooth is taken directly from a living, perfectly healthy individual, and placed at once, under antiseptic precautions, into the alveolus.

In all other cases it is better first to remove the pericementum, since it must be devitalized in the process of sterilization, and the dead pericementum can act only as an irritant, and delay the healing process. For implantation, chiefly old dry teeth have been made use of, and in such cases the pericementum is naturally already dead before beginning the disinfection.

The usual method of disinfection, placing the teeth in dilute solutions of bichloride of mercury for a few minutes or even hours, gives no guarantee that the teeth are made absolutely sterile. How are we to know whether the solution penetrates into the microscopic spaces of the tooth, the cement-lacunæ, channels of chance blood-vessels, dentinal tubuli, etc., which are filled with air? Dry teeth placed for a number of hours in watery solutions of coloring-matter show no penetration of the coloring-matter worthy of mention.

Under high pressure the permeation of the external layers of the tooth with the solution might probably be accomplished. A certain sterilization, however, can be effected by heat alone, either by boiling water or by steam at 100° C. In order to devitalize such spores as may be present, it will be necessary to repeat the sterilization process two or three times, at intervals of about twelve hours. A large number of teeth might be sterilized at one time in a flask closed with cotton, and in this shape put away for later use.

PART II.

THE PATHOGENIC MOUTH-BACTERIA,

AND

THE DISEASES WHICH THEY PRODUCE.

CHAPTER X

THE BUCCAL SECRETIONS AS CARRIERS OF TOXIC SUBSTANCES AND OF PARASITIC EXCITANTS OF DISEASES.

It is a well-known fact that the inflammatory processes in the tooth-pulp, pericementum, and gums, brought about by a diseased condition of the human teeth, lead not only to obstinate neuralgias, but also to severe diseases of the eye and ear, to eruptions of the skin, spasm of the muscles, etc.

Cases of spasms of the facial muscles, lockjaw, convulsions, spasm and paralysis of the ciliary and other muscles of the eye, strabismus, ptosis, lagophthalmus, epiphora, ectropium, asthenopy, amaurosis and amblyopia, mydriasis, myosis, glaucoma, cataract, keratitis, retinitis, conjunctivitis, panophthalmitis, etc., otitis, thrombosis of the sinuses of the brain, eczema of the face, indigestion consequent on imperfect mastication, nervousness, epileptic attacks, paralysis, etc., proceeding from decayed teeth, come to our notice, many of them repeatedly, in dental and medical literature. These are secondary affections caused by reflex action, in which the mouth-bacteria participate only in so far as they are to be regarded as the excitants of the primary diseases of the mouth. As is well known, similar phenomena very frequently occur during dentition, in obstructed eruptions of wisdom-teeth, in exostosis of the cement, formation of pulp-stones, etc.

The intimate connection of the quintus through the ganglia ciliare, spheno-palatinum, oticum et submaxillare with other cranial nerves and with the sympathicus, easily accounts for them.

We have, however, at present to occupy ourselves with the

infectious diseases of the oral cavity itself, and with those that are called forth by a migration of pathogenic micro-organisms from the mouth to more remote parts of the body.

TOXIC PROPERTIES OF MIXED HUMAN SALIVA.

The belief that the human saliva may under certain circumstances have a poisonous effect upon the animal body is by no means of recent origin. Habdarrhamus, Ægyptus, Aëtius (De re med. 2. 107), Ælianus, and many others were aware that the saliva of a person with an empty stomach is fatal to scorpions, and the celebrated Galen himself saw a scorpion killed by saliva without the use of magic. Aristotle observed a girl whose bite was as poisonous as the most fatal snake-bite; an arrow dipped in the saliva invariably killed anyone wounded by it (Stricker). Various other celebrated authorities of olden times who bear evidence to the poisonous character of the human saliva will be found in the work of Stricker,[140] from whom the above notes are taken. In modern and in very recent times the saliva has been the subject of repeated experiment on the part of both physiologists and pathologists.

Eberle[141] maintained that the saliva of persons excited or enraged or suffering pain acquired poisonous properties, which he accounted for by an increased formation of sulphocyanide of potassium. Eberle was actually able, as he thought, to detect an increase in the amount of this salt in his own saliva during rage or anger.

Senator[142] made subcutaneous injections of purulent sputum in dogs, and saw the animals soon sicken; they manifested high temperatures, chills, diarrhœa, etc., and perished without exception.

Wright observed that the injection of his own saliva into the stomach of dogs was invariably followed by sickness and vomiting. Since, however, Wright and others who followed him smoked tobacco in order to excite the flow of saliva, the toxic action is in this case to be attributed to the tobacco alone. When the experiments were repeated without the use of tobacco, no vomiting occurred.

Moriggia and Marchiafava (1878) demonstrated that an injection with the saliva of children who had died of lissa proved fatal to rabbits.

The first authors who referred the poisoning caused by the injection of mixed saliva to the presence of micro-organisms were, as I believe, Raynaud and Lannelongue.[143] They vaccinated rabbits with the saliva of a child afflicted with hydrophobia, and saw the rabbits die within forty-eight hours. Injections with the blood as well as with the buccal mucus of the dead child had negative results.

At the same time Pasteur[144] reported on experiments which he had made together with Chamberland and Roux, with the saliva of the same child. Two rabbits inoculated with it died after thirty-six hours. The micro-organisms from the blood, cultivated in bouillon, appeared as rods 1μ in diameter, contracted in the center, resembling the figure 8. They were surrounded by a gelatinous capsule. At first Pasteur thought he had discovered the cause of hydrophobia in this microbe, although Colin at once expressed the opinion that the disease called forth in rabbits by the experiments of Raynaud was not hydrophobia, but rather showed much more similarity to septicæmia. The rapid progress of the disease particularly spoke against the former supposition. Colin was accordingly the first to obtain an insight into the true nature of the affection following the injection of human saliva.

Vulpian[145] soon after reported that he had produced the same disease by vaccinating animals with the saliva of healthy persons. By subcutaneous injections of minute quantities of blood the disease could be transmitted from one animal to another. In the blood of these animals Bochefontaine and Arthaud found microbes which morphologically coincided with Pasteur's.

Sternberg[146] and Claxton, quite independently of the foregoing, corroborated Vulpian's statements, while Griffin[147] showed that pure parotid saliva is altogether harmless. In his opinion, the local and general phenomena which appeared after an injection with mixed saliva were caused by soluble or insoluble substances formed in it by putrefaction.

G. Gaglio and di Mattei[148] concluded that human saliva as such exerts no toxic influence, but gains its poisonous property by admixtures from the oral cavity. Boiled saliva exerts no, or but a comparatively insignificant, action.

A. Fränkel[149] further substantiated Vulpian's observations, and especially emphasized the remarkable fact that the microbes in question may be present in the saliva of one and the same individual at certain times and at others not.

Fränkel, as well as other observers, found rabbits best adapted for these experiments; mice and guinea-pigs also proved susceptible, whereas chickens, pigeons, and dogs were refractory. I[150] obtained the same results by inoculating mice and rabbits with the saliva of a woman afflicted with mycosis tonsillaris benigna. The saliva mixed with bouillon was allowed to stand for a number of hours at blood temperature, and then injected into the lungs of two rabbits and two mice. The death of all the animals resulted within thirty hours; in the blood I found numerous cocci and diplococci, most of them enveloped in a gelatinous capsule.

I furthermore isolated a micrococcus from decayed dentine which exhibited unquestionable pathogenic properties.

Klein[151] and others also call attention to the infectious properties of human saliva, particularly under diseased conditions. It was established by these numerous investigations, beyond doubt, that a group of micro-organisms belonging to the coccus form occurs almost invariably in the buccal juices, which, when brought into the circulatory system in sufficient numbers, may provoke the most dangerous diseases. Of late years, by the cultivation of mouth-bacteria on artificial media and in the animal body, the pronounced pathogenic properties of a large number of them have been conclusively demonstrated. The most important of these will be discussed below.

PATHOGENIC BACTERIA OF THE HUMAN MOUTH.

Not for the less dangerous ferment-bacteria alone, but for micro-organisms of a pathogenic nature as well, the oral cavity presents in point of temperature, moisture, nutritive materials, etc., an almost perfect breeding-place.

From this reason it is to be expected that among the many

pathogenic micro-organisms entering the mouth from time to time some may obtain at least a temporary foothold, or may propagate themselves for a certain length of time, as long as the conditions remain favorable, or finally may establish themselves permanently.

The observations of many bacteriologists have led to the unanimous conclusion that there is a large number of well-characterized mouth-microbes which will not grow on any of the artificial nutrient media now in use. The thought therefore suggests itself that there may be other bacteria in the mouth, which, possessing no striking morphological features and not growing on artificial media, have thus far escaped detection, and which, nevertheless, may possess pathogenic properties which they may unfold under propitious circumstances.

For the present, therefore, we distinguish two groups of pathogenic mouth-microbes, the non-cultivable and the cultivable.

1. Non-cultivable Pathogenic Mouth-Bacteria.

As has been stated above, there is a considerable number of species of bacteria in the mouth which do not appear to grow on any of the media at present in use; among others, Leptothrix innominata, Bacillus buccalis maximus, Jodococcus vaginatus, Spirillum sputigenum, and Spirochæte dentium. These occur in every mouth, the last-mentioned sometimes even in almost pure culture. Nevertheless, all attempts at cultivation, and thousands of them have been made, proved futile. For some years I myself made hundreds of experiments with diverse solid and liquid nutrient media, in order to obtain a pure culture of Spirillum sputigenum and Spirochæte dentium, but in vain. Up to the present, no one, as far as I know, has been more successful than I.

Since these well-known microbes will not grow outside of the mouth, we may suspect that there are other organisms in the mouth, less known or wholly unknown, pathogenic as well as non-pathogenic, which are not cultivable. This, of course, renders it difficult, if not impossible, to acquire a knowledge of their properties.

An important contribution to the study of this group of mouth-bacteria has been furnished by Kreibohm,[152] in the hygienic institute of Göttingen. He found two pathogenic bacteria in the mouth, which were characterized by the fact that they would grow on none of the usual artificial media.

"The first kind was twice obtained by injecting mice with scrapings from a coated tongue; the mice died after a few days, and showed great quantities of uniform bacilli in the blood. The rods are very like those of rabbit septicæmia, perhaps somewhat longer and more pointed; they are not contracted in the middle, take up coloring-matter at the extremities only, consequently display a light central zone. In the blood they lie singly or in small groups, seldom arranged in threads by twos or threes. Blood containing these bacilli inoculated into mice in quantities of one drop invariably gave rise to the same disease in thirty successive generations. On the first day no change in the inoculated animals was perceptible, on the second day they became sluggish, sat with their backs drawn up, the eyes glued together; usually after two to three days, sometimes only after five days, death ensued.

"The autopsy showed only a greatly enlarged spleen and less enlarged liver. In sections of all the organs small heaps of bacteria were found within the capillaries, but they did not occur in great numbers, except in the lungs. Rabbits were comparatively little susceptible. After inoculation with small quantities of blood, they became only temporarily ill. After a subcutaneous injection of larger quantities of blood, the animals died in the course of two or three days, and showed the same distribution of bacilli as mice. Field-mice were very susceptible. The inoculation of a chicken had a negative result.

"Cultures on diverse solid and fluid media were tried at various temperatures; all of them, however, remained sterile."

"The second species was isolated in the same manner, through the animal body (mice) from the coating of the human tongue. They presented short rods, rounded at the extremities and slightly contracted in the middle. After coloration, which in this case also is more intense at the extremities, they resemble the figure 8, and are also surrounded by a light halo, on the whole most like the bacilli of chicken-cholera. The rods were contained in great numbers in the heart-blood of the dead mice. In sections of the organs they were found within the capillaries, but generally in isolated heaps, and not more plentifully in the lungs than in other organs. By means of minute quantities of blood it was possible to transfer the disease to forty to fifty generations of mice; death ensued more rapidly than from the bacterium described first, often after but eighteen, at most after forty hours.

"Rabbits were completely refractory. Culture experiments yielded an increase of bacteria only in the blood transferred to the first medium; in further inoculations no increase ever occurred."

While experimenting with the bacteria of the gangrenous pulp (*Dental Cosmos*, April, 1888) I discovered a microbe, which, subcutaneously injected into mice, excited a gangrenous process. Twenty-four hours after the infection a pea-sized swelling had formed, which when lanced emitted a stinking pus mixed with gas-bubbles. By inoculating small quantities of this matter from one animal to another the infection was transferred through several generations. The bacteria cultivated from such abscesses did not possess this characteristic effect, from which fact I concluded that the specific bacterium is uncultivable.

I do not doubt that continued study will discover other members of this group of uncultivable pathogenic mouth-bacteria.

2. Cultivable Pathogenic Mouth-Bacteria.

a. Micrococcus of Sputum Septicæmia.

Of the many pathogenic bacteria which have of late been obtained in pure culture from the mouth, the micrococcus of sputum septicæmia is perhaps the most important. It is probably the same micro-organism which Pasteur, Raynaud, Lannelongue, Vulpian, Moriggia and Marchiafava, Sternberg, Klein, myself, and many others had to do with in the experiments on the infectious nature of healthy as well as diseased human saliva.

Klein [151] was, it appears, the first who succeeded in obtaining a pure culture of the coccus of sputum septicæmia, using blood-serum and agar-agar peptone at 38° C.

A. Fränkel[153] also obtained pure cultures of the same organism from the blood of a rabbit which had just died. He used agar-agar dissolved in calf's or beef broth, and added ½ to 1 per cent. grape-sugar or an equal quantity of the double tartrate of potassium and sodium. A culture on coagulated beef-blood serum proved still more successful. Optimum of temperature, 35° to 37° C.

"Within twenty-four hours, at 35° to 37° C., the culture grew in the shape of a nearly transparent grayish-white, gelatinous coating upon the surface. Viewed by reflected light, it resembled a dew-drop.

"When scraped together with the needle, the coating presents a yellowish-brown appearance."

Flasks of bouillon exposed to a temperature of 30° to 35° C. become equally clouded throughout twenty-four hours after the infection; later the culture sinks to the bottom as a peculiar, granular, sandy precipitate, while the liquid above it becomes clear.

The coccus of sputum septicæmia grows only between 22° and 42.5° C., no development taking place either below the former or above the latter temperature. Its cultivation is difficult under all circumstances. Above all, the nutrient medium must not be too concentrated (according to Weichselbaum, 1½ per cent. of peptone, 1½ per cent. of grape-sugar, 1½ per cent. of common salt in 1½ per cent. solution of agar-agar), and must be exactly neutralized.

FIG. 111.

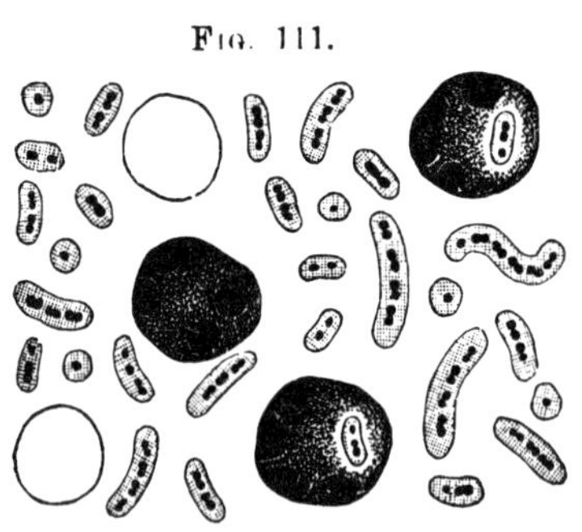

CAPSULE COCCI from pneumonic exudation in man. (After Baumgarten.) 1500 : 1.

This bacterium appears in the form of oval cocci, sometimes single, oftener in pairs, as diplococci, or in short chains (Fig. 111). The separate cells, as well as the chains, are surrounded by gelatinous capsules, which become visible even under 300 to 400 diameters, and may be stained by the method of Friedländer. The specimens are placed for two minutes in a concentrated solution of gentian-violet in aniline water, then treated with alcohol (from one-quarter to one-half minute), and rinsed with water. They may be examined in water, or after being mounted in Canada balsam.

Injections of pure cultures into the subcutaneous connective tissue, or into the abdominal or thoracic cavities, or directly into the lungs, provoke the same symptoms as injections with saliva. Death ensues within twenty-four to thirty-six hours, under phenomena resembling septicæmia. The autopsy reveals large quantities of capsule-cocci in the blood and in the different organs, large tumor of the spleen, often also peritonitis with or without slight exudation. But little reaction occurs at the point of infection. Mice and rabbits were highly susceptible; pigeons, chickens, dogs, refractory; guinea-pigs variously disposed.

The blood of the deceased animals is highly infectious. *Animals which had survived one severe infection did not react a second time.*

An exposure of forty-eight hours in a liquid culture medium to a temperature of 42° C. was sufficient to destroy the pathogenic properties of the coccus of sputum septicæmia. Cultivated in milk, it is said to lose its virulence in a short time.

If the micrococcus of sputum septicæmia has been repeatedly found in the oral cavity of healthy persons, its occurrence in the mouths of those suffering from pneumonia is almost constant. In genuine croupous pneumonia Fränkel found it twelve times out of fourteen, and Weichselbaum eighty-one times out of eighty-eight.

When we take into consideration the fact that this coccus is not easily cultivable, we may readily suppose that its absence in the two and seven cases respectively may have been due to faults in the method of cultivation.

If, now, the view held by Fränkel, Weichselbaum, etc., to which also Baumgarten[154] adheres, that the coccus of sputum septicæmia is to be regarded as the most frequent, if not as the sole, excitant of lobar pneumonia, be correct, then we may with sufficient reason assume that the infection, at least in many cases, most probably proceeded from the mouth. The oral cavity serves as a gathering-point for this microbe, which from time to time is carried into the lungs with the air until at last, at some weak point, or as the result of some slight inflammatory action in the lungs through which their power of resistance is impaired, it obtains a foothold in the lungs themselves. For this reason, therefore, among many others, the neglected oral cavity furnishes a most dangerous source of infection, which has by no means received the attention which its importance demands.

b. Bacillus crassus sputigenus.

Kreibohm[155] found twice in sputum and once in the coating of the tongue a cultivable bacterium which he termed Bacillus

FIG. 112.

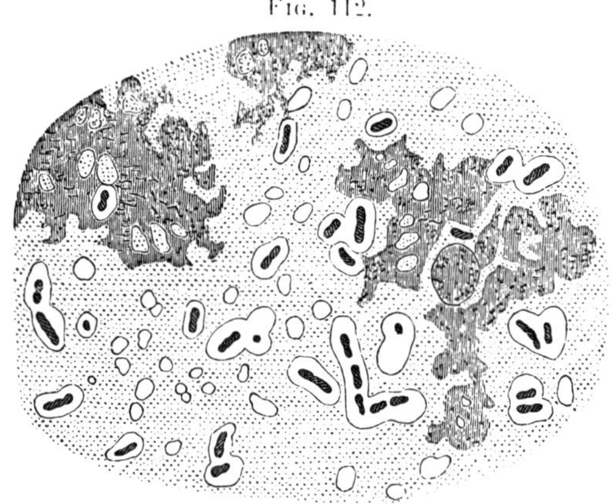

BACILLUS CRASSUS SPUTIGENUS.
Cover-glass preparation from the heart-blood of a mouse. (After Flügge.) 700 : 1.

crassus sputigenus, which possesses distinct pathogenic properties.

"Short, thick bacilli, representing oblongs with rounded corners, often curved or twisted like a sausage. Immediately after fissation the longitudinal diameter exceeds the transverse only by about one-half; afterward the former becomes much longer, so that before a second fissation the bacilli are three or four times as long as they are thick (Fig. 112).

"We often see bacilli in a state of fissation, or still adhering to each other after fissation; long pseudo-threads are, however, wanting. Specimens prepared from blood, as well as from cultures, reveal bacilli with swollen extremities or irregular outlines (involution forms), here and there transformed into shapeless masses. The bacilli are easily stained, and retain their color even after the application of Gram's·method. At a higher temperature they appear to form spores.

"These bacilli may be cultivated on various nutrient media. On gelatine-plates they form (after thirty-six hours) distinct grayish-white dots, which soon rise above the surface and then form large greenish-white, round, slimy drops, rising quite high above the level of the gelatine. Under a weak power the youngest colonies appear circular, of grayish-brown dark color, and their entire surface covered with dark dots or with short, dark lines and flourishes (Schnörkeln). The larger superficial colonies appear much lighter, irregularly outlined; the surface distinctly granular, especially at the margin.

"Puncture-cultures develop very quickly (in about twenty-four hours), and show a typical nail-shaped growth. On potato slices a thick, grayish-white, moist, shining coating is formed."

"Mice die about forty-eight hours after inoculation with small quantities of the culture; numerous bacilli are found in the heart-blood and in all the capillaries, most abundantly in the liver. Rabbits are not perceptibly affected by small inoculations; but after intravenous injections of small doses they perish from blood-poisoning within forty-eight hours, and show great masses of bacilli in the blood.

"Large quantities of the culture injected into the veins caused in rabbits, and in a more pronounced degree in dogs, diarrhœa, sometimes bloody stools, and death within three to ten hours; the autopsy revealed also the characteristics of an acute gastro-enteritis."

c. Staphylococcus pyogenes aureus and albus. Streptococcus pyogenes.

It cannot for a moment be doubted that these typically pyogenic organisms, which are very widespread in nature, frequently gain access into the mouth. It would also seem very probable that the conditions existing in the oral cavity favor their growth, although no attempt has as yet been made to establish the accuracy of these two suppositions experimentally.

All results obtained from culture-experiments coincide in this, that the two micro-organisms first named actually occur in the mouth, whereas the statements concerning the frequency of their occurrence greatly diverge.

Black[156] examined the buccal juices in regard to pyogenic micro-organisms, and found them in many cases. In the saliva of ten healthy persons he found Staphylococcus pyogenes aureus seven times, Staphylococcus pyogenes albus four times, and Streptococcus pyogenes three times. The material was obtained by scraping the back of the tongue or any part of the mucous membrane with a sterilized platinum wire. In some cases Black found staphylococci in all parts of the mouth, in others he did not succeed in finding them, but believes that they might be discovered in almost all mouths if the latter were examined with sufficient care. Black but seldom found other pyogenic bacteria in the mouth.

"As dentists," he continues, "we must take into consideration that the pyogenic bacteria are generally present in the oral cavity and endanger every wound which we make in it."

Other bacteriologists who have examined the buccal juices have not succeeded in finding the above-named bacteria so constantly. Vignal[59] found Staphylococcus aureus and albus but rarely in the mouth; Streptococcus pyogenes never. Netter found Staphylococcus pyogenes aureus seven times in one hundred and twenty-seven cases. During the many years in which I have occupied myself with the study of mouth-bacteria I have met these species comparatively seldom; in suppurative processes five times in twenty-two cases, in healthy mouths more rarely. I have, however, made comparatively few experiments for the sole purpose of determining the presence or non-presence of these organisms, and consequently do not attach very much importance to my own work on this point. The results of Vignal and Netter are not so easily disposed of. Further experiments must consequently determine whether pyogenic bacteria really occur in the saliva of healthy persons as often as Black's observations would lead us to suppose.

d. Micrococcus tetragenus.

This micro-organism has been repeatedly mentioned as an inmate of the oral cavity. I myself have found it quite often, but unfortunately took no notes concerning its frequency. Biondi found it three times out of five.

It occurs in the form of cocci, about 1μ in diameter, which by fissation in two directions form groups of fours (Fig. 113). The cells are inclosed and held together by a gelatinous disk.

Fig. 113.

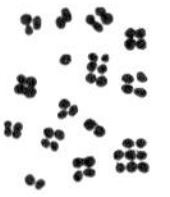

Micrococcus tetragenus. 600 : 1.

It grows on gelatine-plates, without liquefying the gelatine, in the shape of small, white, dot-like colonies, which, under weak power, appear finely granular and have a peculiar glass-like brilliancy (Eisenberg).

White mice and guinea-pigs inoculated with Micrococcus tetragenus perish in from three to ten days. According to Biondi, even the injection of saliva which contains this microbe proves fatal in four to eight days. The cocci are found in the blood as well as in all organs.

Micrococcus tetragenus was first found by Koch[157] and Gaffky[158] in the lungs of a consumptive. It frequently occurs in lung-tuberculosis, but the part it plays in this disease has not yet been ascertained (Flügge).

Biondi's Mouth-Bacteria.

A valuable contribution to our knowledge of pathogenic bacteria of the mouth has been furnished by Biondi.[159] He isolated from human saliva five different pathogenic micro-organisms, to which he gave the following names:

Bacillus salivarius septicus.
Coccus salivarius septicus.
Micrococcus tetragenus (mentioned above).
Streptococcus septo-pyæmicus.
Staphylococcus salivarius pyogenes.

e. *Bacillus salivarius septicus.*

Of these, Bacillus salivarius septicus is said to occur most frequently in the saliva of healthy as well as of sick persons. It forms very short elliptical rods with somewhat tapering extremities and comparatively thick bodies, and grows but poorly on common neutral media.

"Mice and rabbits injected with one-half to one cubic centimeter of such saliva generally succumbed within twenty-four to forty-eight or seventy-two hours. The autopsy revealed œdema, hemorrhage, tumor of the spleen, and micro-organisms in the blood. This bacillus acts most intensely at the point of infection, without showing a special predilection for any particular organ. At first it proliferates at the point of entrance, is then carried through the blood- and lymphatic vessels to the rest of the body, and multiplies in these channels until death is caused." Passage through the body of a refractive animal, high temperatures, etc., diminish the virulence of this micro-organism. Animals infected with weakened material proved resistant to virulent inoculations.

f. *Coccus salivarius septicus.*

Coccus salivarius septicus was found but once, and is therefore hardly to be regarded as a mouth-bacterium, but rather as an accidental contamination of the saliva, particularly as the patient in whose mouth it was found suffered from violent puerperal septicæmia.

"Subcutaneous injections with this saliva in mice, guinea-pigs, and rabbits proved fatal after four to six days. The only and constant result of the autopsy was the presence of the cocci in the blood and the tissues."

This microbe is easily isolated from the blood, and grows well on the usual culture-media. The colonies within the gelatine of plate-cultures are perfectly round, and of white-grayish color, sometimes merging into black.

g. *Streptococcus septo-pyæmicus.*

"When subcutaneously injected in quantities of ½–1 c.cm., the saliva containing this streptococcus proved pathogenic for guinea-pigs, rabbits, and mice, although not constantly. Often also two different forms of disease are caused by it.

"Rabbits frequently perished after fifteen to twenty days, showing symptoms of chronic septicæmia,—increase of temperature, general debility, gradual emaciation, etc. At the point of infection nothing characteristic was found, sometimes only a circumscribed infiltration with suppurating center; the internal organs revealed intense anæmia; the blood and the organic juices contained but few cocci, which were usually arranged in short chains. Inoculations with the blood of the diseased animals were without result.

"In guinea-pigs and mice which had been subcutaneously injected with saliva, pus formed at the point of vaccination, and had the tendency to spread into the subcutaneous connective and muscular tissues. Guinea-pigs often survived this suppuration, mice generally died.

"Infections with pure cultures of this bacterium also had the same effect.

"This streptococcus cannot be distinguished from that of erysipelas, phlegmon, and puerperal metritis. Their colonies have the same appearances, their development is equally slow, and the results of experiments made with them on animals are identical."

Vaccination on the scarified ear of rabbits usually led to the characteristic symptoms of erysipelas.

h. Staphylococcus salivarius pyogenes.

Staphylococcus salivarius pyogenes was likewise observed but once, in the contents of an abscess of a guinea-pig which had been inoculated with the saliva of an individual suffering from angina scarlatina. It was cultivated in milk, bouillon, blood-serum, agar-agar, potato, beef-water and wheat-infusion gelatine. The latter was liquefied. Milk was precipitated in large flakes. In twenty-four hours bouillon at 37° C. became very cloudy, afterward the growth was precipitated as a white, dense deposit. This micro-organism is easily obtained in pure culture from the contents of such abscesses, by making the usual cultures from a drop of pus. Cultivated on gelatine at room temperature, the growth does not become apparent until after two or three days. The separate colonies, especially when lying at some distance from each other, reach the maximum of their development on the fourth to sixth day, and then slowly commence to liquefy the surrounding gelatine. Colonies within, as well as on the surface of the gelatine, observed at this time, appear perfectly round, with clearly-defined margins, and of a whitish opalescent color.

"It was immaterial whether the animal was inoculated subcutaneously with very minute quantities of material obtained from old cultures, or with one-tenth of a drop of matter; all animals infected with these micro-organisms reacted by abscess-formation at the point of inoculation."

In the pus these small cocci almost always appear singly, neither united, as diplococci, nor in chains, nor in clusters. Abundant quantities brought into the jugular vein caused general infection and death. Injected into the abdominal cavity they produced peritonitis.

Original Investigations on Pathogenic Mouth-Bacteria.

Although much attention has of late years been given to the study of the pathogenic micro-organisms of the mouth, and our knowledge concerning them has been essentially increased by the investigations of Kreibohm, Biondi, and others, much yet remains to be done before the subject will be but in some measure exhausted.

I have occupied myself with the study of the pathogenic mouth-bacteria for a number of years, and obtained some results which may, perhaps, contribute somewhat to our knowledge of them.

I have experimented with forty-two pure cultures, two mixed cultures, and twenty-two gangrenous pulps, and have made ninety-three subcutaneous inoculations of mice in pockets, using pure cultures, ten subcutaneous injections of pure cultures, fifty-eight pocket inoculations with pieces of gangrenous pulps, or with pus arising from such inoculations, sixty injections of pure culture into the abdominal cavity of mice, rabbits, and guinea-pigs, twenty-two injections into the thoracic cavity, besides a number of mixed infections.

The pockets were made in the customary manner, at the root of the tail, and the material for inoculation was usually taken from an agar-agar culture one to two weeks old. Injections were made with the sterilizable subcutaneous syringe, cultures in beef-extract-peptone solutions from two to four days old being used. For mice, 0.05 to 0.1 cc.; for rabbits and guinea-pigs, 0.25 to 0.5 cc. were injected. The mice were always etherized before making the injection. The etherization renders the operation much easier and surer; it may be accomplished in fifteen seconds by taking the mouse by the tail and holding him in a wide-mouthed ether-bottle.

In 18.8 per cent. of the pocket inoculations a severe local reaction followed, resulting in the formation of a small abscess, generally remaining superficial, but occasionally penetrating into the subcutaneous tissue. In eight cases the inoculation was followed by death, the mice showing, in three cases, symptoms of blood-poisoning, the micro-organisms being also present in the blood and different organs. In a number of cases necrosis of the skin around the pocket occurred, a piece of skin one-fourth to one-half inch in diameter being thrown off. In 50 per cent. the reaction was light, nothing more than a slight local redness and formation of a very minute quantity of pus being observed. In 31.2 per cent. no reaction whatever could be detected, the wound healing rapidly, without either suppuration or swelling. Of the subcutaneous injections, 24 per cent. produced violent reactions, resulting either in the death of the animal from septicæmia, peritonitis, pleuritis, etc., or in extensive suppuration and abscess-formation. Slight reaction was produced in 32 per cent.: temporary sickness, from which the animals soon recovered, or slight swelling at the point of injection; in 44 per cent. no effect could be detected.

Subcutaneous inoculation with portions of gangrenous pulps produced comparatively severe symptoms in 36.8 per cent. of the pulps experimented with, slight effects in 47.4 per cent., and no apparent reaction in 15.8 per cent.

It appears from these results that inoculation with portions of gangrenous pulps is more dangerous than inoculation with pure cultures from the same pulps, which is as we should naturally expect it to be. I intend, however, later (Chapter XI) to discuss the question of infection through foul pulps at length, and pass the subject here with this brief mention.

The mixed infections invariably resulted in the death of the animal.

During these studies I have found in the oral cavity a number of bacteria which possess more or less pathogenic action, four of which I have examined more in detail, and named as follows:

Micrococcus gingivæ pyogenes.
Bacterium gingivæ pyogenes.
Bacillus dentalis viridans.
Bacillus pulpæ pyogenes.

FIG. 114.

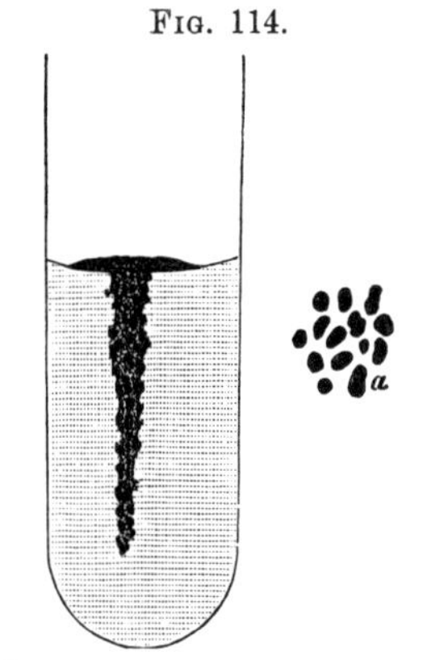

MICROCOCCUS GINGIVÆ PYOGENES. Culture in gelatine, 8 days old. *a*, separate cells. 1100 : 1.

i. Micrococcus gingivæ pyogenes.

I found this organism in a case of pyorrhœa alveolaris three times in the same mouth, at intervals of three months; also in a very filthy mouth, in the deposit around the teeth. It appears as irregular cocci, or very plump rods, singly or in pairs (Fig. 114, *a*). In gelatine plate-cultures it grows rapidly at room temperature, forming round colonies, with a distinctly sharp margin. At first the colonies appear very slightly colored under the microscope; as they become older they grow very dark, especially where they lie far apart. Line-cultures on agar-agar present a moderately thick, grayish growth, having a tinge of purple by transmitted light. Under the microscope they appear as a homogeneous, nearly colorless matrix, interspersed with darker figures of various irregular shapes.

Puncture- (*stich*) cultures in gelatine have, when eight days old, the appearance seen in Fig. 114. The gelatine does not become liquefied. Cultures in beef-extract-peptone-sugar solutions show a strong acid reaction and develop considerable quantities of gas. Subcutaneous inoculations of mice were followed by abscess and necrosis of the skin, occasionally resulting in the death of the animal. Injections in the abdominal cavity invariably produced the death of the animal in twelve to twenty-four hours, the autopsy revealing immense numbers of bacteria in the abdominal cavity, a considerable quantity of a serous exudation, peritonitis, etc. Only a very limited number of larger animals —two rabbits and two guinea-pigs—were inoculated. The animals appeared sick for a time, sitting quietly in the corner of the cage and refusing to eat. After two or three days, however, all symptoms disappeared.

k. Bacterium gingivæ pyogenes.

This bacterium was found in the same mouth with the micro-organism just described, and also in a suppurating tooth-pulp of a second person. It appears in form of thick, short bacteria with rounded ends, one and a half to four times as long as thick. (See Fig. 115, *a*.) In plate-cultures it grows very rapidly, even at room temperature, the colonies being clearly visible to the naked eye in twenty-four hours. Under the microscope they appear as beautiful, perfectly round, yellowish colonies, with a sharp, dark border. The gelatine becomes rapidly liquefied, so that in forty-eight hours the first dilution is completely melted.

Fig. 115.

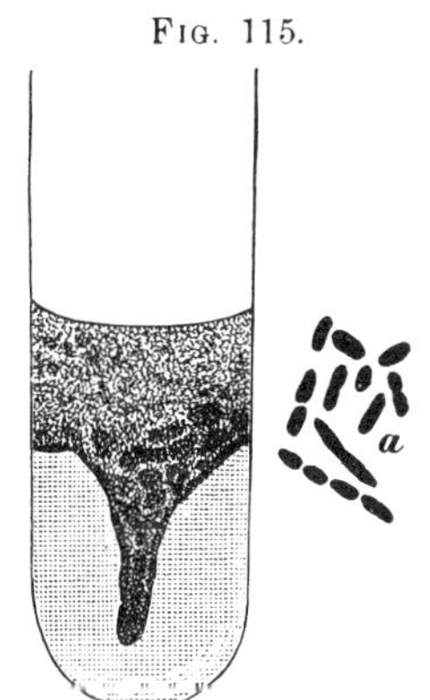

Bacterium gingivæ pyogenes.
Culture in gelatine, 8 days old. *a*, single cells under 1100 : 1.

Line-cultures on gelatine appear in fifteen hours as a trough of melted gelatine $1\frac{1}{2}$ mm. broad, the side of the trough being cloudy and the bottom marked by a line of white sediment.

Line-cultures in agar-agar present a thick, moist, slightly grayish growth by transmitted light, having a slight greenish-yellow tinge under the microscope, colorless at the margin, yellowish brown toward the middle, and presenting a fibrillated structure.

Puncture-cultures in gelatine, eight days old, have the appearance seen in Fig. 115. The gelatine rapidly melts in form of a funnel, while the masses of bacteria sink to the bottom, the melted gelatine, however, remaining cloudy.

Injections of this bacterium into the abdominal cavity of white mice produced death in ten to twenty-five hours. During their sickness the mice sat drawn up, with bent back and eyelids glued together. The autopsy showed peritonitis, and in some cases purulent exudation. Micro-organisms were found only in very small numbers in the blood.

Fig. 116.

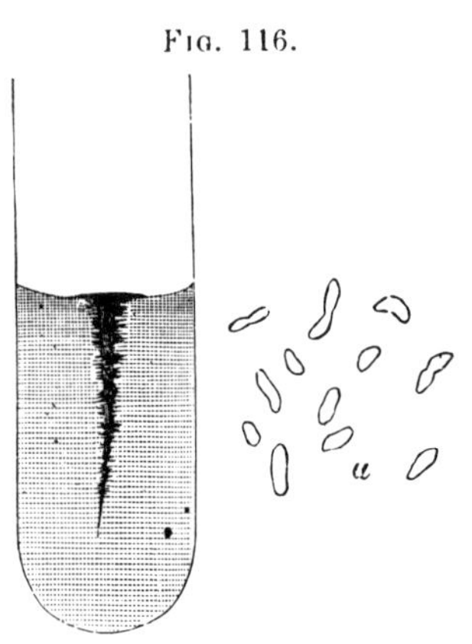

Bacillus dentalis viridans.
Gelatine culture, 8 days old. *a*, single cells. 1100 : 1.

Injections of 0.25 into the abdominal cavity of rabbits and guinea-pigs produced identical results. Injections into the lung produced death in less than twenty-four hours. Subcutaneous inoculation (injections) of mice resulted in extensive abscess-formation.

l. Bacillus dentalis viridans.

This organism was found in the superficial layers of carious dentine. It appears as slightly curved, pointed rods, singly or in pairs (Fig. 116, *a*). It grows well in plate-cultures at room temperature; the colonies under the microscope are nearly colorless, having but a slight yellow tinge; they are perfectly round, with a sharp contour, and show, when they do not lie too close together, two or three concentric rings. This bacterium is characterized by the production of a beautiful opalescent green coloring-matter, which it imparts to the gelatine; the cell itself is not colored.

Line-cultures on agar-agar produce a very thin growth, with irregular margins, bluish by transmitted light, greenish gray by reflected light, and colorless under the microscope.

Puncture-cultures on gelatine, eight days old, present the form seen in Fig. 116.

Subcutaneous applications from pure cultures of this bacterium produced severe local inflammation and suppuration, and in one case death by blood-poisoning, the bacteria being found in large numbers in the blood and tissues.

Injections into the abdominal cavity of white mice and guinea-pigs produced death in 60 per cent. of the cases, in twenty-two hours to six days, from peritonitis. Bacteria could not be found in the blood microscopically, but cultures made from the blood of the heart developed pure cultures of the bacterium injected.

The fourth micro-organism with pronounced pathogenic action,

m. Bacillus pulpæ pyogenes,

was found in a gangrenous tooth-pulp. It occurs as bacilli, often slightly curved and pointed, either singly, in pairs, or in chains of four to eight (Fig. 117, *a*). It grows moderately well in gelatine plate-cultures, the colonies appearing large and round, dark, yellowish brown, with distinct margins.

FIG. 117.

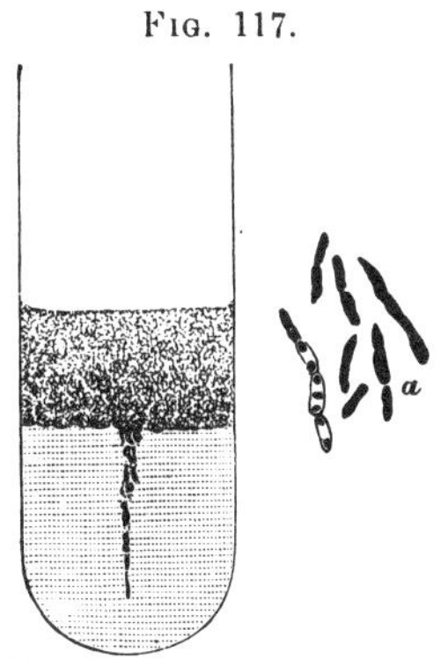

BACILLUS PULPÆ PYOGENES.
Gelatine culture, 8 days old. *a*, single cells. 1100 : 1.

Line-cultures on gelatine begin to melt in eighteen to twenty-four hours, up to that time appearing as grayish, shining lines, slightly elevated above the surface of the gelatine, and about 1 mm. wide.

Line-cultures on agar-agar produce a moderately extensive growth, bluish white, glistening by transmitted light, gray by reflected light; under the microscope granular, sometimes fibrillar in structure, gray, or in older colonies, yellowish.

Puncture-cultures in gelatine, eight days old, present the appearance seen in Fig. 117, the gelatine melting with about equal rapidity on the sides and in the middle of the tube. Injections of 0.05 into the abdominal cavity proved fatal to mice in eighteen to thirty hours.

CHAPTER XI.

ENTRANCE-PORTALS OF THE PATHOGENIC MOUTH-BACTERIA.

THE diseases caused by the pathogenic bacteria of the mouth may be considered under six heads, according to the point of entrance of the infection:

1. Infections caused by a breach in the continuity of the mucous membrane, brought about by mechanical injuries (wounds, extractions, etc.). These lead either to local or to general disturbances.
2. Infections through the medium of gangrenous tooth-pulps. These usually lead to the formation of abscesses at the point of infection (abscessus apicalis), but also sometimes to secondary septicæmia and pyæmia with fatal termination.
3. Disturbances conditioned by the resorption of poisonous waste products formed by bacteria.
4. Pulmonary diseases caused by the inspiration of particles of slime, small pieces of tartar, etc., containing bacteria.
5. Excessive fermentative processes, and other complaints of the digestive tract, caused by the continual swallowing of microbes and their poisonous products.
6. Infections of the intact soft tissue of the oral and pharyngeal cavities, whose power of resistance has been impaired by debilitating diseases, mechanical irritations, etc.

In this connection the possibility of an infection by the accumulation of the excitants of diphtheria, typhus, syphilis, etc., in the mouth must also be taken into consideration.

1. INVASION OF PATHOGENIC MOUTH-BACTERIA FOLLOWING MECHANICAL INJURIES.

Many facts favor the supposition that a considerable number of pathogenic micro-organisms may thrive in the juices of the mouth without showing in their vital manifestations any distinction from the common parasites of the oral cavity, as long as the mucous membrane remains intact. If, however, the soft tissues have been wounded, as in extraction, or if the resistance of the mucous membrane has been impaired, these organisms may gain a point of entrance, and thus become able to manifest their special actions.

Many of the fatal cases of infections following dental operations, which were formerly invariably, and are even now commonly, attributed to infected instruments, are most probably to be accounted for by these auto-infections.

Every extraction not performed under antiseptic precautions may be regarded as an inoculation which, unfortunately, often proves very successful. The severe injuries of the soft tissues and the bone caused by difficult extractions, as well as the open wound left by every extraction, furnish a convenient point of entrance for bacteria. Whoever has examined an unclean mouth, with its broken-down teeth, inflamed gums, thick, smeary deposits with which some of the teeth are wholly covered, will not wonder that inflammation, swelling, suppuration, necrosis, caries of the bone, or even septicæmia and pyæmia may follow upon operations in the mouth, nor, in such cases, without further consideration, accuse the dentist of having used an infected instrument.

Tulpius,[73] as early as 1674, mentions among the consequences of toothache, " disfiguration of the face and certain death." He calls attention to the case of the Amsterdam physician, Gosvin Hall, who died from the effects of gum-lancing, performed in a case of impeded eruption of the wisdom-tooth. " Very soon after the gums were lanced he suffered from insomnia, delirium, and died."

Most probably this was a case of septic infection by means of mouth-bacteria, for which the incision furnished an easy entrance.

From this case we see that even as simple an operation as lancing gums may not always be entirely free from danger, and that not only the knife, but also the gums themselves should be thoroughly disinfected before the incision is made. Subsequent to the operation the mouth should be kept as free from micro-organisms as possible by a frequent use of an antiseptic wash.

Leynseele (*Bullet. de la société de Gand*, 1885) describes a case of meningo-encephalitis resulting from the attempted extraction of a tooth. The lower jaw had been fractured at the point of extraction; pus burrowed its way along the bone, laying it bare. From this point it ascended the inner side of the ramus of the jaw as far as the base of the skull, and entered the cranial cavity through the foramen ovale, spinosum, and rotundum, where, spreading along the base of the brain, it became the cause of meningo-encephalitis (Wedl).

Of late years both dentists and physicians have paid particular attention to this fruitful source of most dangerous infections. The cases of fatal infectious diseases proceeding from diseased teeth are now no longer exceptional; not, I think, because they occur more frequently at present, but because the great influence of the condition of the mouth upon the general health was formerly not appreciated, and cases of this kind were not traced back to their proper source.*

Not only has a large number of pathogenic micro-organisms been discovered and described, but reports have also been made concerning many different cases of general diseases proceeding from the teeth. Zakharevitsch [160] relates the cases of two healthy, vigorous physicians who died, the one on the sixth, the other on the tenth day after the extraction of the left lower second molar. In one case, osteomyelitis supervened; in the other, periostitis and osteitis, with uncommonly severe symptoms. The infection was from the beginning of a septic nature, which, according to the reporter, was due to the use of infected instruments.

Several similar cases have been cited by Baume.[161] A physician had made an unsuccessful attempt to extract the decayed left superior first molar of a student, twenty-four years of age. On the following day a moderate swelling of the affected locality set in; the pericementitis soon extended to the periosteum of

* A case illustrating this fact was brought to my notice some time since. In a workman found dead, the autopsy revealed the cause of death to be a meningitis directly traceable to an abscessed tooth.

the jaw, causing necrosis; the necrotic alveolar process was removed after two weeks. In the progress of the disease the characteristic symptoms of pyæmia appeared,—chills, great debility, and icteritous color of the skin. This was accompanied by pleuro-pneumonia of the right lung. The patient died in consequence of an eruption of pus into the lungs.

In another case, a young man died of pyæmia on the very next day after having a tooth extracted. In this case the patient had suffered from chronic parulis.

Delestre describes several cases "in which meningitis resulted fatally in consequence of spreading inflammations and abscesses after extraction." "A robust man, twenty-seven years old, had a left superior molar drawn; an inflammation followed which spread to the orbit and the brain; the patient died of meningitis."

In a second case, a factory girl, twenty-six years old, died five days after the extraction of the right inferior first molar. Swelling, suppuration, and finally meningitis ensued, causing death.

Von Mosetig-Moorhof[162] noticed four cases of inflammation of the jaw-bone with phlebitis suppurativa, leading to a fatal pyæmia, which had been caused by diseased roots; moreover, many cases of acute sepsis occurring after unsuccessful operations or such performed without proper antiseptic precautions. He gives the following account of one case of this kind as an example of many others:

"M. Battista, a woman in the seventh month of pregnancy, went on the 1st of February of the present year to the charitable institute just mentioned in order to have the second right lower molar extracted, which was badly decayed and whose crown was partially wanting. The crown was completely broken off, and the patient sent home without extracting the roots. The pain increased, fever appeared, and on the next morning the face was so much swollen that it was almost impossible to open the mouth; the pain on swallowing was so great that she, in spite of her intense thirst, was scarcely able to swallow a little water. The swelling gradually increased, and finally became so extensive that the totally disfigured patient even suffered from want of breath. On the 3d of February she was transferred to the

Wiedener Hospital. We found particularly the right half of the face terribly swollen, the skin reddened and tense, both eyelids closed by œdema; the infiltration extended across the arch of the jaw, occupied the entire floor of the oral cavity, and continued upon the right side of the neck almost to the clavicle. The whole part was tense and as hard as a board; a disagreeable stench was emitted from the mouth; the jaws could hardly be opened to the breadth of a finger. The cheeks, gums, and base of the tongue were all intensely swollen, and the gums corresponding to the extracted tooth covered with a diphtheritic exudation. Swallowing impossible; respiration somewhat difficult; rattling on account of the inability to expectorate; evening temperature 39.8°. The mouth is syringed with sublimate 1–1000; externally ice-collars employed.

"On the morning of the fourth day we succeeded with comparative ease in removing the broken roots of the right inferior second molar by means of the elevator. Iodoform gauze was placed in the wound, permanganate of potassium used as a mouth-wash and for syringing; evening temperature 40° C. The respiration became more difficult; the patient spent the night in a sitting posture, and gasped for breath.

"On the morning of the fifth day the patient is, if possible, still more swollen; from the nose downward to far below the larynx all outlines are erased; nothing is visible but a hard, stiff, even surface, covered with the dark red skin; no trace of fluctuation. We have here, therefore, an angina Ludovigi septica in optima forma. Breathing is extremely difficult, the face somewhat cyanotic. We bring her into the operating-room, and split the soft tissues in the median line from the chin to below the hyoid bone a distance of about 15 cm. The tissue is stiff from the infiltration, bleeding very slight; a scanty, brown, thin ichor flows from the incision. We make our way preparando to the floor of the tongue, but discover no large center of infection, no accumulation of fluid. Sublimate dressing 1–2000; improvement in respiration; evening temperature 38.9°. On the 6th of February we find fluctuation on the right side of the neck. Another deep, longitudinal incision from the angle of the jaw downward obliquely is followed by a discharge of ichor. The probing finger finds the jaw laid bare; sublimate dressing, syringing with permanganate of potassium every two hours.

"Two more incisions into the cheek and in the region of the ear were necessary. The fever gradually diminished, but up to the present time some of the wounds are not yet closed, for almost the entire cellular tissue in the region of the right side of the neck and lower jaw became necrotic, and was gradually thrown off. Fortunately, the periosteum formed again on the lower jaw, and the case ended comparatively well. But the patient had suffered terribly. Her life was in danger; she had gone through an illness of five weeks' duration, and her face was disfigured by scars. All this was the result of a really criminal omission of all cleanliness and antisepsis, of unskillful operation, and total ignorance of surgical principles."

The *Zahnärztliches Wochenblatt* of September 8, 1888, cites the following case: "About six weeks ago, one Sunday afternoon, a peasant girl, eighteen years of age, called on a dentist to have a tooth extracted; not finding him at home, she sought the aid of a barber. The latter succeeded in extracting the tooth, but was not able, in spite of long-continued efforts, to stop the ensuing hemorrhage, and dismissed the girl with the wound still bleeding. At home the hemorrhage continued, and considerable swelling set in, in consequence of which a physician was sent for, who, however, came when it was too late, as the examination revealed blood-poisoning. A few hours later the girl was a corpse."

A case of septico-pyæmia resulting from the extraction of a tooth is related by Stanislaus Zawadzki.[163] A locksmith, until then in good health, forty-six years of age, whose left lower wisdom-tooth had been extracted fourteen days previously by a barber, suffered on the following day from an exceedingly painful swelling of the corresponding part of the jaw, accompanied by chills and sweats; later he was attacked by deafness of the left ear, and continually increasing headaches. The chills returned again and again, and finally the man lost consciousness and was taken to the above-mentioned hospital, where high stupor, grasping the head, groaning, slight icterus, contracted pupils, high fever (39.9°), small, rapid pulse (ninety per minute), and a slight amount of albumen in the urine, were noted. The region of the angle of the lower jaw on the left side was slightly reddened, hard, swollen, painless, without fluctuation; on the inner side greatly swollen, reddened, and hard. The wound was filled with stinking, discolored matter, which discharged in minute quantities when the gums were pressed. The neighboring lymphatic glands swollen, the spleen greatly enlarged. In the left lower pulmonary region, marked exudation and increased respiratory murmur; cough with thin, stinking expectorations, which contained many pus-corpuscles and streptococci. Intermittent fever appeared, and finally death ensued under convulsions.

The autopsy revealed septic phlegmon of the entire left side of the inferior maxilla and neck, with ichorous periostitis of the affected jaw, cachectic pneumonia of the left lower pulmonary lobe, and a great number of metastatic abscesses in both lungs, further ichorous pachymeningitis of the dura mater, covering the left sphenoid and temporal bone, with ichorous thrombi of the corresponding sinus cavernosus, intercavernosus, and petrosus superior.

"In this case the infectious process, probably caused by an unclean instrument, had begun at the infected wound of the jaw and then continued to spread from the roots of the vena submentalis, sublingualis, pharyngea to the plexus pterygoideus and ophthalmicus, and through the superior sphenoidal fissure to the sinus of the brain."

Another case which belongs to this group of infectious diseases occurred in the surgical clinic of von Mosetig-Moorhof, and has been reported by von Metnitz.[164]

A woman, forty-three years old, who had had several teeth extracted a week previously, was brought to the Vienna Hospital in an unconscious condition. A few days after the extraction she had fallen ill, suffering from continual pain and chills. Three days before her admission delirium, psychical disturbances, and one day before, total loss of consciousness had ensued. Nothing could be ascertained as to any former complaint.

The scalp was considerably swollen, also the left cheek and the malar and temporal regions. The skin of these parts was pale, shining, and tense, both bulbs very prominent, the conjunctiva distinctly yellow and intensely chemotic, the pupils half dilated without reaction. A terrible fœtor was emitted from the mouth; lockjaw existed in the highest degree; the glands of the submaxillary region on both sides were swollen, the neighboring tissues infiltrated; the neck stiff. In the lungs there was nothing especially remarkable. The heart was of normal size, with a slight diastolic murmur at the apex; the abdomen was distended; the uterus could be felt above the symphysis; there was deep stupor, delirium, restlessness, involuntary urination and defecation.

"On the following day delirium, pulse very rapid; in the following night a hemorrhage of the uterus took place, and the digital examination revealed a fœtus, which was removed together with the placenta; the fœtus was 17 cm. long. Death soon followed, in a state of coma.

"On opening into the cavity of the skull the meninges are found thickened, clouded, traversed by numerous densely filled blood-vessels, and on the left hemisphere covered with a layer of pus of considerable thickness. The right hemisphere likewise plainly shows depots of pus along the course of the distended vessels. The substance of the brain is soft, permeated with moisture, and contains numerous ecchymoses. The chamber is much dilated, and filled with a bloody serous liquid. The left middle temporal convolution is yellowish and softened throughout. The base of the brain is covered with a layer of pus, particularly thick on the sella turcica, which may be traced as far as the superior orbital fissure and the optic foramen. The meninges here show the same character as on the convexity of the brain.

"The alveolus of the lower third molar is filled with fœtid pus, the mucous membrane surrounding it is discolored and may be pulled off in shreds. The probe discloses everywhere the rough surface of the bone. All of the muscles inserted on the left side of the lower jaw, as well as the whole of the articular aponeurosis, are infiltrated with pus, at points destroyed, discolored, ichorous; the temporo-maxillary articulation purulent. The submaxillary glands are much enlarged, and also in the interior infiltrated with pus. The bone of the lower jaw is completely divested of periosteum, bicuspids and molars wanting, and the alveolar process consequently much resorbed. The empty alveolus of the third molar is 6 millimeters deep, and communicates through wide openings directly with the marrow-spaces of the bone. The marrow itself is discolored, fatty degenerated, and partly purulently liquefied.

"The neglect of the wound caused by the extraction is without doubt the source of this so violent inflammation in the bone."

According to the cases just cited, the most frequent cause of death, next to blood-poisoning, seems to be secondary meningitis, occasioned by the spreading of inflammation to the pia mater. The inflammation, whether proceeding from the upper or lower jaw, seems in most cases to make its way to the brain through the fossa spheno-maxillaris, fissura orbitalis inferior, orbita and fissura orbitalis superior, less frequently through the foramen rotundum, ovale, spinosum.

Conrad[165] mentions a case of "death by tetanus, caused by the extraction of two teeth." In dental literature, in fact, several cases of tetanus following different dental operations have been recorded.

It may be readily understood that not all infections proceeding from the oral cavity result so seriously. Every gradation may be noticed, from a slight inflammation of the gums to the most severe suppurative periostitis and its consequences. In regard to this point, Ritter[166] writes as follows: "Not only the fœtor often following a simple extraction, but even many accompanying suppurative inflammations, necrosis of the jaw, swellings of the face, etc., are occasioned by the lack of proper antiseptic precautions. I have been able in several hundred cases of suppurative inflammations of the bone to trace clearly the exciting cause of the affection. I have, indeed, seen one case of this kind which terminated fatally, not, it is true, through the local disturbance, but through a general sepsis occasioned by it. I refer to the case of a young man in which the extraction of the first and second inferior left molars was followed by a suppurative periostitis of the lower jaw. The patient died of pyæmia a few days later, in spite of the most careful treatment. I saw frequent cases of necrosis of the lower jaw arising after apparently simple tooth-extractions, some of which ran their course under such septic symptoms as are usually noticed in infected wounds in other parts of the body. In some of these cases which I treated with the assistance of practicing physicians, the sepsis did not remain local, but was accompanied by symptoms of general infection."

Operations in unclean mouths are always attended with more or less danger to the operator himself. Some months ago I saw a case in which a scarcely perceptible injury of the finger by an instrument used in excavating a tooth was followed by severe swelling of the finger and back of the hand, resulting in the formation of a large and stubborn abscess, which did not heal until after several incisions had been made.

A still more serious case occurred some years ago in the clinic of a dental college. A student of dentistry was unfortunate enough to scratch his finger on the sharp point of a diseased root. On the following day severe swelling, redness, and tension, accompanied by intense pain, ensued, which rapidly spread under formation of numerous abscesses to the arm and shoulder; high fever, delirium, and other symptoms of blood-poisoning arose, and only by the most energetic treatment, and after a long period of illness, was the danger of a fatal result completely removed.

In late years the opinion has gradually gained ground that operations in the oral cavity, extractions, lancing, etc., should be performed under antiseptic precautions. Ritter recommends that the tooth to be extracted, as well as the gums, be previously disinfected by a suitable antiseptic, in order to avoid pressing the masses of bacteria into the wound, by which means an infection is undoubtedly often brought about. Sachs regards it as sufficient to dip the beak of the forceps in a five per cent. solution of carbolic acid, and relies upon the action of the antiseptic adhering to the instrument to prevent an infection.

Parreidt[167] gives the following directions for antiseptic extractions: "Simple wounds after easy extractions in cases of pulpitis or a beginning periostitis dentalis require no special treatment. The danger of infecting such wounds is very slight; the tampon of coagulated blood is a sufficient preventive against infection.

Micro-organisms possibly adhering to the forceps, which might be pressed against the gums or into the wound in performing the extraction, are washed away by the flowing blood; moreover, the gums are not especially liable to infections (wounds made by files employed in operating upon decayed roots; Miller's and Galippe's inoculation experiments)."

Parreidt opposes the treatment of the wound with so-called antiseptic bandages, regarding them as more injurious than beneficial. Only in case the wound should give pain a day after extraction should an examination be made to determine whether the thrombus in the alveolus is firm or possibly septical. The latter will sometimes be found to be the case after difficult extractions, or in cases where osteo-periostitis alveolaris or maxillaris was present before the operation. The examination is made by directing a stream of sublimate or carbolic acid solution upon the thrombus, by which means it is readily washed out.

In cases where the protecting thrombus in the alveolus is wanting, the latter should be syringed daily with an antiseptic solution, at first morning and evening, later only once a day, in order to prevent infectious matter from having too long or too intense an action.

Parreidt recommends keeping the instruments as free as possible from germs by first thoroughly cleansing and drying them, then dipping them into carbolic oil (1 : 2) and permitting them to remain moistened with this solution until the next operation. Immediately before using the forceps they should be carefully wiped, and then dipped into a five per cent. watery solution of carbolic acid. Busch[168] recommends that the extraction itself be performed under antiseptic precautions, but regards an antiseptic after-treatment as unnecessary. Cold, clean water is best suited for syringing the mouth until the bleeding stops; the addition of antiseptics is not requisite, and only causes unnecessary complication and expense.

Von Mosetig-Moorhof[162] most energetically demands a strictly antiseptic proceeding in bloody operations in the mouth. "Operative dentistry in its bloody interferences (Eingriffen) is a specialty of surgery; those who practice it must consequently be acquainted with at least the fundamental principles upon which surgery is based. Now, the fundamental principle of the modern science of surgery is antisepsis, and the dentist ought not and dare not practice without it."

Witzel also recommends the cleansing of the mouth before operations, and the requisite after-treatment of the wound or the abscess-cavity.

Not only in tooth-extractions, however, but also in other less serious operations in the oral cavity, removal of tartar, filling of teeth, etc., must the greatest care be taken to keep the instruments clean and aseptic. Years ago I observed a case of the transmission of syphilis by means of dental instruments used in the cleaning of the teeth, and only a few weeks since a severe case of phlegmonous inflammation of the gums, following a careless removal of the tartar. Lanceraux reports on two cases of syphilis, one of which was caused by an infected instrument used in the catheterization of the left tuba Eustachii, the other by dental forceps used in extracting a number of decayed teeth. In this connection I may say that to me it is always a source of wonder that infections do not oftener occur through the repeated use of the coffer-dam for different persons, particularly as it is not always as carefully cleansed as it might be.

2. GANGRENOUS TOOTH-PULPS AS CENTERS OF INFECTION.

Infections through gangrenous tooth-pulps are to be ranked among the most frequent pyogenic infections of the human body; they by no means always have the harmless character commonly ascribed to them. The fact that the point of infection is so deep-seated, and is inclosed by hard, bony tissue, of itself anticipates results of a serious nature. According to Israel, the root-canal furnishes a point of entrance even for the ray-fungus, Actinomyces, and in one case the microscopic examination revealed the elements of this organism in the canal of a pulpless tooth.

If in any way or other (by tooth-decay, mechanical injuries, attempted extraction, etc.) the tooth-pulp be deprived of its natural covering, either totally or to such an extent that but a thin layer of softened dentine remains, a number of different processes may occur which will be discussed here only in as far as is essential to an understanding of the subject under treatment.

In regard to the faculty which the pulp possesses in taking up germs of infection and transmitting them to the tissues surrounding the apex of the root or even to the entire organism, I distinguish the following possibilities:

1. The infection of the pulp begins either on the surface or in the superficial layers; a progressive suppurative destruction of the tissue takes place, gradually spreading towards the apex of the root.

2. An infection of the entire pulp occurs, causing a total purulent inflammation; or, a local septic infection becomes general: for example, a case of pulpitis acuta partialis purulenta develops into a case of pulpitis acuta totalis ulcerosa (Rothmann.)

In both 1 and 2 micro-organisms of a more or less pronounced pathogenic character make their way to the apex of the root, or may even encroach upon the periapical tissue.

3. Necrosis of the pulp occurs without any preceding infection (in cases of total acute inflammation, destruction of the pulp by arsenious acid, etc.). After the death of the pulp has occurred, whether in the manner described in number 1, 2, or 3, an invasion of various bacteria, strictly saprogenic as well as pathogenic, usually takes place: the pulp, or its remains, becomes a stinking, cheesy, or semi-fluid mass (gangrene).

4. We should take into consideration the possibility that micro-organisms may be taken into the circulatory system from a small focus of suppuration in the pulp, such as pulpitis acuta partialis purulenta, etc., thereby leading to diseases of a more serious nature. It is universally known that such a general infection may proceed from alveolar abscesses, as shown by the cases cited below. But, as far as I know, no communications have been made as to the possibility of septicæmia or pyæmia, etc., arising directly from the pulp without the intervening stage of an alveolar abscess, which acts as an accumulator of the poison. A case which may belong under this head is that reported by Schmid (page 291).

5. By way of the circulatory system microbes which acci-

dentally obtain entrance to the blood through slight wounds of the skin, mucous membrane, etc., may enter a diseased pulp or come in contact with a dead one. Finding here a suitable medium, they proliferate, forming a focus of infection which may bring about secondary disturbances at the point of the root. This process may be illustrated by the following observation: A mouse having a wound at the root of the tail was inoculated subcutaneously near the foreleg with a pure culture of a mouth-bacterium; twenty-four hours later this bacterium was found to have established itself in large numbers in the old wound, though it was not to be found in other parts of the body. If the mouse had had a tooth with a dead pulp, I have reason to think that the bacterium would there also have found a suitable nutritive medium. The infection of the periapical tissue is usually occasioned either by the micro-organisms working their way into it independently from the pulp, or by the mechanical forcing of infected material (remains of pulp, etc.) through the foramen apicale. The latter may result from the pressure of mastication when the open root is filled with soft contents, or from the pressure of gases accumulating in the canal, or finally from dental operations. The consequences of such an infection depend upon the resistance offered to the advance of the bacteria and upon the virulence and number of the latter. Putrid products, which may be forced through the foramen, intensify the action of the bacteria by exerting a mechanical as well as a toxical irritation upon the tissue. In case the decomposed pulp contains no more living germs, particles of it may be forced through the foramen without causing an infection. In such cases a reaction takes places only in as far as it is produced by mechanical or chemical irritation of the products of putrefaction, which have been forced through the foramen.

Furthermore, apical infection with the harmless parasites of the mouth will, *cœteris paribus*, be accompanied by comparatively slight reaction.

If, on the other hand, living pathogenic bacteria are present in the pulp, an infection will take place whose intensity depends upon the number and virulence of the same.

Where the typically pyogenic micro-organisms, Staphylococcus pyogenes aureus, etc., are present, we may expect severe suppurative inflammation and formation of abscesses.

Parts of the pulp infected with the Bacillus pulpæ pyogenes will also occasion suppurative inflammation.

Infections with various pathogenic micro-organisms (mixed infections) will provoke divers phenomena. The progress of the infection will in all cases materially depend upon the general predisposition of the patient to infections, and upon his momentary state of health. Consequently, apical infections exhibit all transitions from a hardly perceptible reaction to the most dangerous phlegmonous inflammations, accompanied by general symptoms, such as high fever, chills, etc., which, as many instances show, may lead to meningitis, as well as to pyæmic and septicæmic processes, with fatal termination.

The connection between affections of the teeth and severe diseases of the jaw has already been pointed out by Hippocrates. He wrote, "The jaw of the son of Metrodorus mortified in consequence of toothache, and the gums became intensely swollen; the suppuration was moderate. Not only the molar teeth, but even the jaw-bone itself was thrown off."

The following in part fatal infections proceeding from the pulp may also be mentioned. They are almost without exception to be regarded as indirect infections. In all cases, excepting that related by Schmid, a local affection first took place, and only after a considerable quantity of poison had accumulated at the point of infection did the general infection occur.

Mr. Pearce Gould (*Journal of the British Dental Association*, April, 1886) has recorded a case of death from alveolar abscess, resulting in thrombosis of the cavernous sinus. On admittance the patient, aged fifty-seven, presented a sloughy opening in the center of the right cheek. An incision was made from the outside, and six molar teeth were extracted. The trismus was relieved, but œdema of the right temple appeared, and subsequently an abscess above the external angular process of the orbit, and another in the posterior triangle of the neck, but the internal jugular was not thrombosed. The respiration became stertorous, pulse 126, small, temperature 103.8°, and crops of herpes appeared about the lips. Great œdema of the orbit, and chemosis with some proptosis followed, and slight rigors occurred. Death ensued in a state of coma (Tomes).

Porre[169] (International Medical Congress, 1887) reported on eleven cases of chronic pyæmia proceeding from the teeth, all of which were healed by the extraction of the teeth. In one case he mentions the following symptoms:

The patient, male, good constitution and habits, suffered for the last thirty years from neuralgia, besides having constantly recurring furuncles and eruptions in various parts of the body, which would often for months become running abscesses. He experienced burning and itching eruptions of hands and feet, which finally changed to stubborn ulcerations. His bowels were either stubbornly constipated or exhaustingly loose. He suffered from frequent rigors and febrile attacks of varying intensity, profuse night-sweats, retention of urine, serious constrictions of the bowels and urethra. Lancinating pains darted from the maxilla of right side to bowels, bladder, limbs, hands, and feet, or to whatever part was locally affected at the time. This latter peculiarity, together with the discovery of a little pus exuding from the locality of the wisdom-tooth, led to a final correct diagnosis of his case. The tooth referred to was extracted, and a speedy and complete recovery followed.

A case of chronic pyæmia following upon an alveolar abscess has been observed by Mr. Howse. Suppuration occurred in the inferior dental canal, and acute periostitis in the posterior half of the lower jaw, which was denuded of its periosteum; the inflammation extended thence through the pterygoid fossa into the orbit, and thence backward. Ostitis of the vault of the skull followed, and general pyæmia, resulting in the patient's death on the ninth day after the supervention of the acute stage. (Tomes.)

A similar case is described by Baker.[170] Metastatic abscesses formed in different parts of the body. The patient was healed by antiseptic treatment and filling of the root-canal. Baker also reports on a case of fatal pyæmia proceeding from an abscess of a second molar; Poncet[171] on a case of osteitis which, proceeding from a carious tooth, led to a general septical infection, and ended fatally in forty-eight hours. Fripp[172] saw a case of inflammation of the brain proceeding from a dental abscess. Ritter[173] also observed a case of septical blood-poisoning due to a decayed tooth, which resulted fatally.

Coopman[174] noticed a fatal case of blood-poisoning in a boy eight years old, caused by a delay in the extraction of an abscessed tooth. An extensive periostitis accompanied by suppuration supervened. In spite of the extraction of the tooth, which had become quite loose, a metastatic abscess formed at the lower margin of the orbital cavity. The condition of the child grew worse from day to day, and death followed five days after the extraction.

Marshall[175] describes a case of emphysematous gangrene proceeding from an abscessed lower wisdom-tooth, which ended fatally in twelve days after a severe illness characterized by profuse suppuration, swelling, and throwing off of large necrotic masses.

Ed. Pietrzikowski[176] observed in the clinic of Gussenbauer a case of acute osteomyelitis accompanied by necrosis of the articular process of the right lower jaw. The trouble originated in an alveolar abscess.

Harrison Allen[177] reports the following case:

"A young man, in whom the roots of a lower wisdom-tooth had been prematurely filled, was attacked with acute periodontitis, ostitis, and maxillary periostitis, as above described. This was sufficiently severe to excite inflammation in the loose connective tissue between the mylo-hyoid muscle and the jaw. An abscess followed here, and the pus gravitated to form a collection about the hyoid bone, and from that point passed upward upon the face, along the line of the facial artery. The abscess, in addition, pressed directly upward against the floor of the mouth, and caused unilateral glossitis, from the mechanical effects of which upon the organs of respiration the patient died. The duration of the extra-maxillary complication was but four days."

M. Robert also relates a case in which necrosis supervened in an abscess connected with a lower wisdom-tooth; what is described as "purulent infiltration" of the side of the neck followed, and the patient rapidly sank. (Tomes.)

A reference to a case of necrosis of the lower jaw in a boy

seven years old, following an abscess caused by a carious tooth, will be found in the *Dental Cosmos*, vol. xvi, page 614. About one-half of the ramus of the left side was removed through the mouth, after enlarging the fistulous openings.

Schmid [178] gives a full report of a case of partial necrosis of the left half of the lower jaw following upon traumatic septic (gangrenous) pulpitis. The patient had bitten a foreign body into the cavity of an inferior left molar. The following morning the left cheek was so swollen that he was not able to open his mouth. After a long, severe illness, with varying symptoms (intense swelling, recurring abscesses, temperature 40° C., pulse up to 120, insomnia, discoloration of the skin, diarrhœa, etc.), not less than seventy pieces of necrotic bone were thrown off.

I am of the opinion that in this case a part of the septic tooth-pulp was forced through the foramen apicale by the pressure of the foreign body bitten into the pulp-cavity, and that the infection was brought about in this manner.

As is well known, diseased teeth very often occasion severe diseases of the nasal cavity and maxillary sinus. Such cases are too well known to every physician and dentist to necessitate the enumeration of special cases here.

Ritter [179] has of late described sixteen such cases, and thereby essentially strengthened the belief that by far the most cases of diseases of the maxillary sinus and many of the troubles in the nasal cavity are due to diseased teeth.

Galippe [180] also mentions the general disturbances that may arise whenever a secretion of matter in the mouth becomes general and profuse, as is the case in pyorrhœa alveolaris. "We have seen patients afflicted with fever, stiffness, loss of appetite, severe disturbances of the alimentary canal, insomnia, subicteric discoloration of the skin, etc."

Odenthal's [181] investigations have lent probability to the view that the centers of infections formed by decayed teeth manifest their deleterious influence in a manner hitherto but little suspected.

Ungar [182] had previously communicated a case in which a tubercular ulceration of the gums, followed by a swelling of the ymphatic glands, had formed around a badly decayed cuspid.

The circumstances were such as to leave no room for doubt that the tubercular infection of the lymphatic glands of the submaxillary region, consequently the infection of the whole organism, stood in close relation to that observed around the decayed tooth.

Von Bergmann[183] also regards lymphadenitis, the acute as well as the chronic form, as a disease occasioned by infectious germs which enter the lymph-passages from without, and are thence carried into the glands.

Odenthal, prompted by these views and by the investigations of Israel, discussed on page 341, undertook to determine whether decayed teeth were actually often the cause of swellings of the lymphatic glands of the neck. He examined in all 987 children, and found decay of the teeth in 429; in 558 no decay was present. Of the 558 children without decayed teeth, glandular swellings were noticed in 275 cases, that is, in 49 per cent. of all. Of the 429 children with decayed teeth, swellings were noticed in 424 cases, that is, in 99 per cent. Odenthal was also able to establish a constant relation between the extent of the glandular swellings and that of the decay. In such cases where the pulp-chamber was exposed, that is, where there was probably a gangrenous or highly-inflamed pulp, the swelling of the glands was almost invariably more pronounced and extended. Furthermore, the presence of a number of decayed teeth was universally accompanied by very marked glandular swellings. Where there were decayed teeth on both sides of the jaw, there was a corresponding glandular swelling on both sides.

The above by no means exhausts the number of cases reported in the last few years, but what has been said may suffice to show the importance of the subject under discussion, and the necessity of thoroughly examining the oral cavity in all disturbances or diseases the origin of which is not directly apparent. It also shows that the custom of many physicians, to disregard dental diseases altogether as a factor in pathology, is as unjust to their patients as it is discreditable to their profession, and that no physician can afford to be without a thorough knowledge of the pathological processes occurring in the human mouth and their relation to general diseases.

How often cases of this nature occur may be seen from the fact that a pupil of mine, who is making a study of this question, was able to secure the history of no less than twenty-one cases which had come under the notice of two hospital directors within the last five years.

Even leaving these extreme cases recorded above out of account, we find often enough caries and necrosis of the alveolar abscess or of the maxilla itself, chronic pyæmia, large abscesses opening upon the outside, etc., as the consequences of an infected tooth. The course of even the simplest form of alveolar abscess, from the beginning of the pericementitis to the formation of the abscess and the discharge of the pus, is often accompanied by very disagreeable symptoms,—intense pain, swelling, high fever, complete debility, etc. However, the symptoms of alveolar abscesses are too well known to make a further explanation of them necessary in this place.

As regards the etiology of alveolar abscess, we have adopted the universally accepted view that it is caused by bacteria. There can hardly be a doubt of this, particularly as the most careful investigations have proved that suppuration can arise without micro-organisms only in exceptional cases.

Black made the attempt to produce suppuration at the apex of the root by mechanical irritation, and for this purpose several times passed a sterilized steel wire through the foramen of a perfectly disinfected root-canal, but succeeded in causing only a slight temporary inflammation.

According to Arkövy,[184] Rothmann,[185] and others, an infection of the dental pulp may occur while it is still protected by a perfectly healthy layer of dentine, or, in other words, has not yet been reached by the softening of the dentine. Under such circumstances Arkövy repeatedly observed the distinct phenomena of pulpitis, and drew therefrom the conclusion that acute pulpitis must be referred to a much earlier stage of dental decay and of dental infections in general than heretofore supposed. The microscopical examination revealed numerous micrococci in the connective tissue at the base of the odontoblast layer, on the nerves, etc. (Fig. 118). Comparative examinations of intact pulps revealed no invasion of micro-organisms. On the strength of these facts Arkövy assumed that a pulpitis due to septical causes is not only possible but actually occurs, and that the name pulpitis acuta septica is appropriately applied.

I regard it as highly probable that bacteria from the decaying dentine may pass through the tubules of a *thin* layer of sound dentine and encroach upon the pulp; that they, however, pass through thicker layers, unless in very exceptional cases, seems to me doubtful; that they may pass through the entire thickness of the solid dentine is quite out of the question.

Any doubts which might still be entertained concerning the infectious nature of the germs contained in putrid pulps have been completely removed by a series of culture and infection experiments which I made during the year 1888, and which prove beyond doubt that purulent and gangrenous tooth-pulps represent a very fertile source of infection.

FIG. 118.

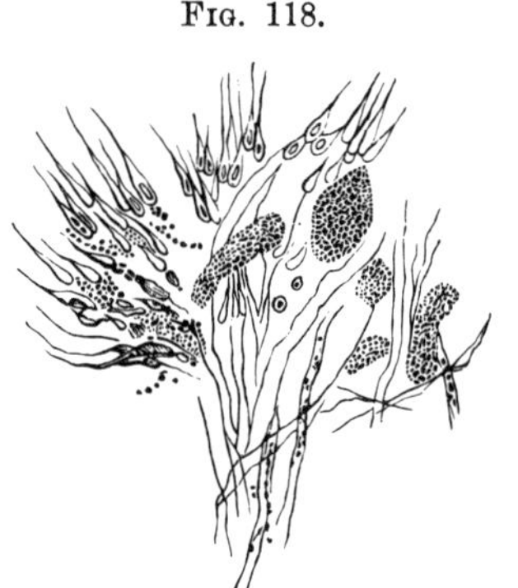

Infection of the pulp with micrococci in pulpitis acuta septica. (After Arkövy.)

Small particles of such pulps brought under the skin of mice, occasioned after twenty-four hours in the majority of cases inflammation and swelling surrounding the point of infection. At the end of the second or third day a small abscess was generally found, which, when opened, discharged a drop or two of pus.

In all, fifty-eight subcutaneous infections were made in this manner. In 36.8 per cent. the infections were accompanied by severe symptoms, in 7 per cent. the disease resulted fatally, in 47.4 per cent. the infection was insignificant, and in 15.8 per cent. no reaction was discernible.

As a rule, the reaction is not so violent following such inoculations as when a human being is infected by forcing particles of gangrenous pulps through the foramen apicale, for the reason that in the latter case the point of infection is more deeply seated, and at the same time surrounded by unyielding tissue. In one case especially, interesting and characteristic phenomena appeared. In twelve to fifteen hours a blackish or bluish-black spot had formed around the pocket; in twenty-four hours some swelling was noted, and also a slight fluctuation, *i.e.*, a slight formation of pus. At the end of the second day a tumor about the size of a pea had developed, which, on being punctured, evacuated a considerable quantity of pus mixed with gas and emitting an extremely strong and offensive odor. A second mouse inoculated with a small quantity of this pus developed exactly the same symptoms; likewise a third inoculated from the second, and so on to the twelfth generation. At this time I was obliged to leave Berlin for a few days, during which the mouse last inoculated died, and with it this series of inoculations. The specific bacterium of this strictly gangrenous process I was unable to cultivate, for the reason that it, like many others of the oral bacteria, does not grow upon artificial media.

Pure cultures from gangrenous, as well as from suppurating pulps, revealed besides the pyogenic staphylococci other microbes of considerable pathological action, one of which, Bacillus pulpæ pyogenes, is described at length on page 273.

These few experiments suffice to show how dangerous a source of infections the pulp represents. It is highly desirable that this subject be investigated as thoroughly as its importance demands.

3. COMPLAINTS CAUSED BY THE DIRECT ACTION OF BACTERIA UPON THE MUCOUS MEMBRANE OF THE MOUTH AND PHARYNX.

We know that under certain circumstances Saccharomycetes may directly colonize in the mucous membrane of the mouth, and that in the mouths of enfeebled individuals bacteria also may occasionally obtain a foothold. The mucous membrane of the mouth and pharynx is especially susceptible to the action of certain germs of infection (those of diphtheria, syphilis, etc.), and large portions of the mucous membrane and the submucous tissue may be wholly destroyed by parasitical influences.

The question now arises: May not the constant contact with

bacteria and their fermentative products exert a deleterious influence even upon the normal mucous membrane and upon the entire organism by impairing its condition, lowering the sensation of taste, spoiling the appetite,—in other words, by producing a condition of the mouth which corresponds to that condition of the stomach denominated as "disordered stomach"? May not the "coated tongue," the "pappy taste," etc., which are concomitants of the disordered stomach, be conditioned, independently of the stomach, by fermentative processes in the oral and pharyngeal cavities? Indeed, the "spoiled mouth," as well as the "spoiled stomach," deserves a place among the diseases of the digestive tract, and many complaints of loss of appetite and of bad smell, which are said to come from the stomach, no doubt have their origin in the neglected condition of the oral cavity.

As early as 1756 Pfaff[86] had recognized the importance of putrefactive processes in the mouth. "It is necessary," he writes, "to remove the tartaric matter, because it is a heavy body and daily accumulates mucus, which alters the fine color of the teeth, gradually putrefies, attacks the gums, or even destroys their connection with the teeth. The teeth consequently become loose, a very disagreeable odor is emitted from the mouth, which is often falsely attributed to the innocent stomach."

The investigations of von Kaczorowski[133] have furnished a satisfactory solution of the above question. He had long held the belief that the nature of most inflammatory processes of the gums consisted essentially in an infectious process brought about by micro-organisms, and was strengthened in this belief by the observation that a frequent disinfection of the inflamed gums or oral cavity of teething children removed in a remarkably short time not only the inflammation, but also the concomitant catarrh of the mucous membrane of the respiratory and digestive tracts, the feverish excitement, convulsions, conjunctivitis, eczema, etc.

Not in children alone, however, but also in patients of every age has this fact been repeatedly observed. Von Kaczorowski justly opposes the view that the tongue is an indicator of the condition of the stomach, and that the latter is always responsible for the want of appetite. On the other hand, according to him, the appetite is chiefly determined by the condition of the mucous membrane of the tongue and of the oral and pharyngeal cavities. When the tongue is clean, even fevering patients retain their appetite, while, on the other hand, the digestive process may go on perfectly while the appetite is impaired. This is proved by the favorable results of stomach-feeding even of such patients who are not able to take food on account of the retching produced as soon as the attempt is made to swallow it.

The nausea is consequently not due to the stomach, but to the diseased throat; and the antipathy to taking food, which is caused by the condition of the throat, may be removed by frequent disinfection of the oral and pharyngeal cavities.

What far-reaching disturbances of the general health may be obviated by the simple sterilization of the mouth is shown by the following case: "A lady, fifty years old, who was afflicted with a long-standing insufficiency of the aorta, but otherwise in good health and enjoying a vigorous digestion, began after a heavy sorrow to lose her appetite, complained of cardialgia (which set in after every meal), belching, and heartburn, until she could take but slight liquid nourishment, and finally was compelled to restrict herself to tea. Repeated courses of treatment with Carlsbad water brought but temporary relief. A disagreeable odor from the mouth, especially in the morning, led me to an examination, which revealed swelling and slight ulceration of the gums; besides this, the tongue was heavily coated and the posterior wall of the pharynx somewhat inflamed. Frequent syringing of the oral and pharyngeal cavities with the iodine-myrrh tincture stopped the cardialgia in the course of a few days, and restored the patient to her former appetite.

"As often as the patient, who has a great antipathy to medicines, neglects the disinfection of her mouth for but a single day, the always more or less hyperæmic gums swell again and the old digestive troubles recommence. I have been able now for seven years to watch this play of stomach-complaints in the wake of recrudescent inflammation of the gums."

The connection between bacterial growths in the mouth and severe disturbances of general health is furthermore exemplified by the following case, which occurred a short time ago in my own practice: The patient, forty-five years of age, had complained for months of severe pains caused by eating or even *speaking*, of loss of appetite, indigestion, disordered stomach, etc. These troubles became so burdensome that the patient declared that life had become insupportable. She showed me two envelopes filled with prescriptions both for internal and external use. One glance into her mouth, the odor emitted from it, and the concomitant inflammation and suppuration of the gums, suggested intense fermentative processes. The cleansing of the oral cavity, as well as the use of antiseptic and astringent mouth-washes, caused such a pronounced improvement in a fortnight that the patient could not often enough express her thanks. In this case the source of the trouble was so apparent that I cannot understand why it had not been discovered before.

We frequently meet with persons who, as von Kaczorowski correctly says, carry such filth in their mouths as they would never tolerate on the skin. The physician who must insert his finger into such a mouth is sometimes well-nigh overcome with disgust; the fœtor ex ore is insufferable, the teeth are covered with a thick deposit in a state of active fermentation, the gums intensely reddened, inflamed, suppurating, and where decayed roots are present, which is usually the case, chronic abscesses produced by them continually discharge suppurative and putrefactive products into the oral cavity; and with all this they still expect to enjoy good health! Such patients travel from one bathing-place to another, naturally without finding any relief, whereas the only journey necessary would be to the next hydrant, and the only remedy a strong tooth-brush and a disinfecting tooth-wash, or, at most, a visit to the dentist.

That the relation existing between an unclean mouth and other complaints has not been long ago and repeatedly emphasized is explained by the fact that the mouth as a source of diseases has been very much underrated, as the case just cited most clearly demonstrates.

4. PULMONARY DISEASES CAUSED BY THE INSPIRATION OF GERMS FROM THE ORAL CAVITY.

Comparatively few investigations or observations have been made with regard to diseases of the lungs which may be brought about by the inspiration of mouth-germs. The cases communicated by Leyden and Jaffé, as well as by James Israel, suffice, however, to prove that an infection of the lungs by microbes which have established themselves in the mouth is by no means impossible.

In cases of gangrene of the lungs and of putrid bronchitis, Leyden and Jaffé [186, 187] found elements in the sputum which morphologically, as well as in their reaction upon iodine, were identical with those which occur in the mouth. They formed the opinion that the germs always present in the mouth in such quantities might be carried into the lungs with the inspired air, and there, under favorable circumstances, proliferate. On introducing shreds and larger casts into the lungs of rabbits, they observed in some cases considerable inflammation with gradually progressing contraction of the trachea, and in others severe inflammation, followed by the formation of abscesses.

J. Israel [188] has also furnished striking proof of the correctness of the supposition that pulmonary diseases may be brought about by the inspiration of germs from the oral cavity. In a case of primary actinomycotic infection of the lungs, Israel found a small irregular body, resembling a piece of dentine, which he sent me for examination. It was found to consist of a small fragment of dentine, surrounded by a chalky mass, composed of phosphate and carbonate of lime, presumably tartar. The microscopic preparations of this fragment revealed numerous threads of the ray-fungus, and there can be little doubt that the fragment was the carrier of infection.

Baumgarten [189] also reports a case of primary actinomycosis of the lungs with secondary propagation to the soft tissue of the thoracic wall, caused by inspiration of the specific fungal elements accumulated in the lacunæ of the left tonsil.

On the whole, however, it may be taken for granted that infections of the lungs proceeding from the oral cavity occur more rarely than we might be led to expect, as a very strong inspiration is requisite to detach infected particles from the surface of the mouth and to carry them into the lungs. The very important part probably played by the micrococcus of sputum septicæmia in this connection has been discussed on pages 261, 262.

5. COMPLAINTS OF THE DIGESTIVE TRACT CAUSED BY MOUTH-BACTERIA.

More than thirty years ago the fact was commonly recognized that various disorders of the stomach and intestines owe their origin to local fermentative and putrefactive processes. According to Baginsky,[190] Bednar[191] was the first to give clear expression to this view, in 1854. Bednar expressed the view that indigestion may be brought about *directly* by taking into the stomach any substance already in the state of fermentation; *indirectly*, when the food taken into the stomach undergoes subsequent fermentation on account of its disproportion to the digestive juices.

Henoch[192] favored this conception; he emphasized the fact that a large number of diarrhœas, especially in the case of infants brought up on the bottle or just weaned, depended solely upon fermentative and decomposing processes of the contents of the stomach and intestines, without a material alteration of the mucous membrane of the alimentary canal.

Naunyn[193] and Leube[194] also regarded fermentative processes in the stomach as important factors in the production of gastric complaints: "the very pronounced chemical anomalies of gastric digestion, recognizable through the fermentations in the stomach, go hand in hand with the mechanical insufficiency."

De Bary,[195] on the contrary, concluded from his experiments that the action of bacteria as a factor in the origin of dilatations or other gastric complaints had been overrated.

Frerichs[196] also wrote, "They (the bacteria) neither interfere with nor further the digestive processes, but are harmless inmates."

Ewald,[197] whose examinations of the process of digestion and digestive troubles have met with universal recognition, assigns to gastric fermentations a position corresponding to their importance.

"In diseases of the stomach, which lead either to an insufficient acidification or an abnormally long retention of the food in the stomach, fermentative decomposition of the ingesta readily takes place. In such cases the carbohydrates are decomposed partly into gaseous products, and, according to the ferments present, sometimes the alcoholic or acetic acid fermentation and sometimes the lactic or butyric acid fermentation will ensue.

"My colleague (Rupstein) and myself had opportunity to watch a case in which, as the patient very drastically expressed himself, the vinegar factory alternated with the gas factory. In one case the alcoholic fermentation led to the formation of acetic acid, then the butyric acid fermentation to the evolution of hydrogen and carbonic acid. This case was especially remarkable for the fact that the patient occasionally belched up higher compounds of carbon and hydrogen, such as marsh-gas and possibly olefiant gas, which, on holding a candle to his mouth, ignited and burned with a weak flame."

Escherich,[198] whose examinations into the diseases of the stomach and intestines of infants are probably known to the reader, also recognizes the important part played by bacteria in these diseases, and recommends, besides the administration of antiseptics, as still more important than these, a strict regulation of diet.

It would, however, lead us too far to notice the different views concerning the importance of gastric fermentation for the origin of catarrhs of the stomach, dilatations, etc. The observations of thousands of physicians sufficiently prove the occurrence of abnormal fermentative processes in the stomach; and no one can deny that such processes may appear in stomachs whose functions are otherwise normal as well as in diseased ones. The greater the mechanical or chemical insufficiency, the more violent will be the fermentative processes and the more injurious their action on the digestion.

According to Minkowski,[199] the disturbances which are directly caused by the fermentative processes in the stomach may be referred to the following factors:

1. Substances may be formed which irritate the mucous membrane of the stomach and bring about a state of catarrhal inflammation.

2. Considerable quantities of gas may be formed which cause subjective complaints and heighten the already existing mechanical insufficiency of the stomach.

3. The fermentations may lead to the production of substances possessing toxic properties.

4. In fermentations of albuminous substances alkaline products may arise which occasion neutralization of the gastric juice.

5. The gastric fermentations may further exert a great influence on the functions of the intestines.

We have now to consider the following question: What part may be assigned to the oral cavity as a breeding-place or starting-point for the infection of the digestive apparatus?

There can be no question that microbes are carried from the mouth into the stomach and intestines every time that food is taken. The view formerly held, that the swallowed germs perish in the stomach, is entirely erroneous, as I myself[200] have shown, and as has since been corroborated by MacFadyan,[201] Sucksdorf,[202] and others. Baumgarten[203] had previously established the fact that in the case of the tubercle-bacillus the normal gastric juice does not destroy its virulence. Sucksdorf undertook to ascertain by experiments to what extent our food and drink are responsible for the regular importation of bacteria into the stomach and intestines, and in how far their quality and composition and the manner of their preparation influence the growth of germs found in the intestinal tract. As result of these investigations, it was found that the number of bacteria in the fæces was considerably diminished by partaking of sterilized food only. In mixed food Sucksdorf found on an average 380,000 cultivable germs in one milligram of fresh fæces. If the food was sterilized before the meal, only 10,390 colonies on an average developed. These results show very clearly that the number of bacteria in the intestinal tract depends in a high degree on the number continually reimported with the food.

Nothing is said in Sucksdorf's experiments as to the condition of the oral cavity, and nothing concerning the manner in which the food was preserved. Besides, the experiments were made at a season which is most favorable to the development of bacteria in foods.

When, therefore, Sucksdorf concludes that out of one hundred bacteria found in the fæces ninety-seven must be considered as derived from the food and drink and only three from the oral cavity itself, this conclusion may possibly be correct in the case of a healthy, well-cared-for mouth and badly preserved food; in general, however, I do not think that it is so, as is shown by his experiments on a second person, where 30 per cent. of the bacteria present in the fæces must be regarded as derived from the mouth.

From neglected mouths, such as repeatedly come under the notice of dentists, enormous quantities of bacteria must reach the intestinal tract in spite of the sterilization of the food. In a very unclean mouth examined for this purpose I estimated, by culture methods, the number of cultivable bacteria at 1,140,-000,000; many of these were doubtless carried to the stomach during every meal, to be replaced by others developing between meals and over night.

The following case, among many communicated by von Kaczorowski, proves clearly enough that the micro-organisms in an unclean mouth, quite independently of those introduced with food and drink, suffice to produce intense fermentative processes, chronic dyspepsia, etc., in the stomach.

" A hale and hearty landed proprietor, fifty years of age, who, according to his statement, had never been ill, nevertheless complained for some years of a troublesome inflation of the stomach after meals, which did not subside for hours. The examination revealed an artificial plate of the upper jaw, which the patient had not touched for two years. After removing it, I observed an intense redness and sponginess of the gums and hard palate. After the patient had become accustomed to removing his artificial teeth after every meal, and to disinfecting his mouth, the digestive troubles ceased without the use of remedies, and after four weeks, when I saw him again, a swelling of the liver with which he had been affected for some time had also disappeared."

During 1885–86 I made some experiments in order to determine the relation of mouth-, stomach-, and intestine-bacteria to each other, and also concerning certain disturbances in the stomach and intestines caused by them, the results of which I have communicated in the *Deutsche med. Wochenschr.*,[204] and here recapitulate:

"Of twenty-five different kinds of bacteria which I have isolated from the secretions of the human mouth, twelve are cocci and thirteen bacilli or bacteria. It was not possible in all cases to make a distinction between bacilli and bacteria, since so many kinds produce at the same time long rods (bacilli) and short rods (bacteria).

"Twelve of the mouth-bacteria I found again in the fæces, and eight in the contents of the stomach. In the latter case the material for the investigations was furnished by a gentleman who could evacuate his stomach at will an hour or two after partaking of a small quantity of fruit, particularly strawberries. Each time the oral cavity was carefully cleaned and sterilized with sublimate (1–1000), in order to prevent the intermixture of bacteria from the mouth. That the micro-organisms really came from the stomach, and not from the mouth or œsophagus, could readily be seen by their large numbers. I have satisfied myself by repeated experiments that in plate-cultures from the saliva of a mouth which has been treated as stated above, very few, or no colonies at all, will be developed, while in the cultures from the contents of the stomach a small drop in 5.0 cc. of gelatine would produce colonies so numerous that the separate ones were indistinguishable. Again, all organisms which were represented by only a few colonies were excluded.

"It is, perhaps, allowable to take for granted that all the stomach-bacteria enter the stomach along with the food; it is much less probable that they find entrance from the duodenum, although the possibility cannot be entirely excluded. It would not be permissible to assume that the intestinal bacteria all came from the stomach, since an entrance per anum is not to be overlooked, and since the stomach is supposed to present an impassable barrier for most micro-organisms. The results obtained from the experiments to be described indicate, however, that the latter is not the case, but that any bacterium, under a variety of conditions, may readily pass the stomach without losing its power of development. The resistance of many micro-organisms to the action of the gastric juice may be seen from the following experiment:

"About three hours after a moderate meal, 70 cc. of the contents of the stomach were evacuated and placed in the incubator under exclusion of air-germs. Three hours later, by means of plate-cultures, I found three kinds of bacteria, and ten hours later one kind. Not till after the lapse of fourteen hours were all bacteria missing. The fact that a bacterium in an artificial gastric juice (containing 0.2 per cent. HCl) may lose its vitality in a short time, is no proof that it may not safely pass through the stomach, because—

"1. The microbes which are swallowed at the beginning of a meal do not pass into a stomach filled with gastric juice, but into an empty stomach having a neutral or alkaline reaction, where free hydrochloric acid, in detectable quantities, does not appear until after the lapse of one-half to one and one-half hours.

"2. The micro-organisms are often imbedded in solid particles of food, thus escaping for a while the action of the juice.

"3. Liquid substances do not remain long in the stomach, but soon pass into the duodenum, and carry with them the bacteria before any considerable quantity of gastric juice has been secreted. In a case of fistula in the upper part of the duodenum, Busch saw the first portions of food appear fifteen or twenty minutes after the beginning of the meal (*vid.* Hoppe-Seyler, 'Phys. Chem.,' page 326). In case of soft liquid food, the transit may begin still sooner. The experiments of Watson Cheyne, and others, in connection with this subject, do not appear to me to be conclusive, because made under conditions too unlike those actually present in the stomach. Cheyne added material containing micro-organisms to a comparatively large quantity of artificial gastric juice, and observed that they were destroyed in a short time. Such experiments simply show that the normal gastric juice has antiseptic properties sufficiently strong to devitalize certain bacteria within a certain time. They give us, however, very little information as to the real occurrences in the stomach itself.

"In order to reproduce as nearly as possible the conditions present in the normal stomach, I chewed up a quantity of bread and meat, added a small quantity of liquid (milk), and divided the mixture into portions of 26.0 cc. each. These portions were brought into small flasks, sterilized, and then infected, some with a very sensitive vibrio, the others with hardy ferment-bacteria from the stomach. To each portion was now added, every ten minutes, 2.0 cc. of an artificial gastric juice containing 0.4 per cent. HCl (1.6 cc. HCl solution of sp. gr. 1.1233), so that, at the end of the second hour, the mixtures contained each 0.2 per cent. HCl, corresponding to the most active point of normal gastric digestion, which has been determined to be at about the end of the second hour or a little later, when the acidity of the stomach has reached its highest degree. Cultures made from time to time, during the course of the experiments, from the different flasks showed that the least resistant of the micro-organisms experimented with retained their vitality till the end of the third half-hour, sometimes even longer, and that the less sensitive ferment-bacteria showed no diminution in number at the end of the experiment, and in many cases some of them were still found six to eight hours later. Inasmuch as portions of food pass into the duodenum in less than half an hour after entering the stomach, these experiments seem to indicate that any micro-organism swallowed at the beginning of a meal might readily pass through the stomach alive. The case is somewhat different, however, if the bacteria are swallowed when the digestion is at its most active stage (second and third hour). Experiments representing this stage of digestion showed that very sensitive putrefactive bacteria may thus be destroyed within ten minutes, while the hardiest ferment-bacteria may resist for hours.

"From these experiments the conclusion appears warranted that all bacteria which are swallowed at the beginning of a meal may pass alive into the intestines, while of such as are swallowed in the second or third hour, only those which are less sensitive to the action of acids retain their vitality. If we furthermore take into consideration the various and numerous affections in which the quantity of gastric juice or its percentage of HCl is abnormally small, it will appear as though the stomach affords almost no protection whatever against the entrance of pathogenic organisms into the intestinal canal, and that the condition of the intestines themselves must be looked upon as the factor which determines whether a pathogenic micro-organism which has entered the alimentary tract shall or shall not come to development or manifest its characteristic action in the intestines. We have an exact proof that such is the case with the cholera-bacillus. Koch [205] found that in order to make guinea-pigs susceptible to the cholera poison it did not suffice to secure the passage of cholera-bacilli into the duodenum by neutralizing the contents of the stomach, but that it was necessary first to induce an atonicity of the intestines themselves, with cessation of the peristaltic action.

"It is worthy of mention that, although particles of food take up the acid with avidity, they nevertheless often appear to afford a certain protection to the micro-organisms. I have repeatedly observed in plate-cultures that muscular fibers in particular were lined with colonies, while on other parts of the plate very few were to be seen."

Some further questions of interest in this connection are the following: At what stage in the process of digestion, or at what percentage of acid in the contents of the stomach, does fermentation cease? How much of a given antiseptic—hydrochloric acid, salicylic acid, etc.—must be administered in order to bring about a cessation of an abnormal fermentation in the stomach? I attempted to effect a solution of these questions through the following experiments:

I chewed up a portion of meat and bread, and added a small quantity of sugar with sufficient milk to make a thick paste. I then infected this mixture richly with three kinds of stomach-bacteria which are characterized by the large quantities of gas that they produce, and added to it an equal quantity of 4 per cent. peptone-sugar gelatine. After it had stood for an hour in the incubator, it was divided into a number of portions of 20 cc. each. To each of these portions I added hydrochloric acid in increasing quantities, so that the first received 4 parts of HCl to 10,000, and the last 2 to 1000. After this they were poured into test tubes, and the level of the mixture in each tube accurately marked. The portions being kept at 20° C. soon solidified, and after eight to twelve hours, in all the tubes where fermentation took place an elevation of the surface of the gelatine was observed, due to the formation of bubbles of gas, and in those tubes containing the smallest quantity of HCl the mixture was in part driven quite out of the tube. I found that not till the proportion of HCl reached 1.6 to 1000 did the surface of the mixture remain at a constant level, or, in other words, did the fermentation cease. Salicylic acid effected the same in the proportion of 0.4 to 1000. If, therefore, in a food mixture we wish to prevent fermentation, or to arrest it when once begun, we must add 1.6 grams HCl or 0.4 gram salicylic acid to each 1000 grams of the mixture.

In the human stomach, however, we have to deal, not with a total lack of HCl, but rather with a diminution in the quantity of the same, so that we require only to supplement the acid already present. When digestion is at its most active stage, the proportion of HCl in the contents of the stomach under normal conditions is about 2 to 1000, and since fermentation does not take place till this proportion has been reduced to 1.6 to 1000, we must, in cases of continued fermentation in the stomach, suppose a lack of HCl equal to at least 0.4 gram per liter of stomach contents, and this quantity must be administered in order to restore the normal condition.

According to the determinations of Bidder and Schmidt, ten to twenty liters of gastric juice are secreted daily. If we consider this estimate as two to four times too high, and take five liters as the real quantity, we still have ten grams HCl (forty grams HCl solution of sp. gr. 1.1233) which are daily poured into the human stomach. Under such circumstances we can hardly expect to produce much impression by the three- to ten-drop doses recommended in text-books. The quantity of any given antiseptic which is necessary to suspend fermentation in the human stomach depends upon the intensity of the fermentation and the quantity of the stomach contents; in any case we must calculate upon large and repeated doses of HCl if we wish to produce a marked impression. In case of the ordinary lactic-acid fermentation outside of the stomach the process will, in a few hours, be retarded by the antiseptic action of the acid which is produced. In the stomach this action loses its significance, from the fact that the acid produced is speedily absorbed, and the contents of the stomach are replaced a number of times daily by neutral material. These experiments also show how small a change in the quantity or quality of the gastric juice may suffice to render a permanent fermentation (*dyspepsiă chronica*) in the human stomach possible.

The objection may be urged against these experiments that, in the solidified condition of the mixture, the HCl could not have its full effect. The control experiments, however, made at the temperature of the human body (at which the mixture of course became liquid), confirmed the accuracy of the previous results. It may be further said that a portion of the HCl disappeared in combination with bases in the mixture, but I am satisfied, from experiments not here described, that the loss from this source must have been very small, and was compensated for by the acid present in the mixture at the beginning of the experiment, the reaction in each case being clearly acid.

I next attempted to determine the action of these micro-organisms on carbohydrates, particularly their acid-producing power, being anxious to find the source of the acids of the human mouth. For this purpose I cultivated them in beef-extract-sugar solutions, in peptone-sugar solutions, and in milk. Sixteen of the mouth-bacteria produced an acid reaction, four an alkaline, and five gave inconstant results. The corresponding numbers for the stomach-bacteria were nine, two, and two; for the bacteria of the intestines, six, five, and three. The proportion of the acid-forming bacteria in the mouth and stomach is, according to these results, much greater than in the intestines. Whether this condition is constant or not, could be determined only by a large number of series of experiments. The cultures in sterilized milk gave results slightly different from the above. It was, furthermore, not possible to draw a sharp line between those bacteria which produced an acid and those which produced an alkaline reaction, since in some cases the reaction was only slight and changed with time, while in other cases it was altered by a change in the amount of sugar present. One bacillus which I tested in reference to this question, cultivated in 3 per cent. beef-extract solution, left the reaction neutral when one-tenth per cent. sugar was present; if the amount of sugar was increased, the reaction became acid; if it was diminished, the reaction became alkaline.

It is equally difficult, I think, to draw a sharp line between putrefactive and fermentative organisms, since many ferment-organisms are capable of decomposing albuminous substances with development of putrefactive products, while on the other hand many organisms which pass as putrefactive, when brought into saccharine solutions, give rise to fermentation without the production of a trace of the characteristic products of putrefaction. One of the mouth-bacteria which I examined in reference to this question readily dissolved coagulated albumen with development of bad-smelling gases, among which SH_2 (sulphuretted hydrogen) and NH_3 (ammonia) could be easily detected. It also showed an inverting action, in that it converted cane-sugar into dextrose and levulose. In the third place it split fermentable sugars into lactic acid, with production of CO_2 (carbon dioxide). In the fourth place it gave rise to an acid reaction in a solution of starch, while at the same time the solution acquired the capacity of reducing the oxide of copper; in other words, this bacterium showed also a diastatic action.

In these different fermentations there undoubtedly arise in the later stages various secondary products, so that the changes which may be brought about by this one micro-organism and the products developed under its action make up a very large number. This result affords an explanation of the fact that in an open decomposing substance so many different products may appear, and renders very doubtful the supposition that for every new product in the process of decomposition a new organism must be present. The twenty to thirty different compounds which may be produced in an open decomposing solution are in all probability not produced by one bacterium alone. It is, however, not in accordance with the facts to assume that for every product, or indeed for every stage in the process, a new bacterium must be introduced.

Of the bacteria under consideration I would like to call attention to five which regularly form large gas-bubbles in the gelatine or tear it in pieces, as represented in Fig. 8. One of these, which in albuminous substances also produces considerable quantities of gas (SH_2 and NH_3), was found in the fæces as well as in a gangrenous tooth-pulp. Its possible agency in the causation of dental abscesses has been referred to on page 36.

Three of the other four gas-forming bacteria I found in the stomach, and one in the fæces. It is not difficult to see what disturbances might be produced by an abnormal development of these bacteria in the stomach or intestines.

A further question of interest regards the peptonizing action, particularly of the bacteria of the intestines. By far the greater number of the different species which I have examined grow well on boiled white of egg, and can therefore be said to possess a peptonizing action. In some cases the albumen became completely liquefied by the action of the organisms. Whether they form more peptone than they need for their own nourishment, and whether and to what extent they may thereby be of use to the human body, is a question whose solution presents difficulties not yet overcome. In a large quantity of sterilized white of egg infected with a comma-bacillus, I found traces of peptone at the end of the third day.

Very few of the organisms here treated of were found to possess any marked diastatic action. Of nine species which I examined specially with reference to this property, only one gave a decidedly affirmative result. By the action of this bacterium starch was converted into sugar, and this again into acid.

It is generally taken for granted that a bacterium which grows on boiled potato must possess a diastatic action. Such evidence is, however, of little value, because the bacterium is not dependent upon the starch of the potato alone, but may derive sufficient nourishment from the sugar and albumen of the potato to maintain its existence for some time.

Not one, out of more than fifty species that I examined, belonged to that group of micro-organisms called anaërobian; *i.e.*, no one of them grew better or exclusively under exclusion of atmospheric air. On the other hand, I found every gradation, from those which showed no development whatever under exclusion of atmospheric air to those which grew equally well with or without it.

The following conclusions may be drawn from the experiments described above:

1. A large number of the bacteria of the alimentary canal are not restricted to one portion of it alone, but may develop either in the mouth, stomach, or intestines.

2. In by far the greater number of cases, the gastric juice will not prevent the entrance of bacteria into the intestines. All bacteria which I have examined may pass the stomach without losing the power of development, provided they are swallowed at the beginning of a meal. If, on the other hand, digestion is at its most active stage (two or three hours after the beginning of a meal), then those bacteria more sensitive to the action of acids will be destroyed before they reach the intestines.

3. Lactic-acid fermentation may continue in the stomach until the percentage of HCl reaches 1.6 to 1000. If too little HCl is secreted, or too much food taken at once, the fermentation may become permanent. Diseases of the stomach, general disorders of health, fever, etc., accelerate the fermentation by interfering with the normal secretion of gastric juice.

4. Fermentation in the stomach may be more readily arrested with salicylic than with hydrochloric acid.

5. A large number of the bacteria of the alimentary canal cause lactic-acid fermentation in solutions of carbohydrates, whereby the frequent appearance of lactic acid may be accounted for. Other ferment-acids, acetic, butyric, etc., I have observed less frequently and in smaller quantities.

6. Five of the species examined caused fermentation with formation of large quantities of gas, chiefly CO_2 and H.

7. It is impossible to make an exact division between those bacteria which produce an acid and those which produce an alkaline reaction in a given solution; also between ferment and putrefactive bacteria.

8. The majority of the bacteria which I have examined manifested a peptonizing, very few a diastatic action.

Gas-Forming Bacteria of the Stomach.

Reference has been made above to five kinds of bacteria, which are characterized by the very considerable quantities of gas which they produce in starchy and saccharine substances, and further by the marked resistance which they possess to the action of the gastric juice.

In view of the great importance which a thorough knowledge of the physiology of these micro-organisms has in the therapeutics of many disorders of the stomach, and especially in the dietetic treatment of such troubles, the results of a series of experiments made in connection with this subject may not be without value.

Two questions in particular appear to me to require a solution: 1. Are the micro-organisms which are taken into the stomach at any meal passed out or devitalized before the recurrence of meal-time, or does the stomach, of dyspeptics in particular, contain bacteria at all times? 2. In what manner is the quantity of gas generated by these bacteria influenced by the kind of food taken?

Respecting the first question, practical experience would incline us to the belief that the diseased or impaired stomach contains micro-organisms at all times, otherwise how are we to explain the fact that many patients almost immediately after taking starchy or saccharine foods are troubled with the distention of the stomach from formation of gas? I have demonstrated by various experiments that the bacteria which may be swallowed with a piece of bread are alone certainly not capable of bringing about this distention. Nevertheless, it appeared desirable to test the correctness of this supposition experimentally; and since the proper experiments could be performed on the human subject only with great difficulty, I chose dogs as the subjects, as they have a digestive process very similar to that of human beings. Up to the present but six dogs have been experimented upon, but as the results were the same in every case, they are entitled to consideration.

Four of these dogs, all healthy, were fed for two days on a mixed diet of meat, bread, milk, and sugar, richly infected with the gas-producing bacteria referred to. In every case diarrhœa made its appearance in from thirty to forty hours, and in two cases distention of the stomach was very marked. After the last feeding they were muzzled to prevent the possibility of their taking anything into the stomach, and killed after two and a half, six, eight, and nine hours respectively. In every case, except the last, the four kinds of bacteria administered were found in the stomach in great numbers, also in the large intestines; but few were present in the duodenum. In two cases the reaction of the contents of the intestines was strongly sour throughout, in one case slightly sour, and in one only was the reaction neutral or slightly alkaline. The remaining two dogs were treated in the same manner, except that the bread and sugar were omitted; the result was the same as above, only more marked. One of the dogs had profuse diarrhœa in fifteen hours, and the intestines, six hours after feeding, were distended with gas, and the reaction strongly sour. In both cases the bacteria were found in large numbers in the stomach, as well as in the intestines.

It appears from these experiments that these bacteria can maintain their existence, even in the stomach of dogs, for eight or ten hours, and can thereby give rise to disturbance in the intestinal canal; and when we take into account the fact that the gastric juice of the dog is one and one-half times as strong as that of the healthy human subject, and from one and one-half to many times as strong as that of the dyspeptic or stomach-ailing, there is little room left for doubt that living bacteria are constantly present in the stomach, and that many chronic troubles of the stomach are due, not alone to the micro-organisms which are at each meal taken in along with the food, but more particularly to those which are already in the stomach at the beginning of a meal.

It is, consequently, of greater importance to sterilize the stomach before eating than to sterilize the food itself. For example: What is the use of repeatedly boiling milk to free it from every single germ, and then taking it into a stomach containing vastly more bacteria than were in the milk in the beginning? It will furthermore be readily seen that the time for administering antiseptics is not after a meal, or upon the full stomach, but upon an empty stomach, about ten or fifteen minutes before meal-time. In order to determine what action these bacteria may have upon the digestive process when the conditions present are such as to permit of their development, I swallowed a full-grown test-tube culture of the Micrococcus aërogenes immediately after a meal, consisting mainly of bread, potatoes, and milk. A very disagreeable feeling of distention in the stomach and bowels appeared after about one and one-quarter hours, and annoyed me the whole of the next day; after thirty hours I was attacked with diarrhœa, which I aborted by taking sixty drops of hydrochloric acid in water after a light breakfast. The effects of the bacteria did not entirely disappear for some days, and even on the fifth day I still found them in large numbers in my fæces.

I attempted to effect a solution of the second question by the following experiment: I mixed 2.0 grams (30 grains) of the different kinds of food with 3.0 of saliva, added 5.0 grams beef-extract peptone-gelatine, which had been infected with Bacteria aërogene (or, I simply chewed up the food to be tested and mixed it with an equal quantity of the same gelatine). Each mixture was then poured into a separate test tube, the level marked, and placed at a temperature of 22° C. The amount of gas generated in the different tubes would be measured by the rise in the surface of the mixture. After a series of nineteen experiments I succeeded in getting together a table of comparative values, in which bread is used as the unit of comparison. (See Fig. 119.)

As expected, it was found that the carbohydrates are particularly characterized by the production of large quantities of gas, whereas from the albuminous substances only a trace, or no gas at all, is produced. Among the ordinary articles of diet, bread and potato occupy a prominent place as gas-producers, and should be as much as possible avoided by the dyspeptic.

Of those foods which do not appear in the table, and which produce large quantities of gas, I may mention all kinds of sweet desserts, cakes, omelettes, pears, sweet apples, grapes, etc. Cranberries and prunes produce no gas, because they do not furnish a favorable medium for the development of bacteria; if they are

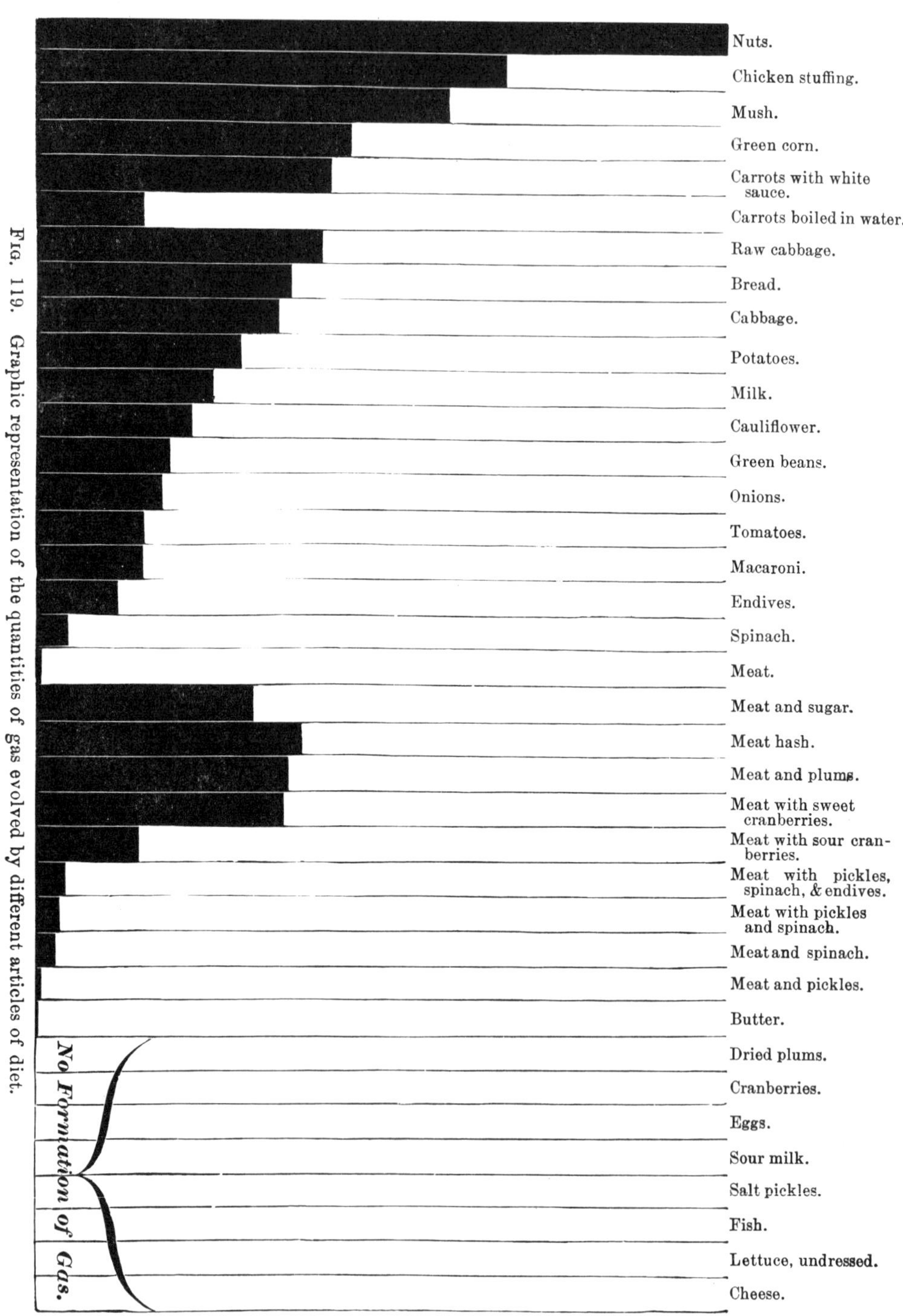

FIG. 119. Graphic representation of the quantities of gas evolved by different articles of diet.

mixed with meat, however, a very rapid development takes place, accompanied by a production of gas.

According to these experiments, a diet for stomach-ailing patients, which should be followed by no production of gas, distention of the stomach, sour eructation, etc., may consist of meat, eggs, fish, spinach, fresh lettuce, and small quantities of endives and sour cranberries.

The administration of an antiseptic before, and a digestive during or immediately after the meal, will materially aid the process of digestion.

I have had abundant opportunity to observe the happy action of the above diet on one who has for years been troubled with indigestion arising from abnormal fermentation in the stomach.

Morphology.

Bacterium aërogenes I. Short rods, single or in pairs, motile; forms on gelatine-plates circular yellowish colonies with distinct outlines. The colony is traversed by dark lines which often radiate from the center and extend close to its margin; it grows rapidly in line-cultures along the whole line with brown-yellow color, and forms a flat grayish-white pappy button; it does not liquefy the gelatine. On agar-agar it forms a grayish-white soft growth with indented irregular margin; grows rather rapidly. In line-cultures it grows as a cream-colored, moist deposit with smooth outlines, and shows under the microscope dark lines, which frequently run from the center to the margin. Growth without access of air somewhat retarded, but numerous gas-bubbles formed under the mica-plate.

Micrococcus aërogenes. Large oval cocci or plump rods, immotile; forms quick-growing, mostly round, but occasionally somewhat indented colonies of dark color, with smooth contour. It is characterized by leprous spots, which are dark or bright according to the adjustment of the microscope; grows in line-cultures like Bacterium aërogenes, but somewhat faster; in old cultures slightly liquefying. Line-cultures are distinguishable by the naked eye from Bacterium aërogenes I by the more undulating course of the borders; under the microscope the dark rays are wanting. Growth on agar-agar and on potato like that of Bacterium aërogenes I, but somewhat more yellowish and less moist; growth without oxygen but little retarded.

Helicobacterium aërogenes. Thin motile rods, single or in chains; grows into long undulating threads which sometimes form Spirulinæ; it develops transparent white or but slightly colored colonies, whose composition of rods and threads is perceptible even under 150 diameters. The colonies are round, oval, snail-, spindle-, or spiral-shaped, in short, show almost every possible form. In puncture-cultures the bacterium grows evenly along the line of puncture with a light yellowish color, and covers the surface after forty-eight hours (though not invariably) with a thin, hardly visible, bluish, dry layer. In line-cultures it also forms a thin, broad growth with very rugged margins; by transmitted light the culture has a flaky or crystalline appearance. Growth on agar-agar not characteristic; grows slowly on potatoes; has an indented margin, dry surface, yellowish-brown (mauve) color; growth without air restricted.

Bacillus aërogenes. Rather small, motile rods of various lengths; forms completely round, homogeneous, transparent, white or slightly yellowish colonies. Older colonies occasionally show a series of concentric rings. In line-cultures it grows evenly along the line of inoculation; is of yellowish color; on the surface it forms a thin, pearl-gray deposit with indented margin; does not liquefy; in older cultures the line of inoculation is dark brown, and surrounded by a peculiar light brown halo; growth on agar-agar shows nothing remarkable; on potato it grows very slowly, forming a dry deposit of bluish-yellow dirty color and irregular margin; growth without air very limited.

Bacterium aërogenes II. Morphologically indistinguishable from Bacterium aërogenes I; on agar-agar, potatoes, and in line-cultures it shows a growth similar to the former. The colonies, however, display essential differences: they are completely round, distinctly defined, yellowish, and, where they are closely gathered, completely homogeneous; where far apart, they show one or many black, irregular fissures on the surface; growth without air very limited; but few air-bubbles form under mica. A very slow liquefaction of the gelatine takes place, forming a funnel (but only after a number of days).

6. POINTS OF ATTACK FURNISHED BY A LACK OF RESISTANCE IN THE SOFT TISSUES OF THE MOUTH.

It is well known that the mucous membrane of the mouth, under certain conditions, loses its normal resistance to parasitical influences.

As a rule, only *weakly* children are afflicted with thrush; in adults the thrush-fungus appears only after debilitating diseases. Other parasitical diseases of the oral and pharyngeal cavities, as, for example, stomatomycosis sarcinica (page 334), mycosis tonsillaris, etc., either accompany marantic processes, or are developed in the course of local inflammations, but are seldom if ever observed when the mucous membrane is intact. The gums are also predisposed to infectious processes by local mechanical irritations.

In short, wherever, by any possible cause, mechanical, chemical, or thermal, local or general, external or internal, the nature of the tissue is so changed as to furnish a suitable culture-medium for certain microbes, a colonization of one or more of the various species in the mouth will take place. The diseases induced in this manner are:

a. Limited suppurative processes at the margin of the gums.

b. Formation of abscesses in consequence of impeded eruption of wisdom-teeth.

c. The affection termed pyorrhœa alveolaris.

d. Stomatomycosis sarcinica.

e. Mycosis (pharyngomycosis) tonsillaris benigna.

f. Stomacace.

g. All inflammations of the gums accompanied by suppurations and abscess-formations.

h. Thrush, occasioned by the yeast-fungus, Saccharomyces albicans. (This disease will be mentioned in the chapter on yeast-fungi.)

a. Limited Suppurative Processes at the Margin of the Gums.

The dentist daily meets with cases of the infections mentioned under *a.* Accumulations of tartar, sharp edges of decayed or filled teeth, pledgets of cotton, protruding fillings, etc., irritate or inflame the gums, thus facilitating or making possible the colonization of pyogenic bacteria. A small degree of suppuration will always be found in such cases; it may, under certain circumstances, extend to the pericementum and lead to abscess-formation.

b. Abscess-Formation resulting from Impeded Eruption of Wisdom-Teeth.

The affection which Arkövy calls abscessus alveolaris diffusus must, in my opinion, as far as it is caused by those difficulties accompanying the eruption of wisdom-teeth, also be assigned to this group.

It is immaterial in these cases whether the disease be seated in the gums,* or in the pericementum, or in the periosteum, or finally in the bone itself. The invasion of the bacteria is in every case made possible by the diminished power of resistance of the soft tissues, caused by long and continued irritation.

The infection by pyogenic microbes, so often accompanying impeded eruption, occasions not only profuse suppuration and abscess-formation in the region of the lower jaw, which are accompanied by pronounced general symptoms, but also often leads to general infection (septicæmia, pyæmia), with fatal result.

Various fatal cases of blood-poisoning occasioned by the impeded eruption of lower wisdom-teeth have been cited on page 289 *et seq.*

The inflammation existing in the pericementum, or in the gums, or in both simultaneously, manifests itself first by swelling, redness, and accompanying soreness of the gums, which in the mildest cases are circumscribed, in more pronounced cases involving a large part of the mucous membrane of the corresponding side of the mouth after inducing severe secondary angina.

The appearance of suppuration is always a bad omen, in my judgment calling for the immediate extraction of the tooth. I have invariably found the formation of pus to begin on the

---

* The difficulties connected with the eruption of wisdom-teeth usually lead to periosteal abscesses, while those arising from suppurative periostitis are generally sub-periosteal. (Arkövy, page 281.)

distal side of the tooth; a bent probe passed under the fold of the gum enters a pocket filled with pus, from which more or less pus exudes on pressure. If extraction is delayed, twenty-four hours may suffice to bring about complete trismus, by which the operation is extremely complicated, or for the time being made impossible. Even in such cases, however, I have seen all the swelling subside and the trismus and its accompanying symptoms disappear without any interference on the part of the dentist. Very commonly, the suppuration not remaining confined to the pericementum causes secondary periostitis and osteitis, involving a large portion of the angle and ascending ramus of the jaw. The bone becomes infiltrated with infectious sanious matter, which in this stage may readily be absorbed in sufficient quantities to occasion general poisoning, or it may make its way to the surface, usually at the outer angle of the jaw (fistula), or the inflammatory process may extend through the fossa pterygoidea, orbita, etc., to the brain, giving rise to a fatal meningitis. The process is accompanied by extensive swelling of the submaxillary region, and sometimes (seldom) by profuse suppuration or even gangrene of the gums. The tooth itself finally becomes exceedingly loose through destruction of the alveolus, and its extraction is accompanied by the discharge of a large quantity of bloody, stinking pus. After the extraction the wound should be thoroughly syringed with a 1–200 solution of sublimate.

c. Pyorrhœa alveolaris.

A disease of probably parasitic nature, which, next to decay of the teeth, has attracted more attention among dental surgeons than perhaps any other disease of the human mouth, and which every dentist has abundant opportunity of observing in his practice, is the so-called Riggs's disease, pyorrhœa alveolaris (loculosis, blennorrhœa gingivæ, periostitis alveolo-dentalis, infectious arthro-dental gingivitis, phagædenic pericementitis, expulsive gingivitis, symptomatic alveolar arthritis, etc.), a chronic suppurative inflammation of the periosteum, with more or less severe inflammation of the gums and necrosis of the alveolar process of the diseased teeth.

The first stage of the disease presents but little characteristic; it manifests itself only as a slight redness of the gums at the neck of the tooth, which cannot be distinguished from a simple gingivitis marginalis, such as is often caused by tartar. In the majority of cases tartar is actually present. The disease at this stage occasions but little or no inconvenience, and is therefore generally overlooked.

Soon, however, distinct and characteristic symptoms appear; the connection between the gums and the root is destroyed by the suppuration of the pericementum, the gums appear more or less swollen or puffed up, dark red or bluish red in color, and but loosely surround the neck of the tooth. Pressure upon the loose gums causes a slight discharge of pus. As the process advances, the margin of the alveolar process becomes involved and gradually broken down.* The gums either become hypertrophied and puffy or gradually recede, exposing a large portion of the root. A loosening of the teeth is now noticeable, which when neglected generally increases until they drop out of their own accord or become so troublesome as to make removal necessary.

The interval of time between the first appearance of the disease and the falling out of the affected tooth varies. I observed a case in which (according to the statement of the patient) three weeks after the commencement of the loosening of the teeth all the superior incisors were irrevocably lost; two fell out spontaneously, the others had to be removed. In other cases, however, the disease becomes chronic and many years elapse before it comes to an end. After the loss of the teeth, the phenomena completely disappear.

Pyorrhœa alveolaris usually attacks adults, by no means, however, exclusively, as many maintain. Some months ago I had an opportunity of studying several pronounced cases of pyorrhœa alveolaris in children of from four to twelve years of age.

By the kindness of Dr. Cass, director of the asylum for rhachitic and scrofulous children at Middelkerk, Belgium, I received permission to examine the mouths of over one hundred patients, and discovered several typical cases of pyorrhœa alveo-

* By many the bone is regarded as the seat of the primary infection.

laris. In the case of a lame boy, nine and a half years old, with remarkably advanced dentition, I found the left inferior first bicuspid so loose that it could be pushed back and forth with the fingers, the alveolus discharging pus profusely under pressure. The superior incisors of a girl four years old were extremely loose; the gums had receded, were very red, suppurating, in short exhibited all symptoms of pyorrhœa alveolaris.

Its etiology is a very much debated question, and at present the greatest differences of opinion prevail concerning it. Some (including Riggs, who first accurately described the disease and whose name it often bears) regard it as an altogether local affection, and consequently advise local treatment only. It cannot be denied that a careful cleansing of the teeth, the removal of accumulations of tartar, etc., may have a beneficial effect in the earlier stages of the disease, although those doubtless go too far who maintain that all cases may be permanently healed by this means. We are never sure that a relapse will not occur; severe cases may be kept within bounds, but not healed; a restoration of the lost portion of the gums is, however, out of the question.

Others, on the contrary, define pyorrhœa alveolaris as a general disorder.

Newland Pedley [206] writes, "The inferences that follow from the points I have enumerated lead to the assumption that pyorrhœa alveolaris is essentially of constitutional origin. In man and in lower animals it is found connected with wasting diseases and depressed conditions of the system. The local exciting cause may be very trivial in nature.

"The weight of evidence tends to place pyorrhœa alveolaris in the category of bone-diseases. The exposed position of the alveolar margin and its intimate relation with organs of such feeble vascularity as the teeth go far to explain why it is this portion of the alveolus that is first affected, and also the usual arrest of the disease by the removal of the teeth. It is not a necessary concomitant of tabes dorsalis."

Bland Sutton [207] indorses the views of Pedley: "The disease is undoubtedly of constitutional origin, but also requires local treatment." He has repeatedly observed the disease in rheumatoid arthritis, mollities ossium, etc.

Taft holds that pyorrhœa arises in consequence of a general disorder of health, and that local treatment is useless unless the general state of health be improved. Others, again, regard it as a disease brought out by some local irritation, but for whose causation a general bodily disorder (predisposition) is necessary. Without both of these factors the disease seldom, perhaps never, appears.

Reeve [208] accuses the use of spirituous liquors, which cause an increased secretion of uric acid. The concrements in pyorrhœa alveolaris, according to him, consist almost exclusively of uric acids.

Patterson [209] examined twenty-four cases, and determined in all the presence of catarrh of the mucous membrane of the nose or pharynx; in many cases both affections. For the most part the patients had the habit of breathing only through the mouth. Patterson is of the opinion that pyorrhœa alveolaris and catarrh are identical, a view to which F. J. Bennett [210] assents.

According to Witzel, pyorrhœa alveolaris is "a marginal necrosis of the alveolus, caused by a septical irritation of the bone-marrow," a view which Arkövy [211] seems to share, since he terms the disease "caries alveolaris specifica." He regards the alveolar margins as the seat of the primary disturbance. "The nature of the disease is a suppurative inflammation, which spreads to all parts lying between the gums and the dentine of the root."

Magitot, referring to the studies of Malassez and Galippe, mentioned below, does not doubt the parasitical nature of the disease; he concludes his remarks with the following propositions:

1. The affection characterized by alveolar suppuration and by the loosening and falling out of the teeth should be designated as a true symptomatic alveolar arthritis, septical and contagious.
2. It generally arises under the influence of certain unfavorable conditions of health and diathesis, also in exanthematic fevers, etc., where it manifests itself either as a complication or as a consequence.
3. The therapeutics should consist chiefly in the application of antiseptics, local alteratives, astringents, or caustics.

Malassez and Galippe have made very careful investigations concerning the etiology of pyorrhœa alveolaris. Galippe considers the disease as undoubtedly of a parasitical nature, "which may be proved by an examination of stained sections, by cultivation and isolation of the parasites contained in the dentinal tubules, by the contagion spreading from tooth to tooth, as well as from individual to individual, as we have observed more than once in persons of different sex, who stand in intimate relations to each other."

Galippe[180] found in the tubules of a tooth attacked by infectious arthro-dental gingivitis a "parasite temporarily designated by the letter η, which shows the form of a very delicate double bubble (Doppelbläschen), and is changed by cultivation into a bacillus, the gelatine melting, and a characteristic rod appearing in the tube of the gelatinous bubble.

"Subcutaneously injected into guinea-pigs it produced, after fifteen days, in the joints of all the paws a series of abscesses, which made all motion impossible; the movements proceeding from the pelvis were extremely painful. Some of the abscesses opened spontaneously, the others were lanced with the necessary precautions. The parasite η could again be isolated from the pus. After several months the guinea-pig recovered from the infection, but the awkwardness and stiffness in the joints remained.

"This parasite showed a preference for the osseous system in a rabbit, into whose abdomen a pure culture of it was injected. After fifteen days the emaciated rabbit manifested a sluggishness of locomotion, and we discovered a considerable abscess in the plane of the left thigh.

"This abscess was lanced; from the pus treated in the usual manner the parasite η was again obtained in pure culture. After a few days the abscess reappeared, and it was observed at the same time that the animal breathed with difficulty. Emaciation and depression increased, and the animal was killed about a month after inoculation. The examination of the heart and lungs revealed nothing particular; the kidneys were sound. The injection had caused no inflammation, either in the digestive organs or on the diaphragm. An enormous abscess occupied the entire posterior surface of the liver. The lower portion of the thigh showed numerous abscesses. On opening them, a fracture of the lower extremity of the femur, about a centimeter from the surface of the joint, was ascertained. Around the fracture the bone was gangrenous, and the point of fracture communicated with the adjacent abscesses. In the neighborhood of the diseased spot we found a number of abscesses, varying from the size of a hazel-nut to that of a walnut. The joint appeared to be sound as far as could be judged from the preparation preserved in alcohol. On the plane of the ribs abscesses were discovered, of which those facing the pleural cavity were especially prominent. The subcutaneous abscesses were less developed; longitudinal sections of the ribs, on a plane with the abscesses, showed that the bone was swollen and much softened, as in certain phases of osteitis. On other ribs, in the plane of the abscesses, fractures were found which communicated with neighboring abscesses.

"According to the view of my teacher and friend Malassez, who examined the lesions, we have here to deal with an osteitis, which brought about the fracture of the bone and the surrounding abscesses. This is the only possible explanation of the fracture of the femur, the care bestowed upon the animal excluding the possibility of a trauma. The same may be said of the fractures of the ribs. The abscesses adjoining them vary in size from a millet-seed to a hazel-nut."

Besides this η parasite, Galippe found still others, on one of which, called β, he lays particular stress; injected under the skin of the abdomen of a guinea-pig, it provoked the formation of well-developed abscesses in the subcutaneous cellular tissue and caused the death of the animal in twenty days.

Direct inoculation with the parasites η and β between the teeth and gums of animals yielded indefinite if not negative results.

"The infectious arthro-dental gingivitis," says Galippe, "is in reality only a local disease." But under certain circumstances (abnormal nutrition, irregular mastication, neglected hygiene of the oral cavity, conditions accompanying locomotor ataxia) "the disease assumes a serious character, which is inversely proportionate to the physical power of resistance of the individual."

Galippe's experiments are doubtless the most extensive and careful that have yet been made to prove the parasitical origin of the disease in question; but notwithstanding the great progress for which we have to thank this eminent investigator, I cannot yet wholly give in my allegiance to the view held by the adherents of the contagion theory.

Although the belief that the disease is hereditary is widely circulated, and might be strengthened by the personal testimony of many dentists (Morgan watched it through three generations), we seldom hear (as far as I know, for the first time in this place) of the transmission from one individual to another by contact.

Pedley energetically denies the possibility of such a transmission. I have myself treated many patients suffering from pyorrhœa alveolaris, but have very rarely met with a case in which husband and wife were afflicted with it; this we should often expect to find if the disease were contagious, inasmuch as the diseased locality is favorably situated for the transmission of the infectious matter. And even should the case be observed, that a person living for a number of years with another afflicted with pyorrhœa alveolaris was also attacked by it, it would be necessary to prove that the second person did not acquire the disease independently before such a case could be regarded as evidence of its contagious nature.

Fig. 120.

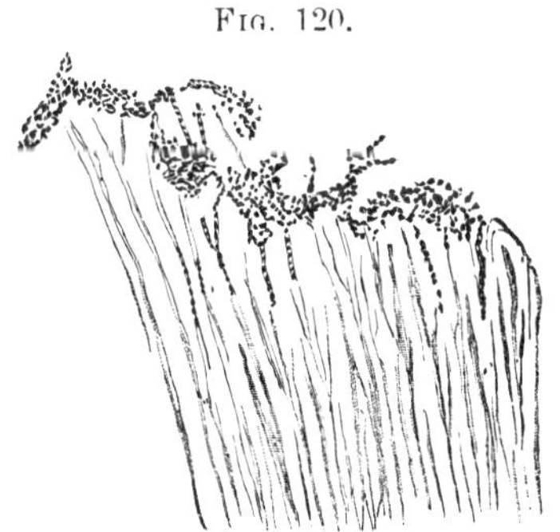

Micrococci penetrating the Canals of Solid Dentine, in a partially absorbed and abscessed but not decayed root. 700 : 1.

The fact also that micro-organisms are found in the dentinal tubules of teeth lost in consequence of pyorrhœa alveolaris hardly justifies the conclusion that they are the excitants of the disease. The invasion of bacteria into the dentinal tubules occurs also in abscessed teeth, particularly when the roots are partially resorbed, so as to expose the open ends of the tubules where there is no trace of the disease. (See Fig. 120.)

ORIGINAL INVESTIGATIONS CONCERNING PYORRHŒA ALVEOLARIS.

Since 1885 I have examined thirty-nine cases of pyorrhœa alveolaris in human beings and six in dogs, in order to determine the presence of bacteria in the pus and in the root. The material for this purpose was obtained in the following manner:

When the disease is so far advanced as to necessitate the extraction of teeth, we first cleanse the crown and neck of the tooth, as well as the adjacent gums, with 5 per cent. carbolic acid, and then, after removing the antiseptic with sterilized cotton, carefully extract the tooth so as not to graze the gums, cheek, or lips with the apex of the root; a small quantity of pure, fresh pus will be found on the root at the border between the dead and the living pericementum. I used this matter, as well as part of the periosteum of the apex of the root, in my culture-experiments. In order to obtain in pure culture the bacteria possibly contained in the cement-corpuscles or dentinal tubules, I placed the tooth for a short time in a sublimate solution of 1–5000 (so as to destroy the germs on the surface). Hereupon it was rinsed in a large quantity of sterilized water, dried with sterilized blotting-paper, and the outer layers removed with a sterilized knife. Small particles from the deeper layers were then scattered on a culture-plate. If extraction is not desirable, we may proceed in the following manner: The neck of the tooth is carefully cleansed and a slight pressure exerted on the gums; by this means the desired pus is pressed out between the gums and the neck of the tooth.

I made dilution- and line-cultures on beef-water peptone gelatine of twenty-seven teeth afflicted with pyorrhœa alveolaris. In two cases no growth took place; in one it was but very stunted. Of the remaining twenty-four cases, twelve grew very rapidly, five but moderately, and seven slowly. The gelatine was liquefied in five cases only. Staphylococcus pyogenes aureus developed but once; likewise Staphylococcus pyogenes albus.

Two formed yellow, one green coloring-matter; the latter is of interest from the fact that it forms no pigment when the access of air is prevented; if, however, the liquefied colorless gelatine is shaken with air, a beautiful deep-green color almost immediately forms. In most cases I obtained but one kind, or one kind so predominated that the rest could be left out of account. In cases 8 and 13, the bacteria cultivated were found to be identical; also in cases 16 and 17. In all the rest they were different; that is to say, twenty-seven cases yielded twenty-two different kinds of bacteria.

From these experiments we might conclude that if there is a specific bacterium of pyorrhœa alveolaris it does not readily grow on gelatine, a result which is of value in so far as it indicates that in further experiments on this subject media should be employed which admit of being kept at the temperature of the mouth. At the same time the thought suggests itself that possibly the bacterium of pyorrhœa alveolaris, like so many mouth-bacteria, is cultivable on none of the artificial nutrient media, which would of course render all experimenting useless.

The few experiments which were made on animals resulted negatively. The gums of healthy dogs (these animals often suffer from pyorrhœa alveolaris) were slightly detached from the neck of the tooth and inoculated with pus, as well as with the deposit on teeth attacked by the disease. Slight inflammation invariably ensued, in one case also a little suppuration, but inside of a week all cases were completely healed. Further experiments are necessary to determine whether positive results may be gained in the case of old or emaciated and sick dogs.

I next made a series of culture-experiments on agar-agar, at blood temperature. Twelve cases of pyorrhœa in human beings and six in dogs were examined. I isolated twenty different bacteria from human beings, and nine from dogs. Among the twenty kinds, Staphylococcus pyogenes aureus was found twice, Staphylococcus pyogenes albus once, Streptococcus pyogenes once. Of the other sixteen, nine subcutaneously injected produced no particular reaction, four a slight, three a severe suppuration in the subcutaneous connective tissue. One of these is more fully described on page 270.

Among the nine species in dogs, Staphylococcus pyogenes albus occurred once. Of the other eight, two subcutaneously injected caused no reaction, five but a slight, and one very profuse suppuration, by which large portions of skin were thrown off.

I succeeded, consequently, in cultivating a large number of bacteria of pyorrhœa alveolaris which possessed pyogenic properties, but was not able to determine the constant occurrence of any particular one which might be defined as the specific micro-organism of pyorrhœa alveolaris. Nor is it evident from Galippe's communication whether he found the η or β bacterium in all cases examined or but once.

The microscopical examination of stained sections revealed masses of different bacteria, cocci and bacilli, more seldom leptothrix, on the surface of the cement, and where there were microscopic cavities in the cement, or the dentinal tubules were exposed in consequence of resorption, the micro-organisms were found to have penetrated for a short distance (Fig. 120).

In my opinion three factors are to be taken into consideration in every case of pyorrhœa alveolaris: (1) predisposing circumstances, (2) local irritations, (3) bacteria.

Every factor must be regarded as predisposing which impairs the power of resistance of the parts in question,—constitutional or local complaints, abnormal composition of the blood, digestive troubles, unfavorable hygienic conditions, etc. Different authors have mentioned as such particularly rhachitis, rheumatism, gout, tuberculosis, scorbutus, scrofula, chronic constipation, exanthematic diseases, malaria, diabetes, tabes dorsalis, dyspepsia, rheuma, syphilis, repeated pregnancy, anæmia, chlorosis and wasting diseases of any kind, bad lodgings, lack of exercise, improper food.

Rhachitis seems to furnish an especial predisposition for pyorrhœa alveolaris. It is well known that the milk-teeth of rhachitic children are shed at an early age. I have seen many rhachitic children of the age of four to six years who had but a few teeth left. When, therefore, authors designate the disease as peculiar to mature age (thirty to fifty years), they are unquestionably mistaken.

During the years 1888–89 I examined twenty-six cases of rhachitis in children under twelve years; seven manifested pronounced symptoms of pyorrhœa alveolaris,—*i.e.*, intensely bluish-red gums, suppurating when pressed, teeth loose, a deep pocket between root and gums, loss of pericementum and alveolar margin, disagreeable odor from the mouth. No symptom was present which would have justified me in designating these cases as anything other than real pyorrhœa alveolaris.

Three other children had previously shown the same symptoms, but were at the time being not afflicted with the disease; the rhachitic symptoms had likewise also considerably diminished in consequence of proper hygienic regulations (sea air, good food, and care). Four children, eleven and twelve years old, who had been cured of severe rhachitis, had perfectly normal teeth and normal healthy gums.

In other diseases of the osseous system, caries, coxitis, osteomyelitis, as well as arthritis, tuberculous inflammation of the joints, tuberculosis, lupus, malum Potti, etc., of which I examined sixty-five cases, I could discover no especial predisposition to pyorrhœa alveolaris. The teeth were also comparatively better than those of the higher classes.

I formerly regarded scrofula as an important predisposing factor in pyorrhœa alveolaris. Its frequent appearance together with rhachitis renders it difficult to distinguish between the effects of these two diseases. After examining over twenty cases of scrofula, not complicated by rhachitis, I concluded that I had overrated its predisposing effect, at least in regard to children.

It is a fact known to every dentist that constitutional diseases are often followed by local expressions on the gums, the pericementum, and the alveolar margin. I need only mention scorbutus, mercurialism, and the gingivitis and pericementitis which accompany exanthematic diseases.

Particularly striking are those affections of the gums that occur during pregnancy, and which lead to swelling, puffiness, and suppuration of the gums at the neck of the tooth, especially between the superior central incisors. These affections bear considerable similarity to pyorrhœa alveolaris, and are asserted by some to result in this disease after repeated pregnancies, although as a rule the symptoms, while yielding to no treatment, completely disappear of themselves after confinement.

As unfavorable hygienic conditions we designate poor quarters, bad food, bad air, want of exercise, etc.

The etiological significance of these factors in the origination of pyorrhœa alveolaris is most easily studied in animals. Wild animals kept in captivity, lap-dogs, especially pugs and other lady's dogs, which have little exercise and eat all kinds of unhealthy stuff, very often lose their teeth, exhibiting symptoms characteristic of pyorrhœa alveolaris, while, as far as I could find out, hunting dogs and such as live under natural conditions are never or but rarely afflicted with it.

Dr. Fröhner, professor at the veterinary high school of Berlin, informed me that particularly dogs that are fed on potatoes, farinaceous food, and sugar are often afflicted with this disease. It also appears in connection with eruptions on the skin, rheumatism, etc.

As regards the local excitation, it can be furnished either by tartar, food-particles, or any other mechanical or chemical agent. Perhaps no other part of the body is exposed to so manifold and lasting excitations (mechanical, chemical, thermal, etc.) as the gums,—accumulations of tartar, particles of food which are wedged between the teeth, strongly-seasoned food and drink, contact with food in a state of decomposition or fermentation, sharp tooth-corners, etc.,—so that the power of resistance of the gums must be very great to avoid being affected.

It is still a matter of debate whether a local irritation be at all requisite to the origination of the disease. I am not able to form any decision regarding this matter, but so much is unquestionably certain that the symptoms are greatly aggravated by local irritations, and that a removal of all such irritations and extreme cleanliness are imperatively necessary in contending against this disease.

As regards the participation of bacteria in pyorrhœa alveolaris, our present knowledge of suppurative inflammations compels us to consider the former as the cause of the suppurations incident to this disease. Micro-organisms which possess pyogenic properties temporarily or permanently inhabit every mouth. If, therefore, the power of resistance of the peridental tissue be impaired by any one of the above-mentioned local or constitutional causes in such a manner as to furnish a suitable culture medium for the bacteria, they will, of course, begin their ravages, and the usual symptoms will follow.

Analogous circumstances are noticed in other parasitic diseases of the oral and pharyngeal cavities.

According to this conception, pyorrhœa alveolaris is not caused by any *specific bacterium*, which occurs in every case (like the tubercle-bacillus in tuberculosis), but various bacteria may participate in it, just as in suppurative processes not only one but generally various species have been found. Besides, as far as we know, there is no bacterium which, inoculated under the gums, is able to provoke the disease in healthy persons.

The pronounced tendency of pyorrhœa alveolaris to recur after it has been apparently healed may be explained by the fact that we are seldom able to determine with certainty the predisposing cause, or, having found it, to remove it. New infections of the wound continually take place from the mouth.

The prognosis is always unfavorable; in the front teeth, however, a marked improvement, if not a complete cure, may be effected. Even in far-advanced cases I have seen the suppuration totally subside after appropriate treatment, and only reappear months after at circumscribed points. I have therefore generally found an after-treatment necessary at intervals of from four to six months, and have in very many cases succeeded in at least retarding the progress of the disease for years, and in restoring the affected teeth, which had been painful and loose, to their former condition of usefulness.

The chance of preserving the molars is exceedingly small.

The local treatment consists in a thorough cleansing of the roots of the teeth, which in all cases anyways advanced can be performed only after making an incision in the gums over and parallel to each root, and extending at least to the line of demarcation between the healthy and diseased tissue. If, then, a tampon of cotton is placed in the incision, the flaps of gums will be pressed apart, and in a few hours the root plainly exposed to view. The mechanical cleansing may be followed by an application of nitric acid (2 to 4 per cent. solution). Finally, astringents, and particularly antiseptics, are to be used. The patient must pay the strictest attention to his mouth, and when there are pockets between gums and roots, syringe them with an antiseptic solution after every meal.

The systemic treatment must be directed against the predisposing cause, and varies therefore according to the history of each individual case.

d. *Stomatomycosis sarcinica.*

The mycosis of the oral and pharyngeal cavities, thus designated, is caused by the colonization and proliferation of sarcina in the shape of "frost-like coatings and deposits on the mucous membrane of the mouth," when its normal power of resistance is impaired by protracted illness, especially in marantic processes, typhus, phthisis, etc. The disease is rare, and is said to occasion no particular annoyance.

e. *Mycosis tonsillaris benigna*

occurs much more frequently. According to my observation, it appears mostly in women and children who suffer from hypertrophy of the tonsils, and are predisposed to chronic pharyngitis. It occurs as a dirty, yellowish deposit, varying in size from the head of a pin to a pea, consisting of numerous bacterial forms and extending deep into the lacunæ of the tonsils. Both or only one tonsil may be attacked, while the tongue and soft palate are more rarely affected. According to Schech,[212] the subjective symptoms consist in tickling, dryness, burning, slight pains in swallowing, inclination to hawking and coughing. In one case he noticed fever with general discomfort; weakness and loss of appetite preceded the appearance of the spots. I myself never observed such disturbances, though many cases have come under my notice, but have seen several in which the mycosis followed an already-existing affection of the pharynx, and concluded that the colonization of bacteria was made possible by the preceding inflammation.

The artificial removal of these deposits is very difficult, and the strongest antiseptics do not seem to exert the least influence on the course of the disease. The deposits, however, usually disappear of their own accord in a few weeks, or as soon as the conditions which made their formation possible are removed.

f. Stomacace.

Stomacace is a disease of the oral cavity or gums, which is usually of a purely local nature. Some authors consider it as an infectious disease, especially since it is often epidemic, and Bergeron was able to communicate it to himself by means of inoculation.

As far as I know, no culture-experiments have been made, nor do we possess any information whatever concerning the supposed bacterium of stomacace.

g. Stomatitis phlegmonosa, ulcerosa, etc.

In all these severe affections of the mouth, accompanied by suppuration, abscess-formation, gangrenous decomposition, sloughing, etc., we designate as chief etiological factors: improper nourishment, unhealthy quarters, severe diseases impairing and weakening the composition of the blood, scorbutus, scrofula, rhachitis, typhus, scarlet fever, etc. At the same time there can be no doubt that parasitical influences must largely affect the aforesaid diseases, if indeed they do not stand in direct causal relation to them. Next to a nutritious diet, antiseptics and disinfectants form the chief remedies in their treatment.

It is not improbable that, under predisposing conditions, the masses of bacteria in an unclean mouth perform the part of a direct etiological factor in these affections.

There are, however, neither clinical observations nor culture-experiments which permit us definitely to conclude what bacteria we have to deal with in connection with these different diseases, or whether possibly each form owes its specific character to the action of a certain bacterium. It is highly probable that various species, pathogenic and non-pathogenic, are present in the later stages of these affections and contribute considerably to the terrible devastations which are frequently consequent upon them.

Diseases of the various tissues of the mouth which are to be classed under this category are very common in domesticated animals; more particularly in sheep. A disease known as scorbutus (Spinola), stomatitis perniciosa (Gips), etc., frequently works terrible havoc in flocks of fine-wooled races. The symptoms of the disease are, consecutively, weakness, loss of appetite, foaming at the mouth, redness of the gums, swelling of the gums and formation of pockets around the neck of the teeth, epithelial defects, ulceration, loosening of the teeth, periodontitis, periostitis and concomitant caries (of the bone), falling out of the teeth (Gips).

The disease appears in the autumn when the animals are put in the stall, attacking chiefly lambs or older animals which are in poor condition, badly fed, anæmic, etc.

Fig. 121.

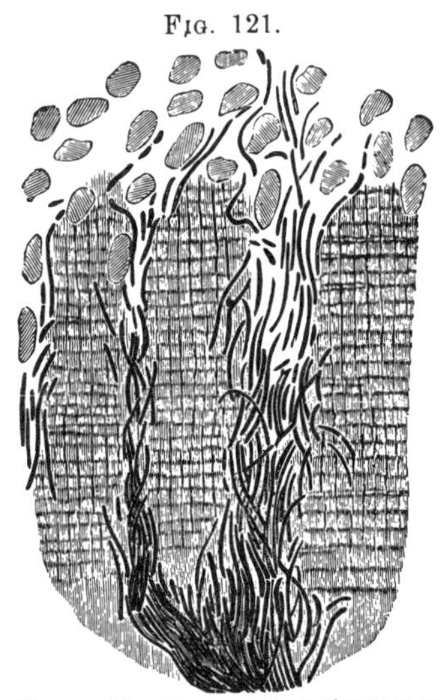

From a Section through Tongue of Calf, ulcerative stomatitis. 700:1. (After Klein.)

Here apparently, as in the human being, predisposing causes play an important rôle.

In stomatitis ulcerosa in the calf, A. Lingard and E. Batt (London *Lancet*, May, 1883) have described peculiar bacilli occurring in the tongue and buccal mucous membrane (Fig. 121). The typical ulcer in advanced cases consists of a sore with free overhanging edges. On section through the sore, the tongue is found necrosed to a considerable depth. "Whenever the sore touches any other part of the mouth or cheek, the disease is communicated and rapidly spreads. In some cases similar necrotic changes had taken place in the lung. The line of junction of the necrotic with the healthy tissues was found to be occupied by a dense mass of bacilli having the appearance of a dense phalanx advancing upon the healthy tissues. The disease has been proved capable of transmission (to the rabbit and mouse) by injection of the bacilli in question, which are equally numerous and virulent after passing through several generations by inoculation." The disease often ends fatally in calves (Klein).

7. INFECTIONS RESULTING FROM THE ACCUMULATION OF THE EXCITANTS OF DIPHTHERIA, SYPHILIS, TYPHUS, ETC., IN THE ORAL CAVITY.

The question naturally follows close upon the above considerations: Does the mouth present favorable conditions for the growth of the specific excitants of those devastating infectious diseases, tuberculosis, cholera, syphilis, etc.? May it serve as a breeding-place for the specific germs of these diseases which may enter it from the air, and thus lead to auto-infections?

We have seen (pages 259–262) that a bacterium identical with the pneumonia-coccus often grows in the mouth of healthy persons, and expressed the view that under certain predisposing circumstances the germs carried from the mouth into the lungs may produce croupous pneumonia.

The occurrence of diphtheria-bacilli in the saliva of a healthy child, as has been observed by Löffler,[213] favors the view that the secretions of the mouth are a suitable nutrient medium for the germs of diphtheria also, and that possibly they appear in the mouth oftener than has hitherto been supposed, reserving their specific action until certain favorable conditions prevail. In such a case the diphtheria-bacillus might also be classed among the mouth-bacteria.

The occurrence of a primary tuberculosis of the oral cavity would seem to justify the hypothesis that the juices of the mouth also furnish the tubercle-bacillus with a suitable nutrient medium. But it must not be forgotten that tuberculosis arises primarily in other localities remote from the oral cavity (testicles, etc.), and that the saliva of healthy persons has hitherto been examined in vain for tubercle-bacilli.

For the syphilis-bacillus the oral cavity seems, as a matter of fact, to be a favorite abode; it is not only particularly preferred by syphilis, but the buccal juices serve also as carriers of the poison, and, leaving copulation out of account, the great majority of infections take place from the oral cavity.

The transmission of syphilitic poison by means of saliva or instruments employed in the mouths of syphilitic patients is, as well known, an only too frequent occurrence.

I have already cited cases of this nature resulting from transplantation of the teeth, on page 248. For most of the following cases I am indebted to the excellent communication of L. Duncan Bulkley[214] on this subject. Dulles[215] reports a case in which the patient, a female domestic of excellent character, developed a chancre of the lip two weeks after the extraction of a tooth by a dentist. Otis[216] saw chancre of the lip develop about three weeks after a morning spent in a dentist's chair. Lanceraux[217] and Giovanni[218] relate similar cases. Leloir[219] and Lydston[220] observed chancre of the gum resulting from cleansing the teeth. Roddick[221] a like affection due to extracting with infected forceps. Parker[222] observed a case where man, wife, and child were all infected with syphilis through a tooth-extraction.

Bulkley furthermore refers to some thirty cases in which syphilis was communicated through tooth-wounds (bites, or blows upon the teeth), as well as to a number of cases in which the dentist had inoculated himself by scratching the finger upon a patient's tooth. It is, moreover, a significant fact that in a recent sitting of the " Conseil d'Hygiène et de la Salubrité de la Seine," it was even suggested to recommend to the proper authorities that measures be taken to prevent the communication of disease in this manner.

Apart from these cases, in which a single individual has become the victim of an often criminal neglect of proper cleanliness on the part of the operator, veritable epidemics have been occasioned by infection with the saliva of syphilitic persons.

I observed the first case in the year 1878, at Philadelphia. A large number of boys had been tattooed by a man who was in the habit of moistening the instrument which he used, with his saliva. This man was syphilitic, as was afterward ascertained. Every one of the tattooed boys became afflicted with syphilis.

I also refer to the recent syphilis epidemic in the Russian province of Wiatka. The belief is said to prevail among the peasants of that region that all affections of the eyes are caused by the presence of foreign bodies. In every case of eye-disease the attempt is consequently made to remove the suspected disturbance by inserting the point of the tongue between the eyelids. Some individuals acquire a certain dexterity with their tongues, and are employed to perform the operation. In this manner thirty-four persons, $6\frac{1}{2}$ per cent. of the entire population, were infected by a single woman, and as many more by other individuals.

The present state of our knowledge of the biology of the germs of these diseases unfortunately makes it impossible for us to determine whether and to what extent the human mouth may serve as a nursery for those which may enter it with the air, and thereby bring about an infection without direct contact with an infected body. The facts given above are, however, sufficient to demand earnest consideration, and present another warning to those who are inclined to underrate the importance of the mouth as a factor in originating and spreading disease.

ACTINOMYCOSIS.

In conclusion, we may mention a parasitical disease occurring frequently in cattle, pigs, etc., but more seldom in human beings. This disease, *actinomycosis*, is caused by the ray-fungus, *Actinomyces*, of Bollinger,[223] and has been for years the subject of numerous investigations. Formerly the ray-fungus was thought to belong to the mould-fungi, Hyphomycetes, but the more recent investigations of Boström,[224] who first succeeded in cultivating Actinomyces on artificial media, have made it probable that the ray-fungus belongs to the most highly developed bacteria, and must be regarded as a species of Cladothrix (perhaps identical with Streptothrix Försteri). Actinomycosis may therefore be properly considered under the bacteritic infections of the mouth.

The ray-fungus, or ray-bacterium, as it should now be called, occurs in the form of spirally curved furcated threads, radiating from a center and dilating into bulbs at the extremities (Fig. 122). These dilations were formerly called gonoids, while Boström pronounced them to be involution forms. It grows slowly on gelatine, quicker on agar-agar and beef-blood serum. According to Boström, the optimum of temperature lies between 33° and 37° C.

"On the lower jaw of cattle tumor-like neoplasms sometimes

occur, which proceed from the alveoli of the molars or from the spongiosa of the bone, inflate the latter, corrode it, and finally, after having loosened the molars and destroyed the normal tissues which impeded their growth, break through the skin externally or into the oral or pharyngeal cavities.

Fig. 122.

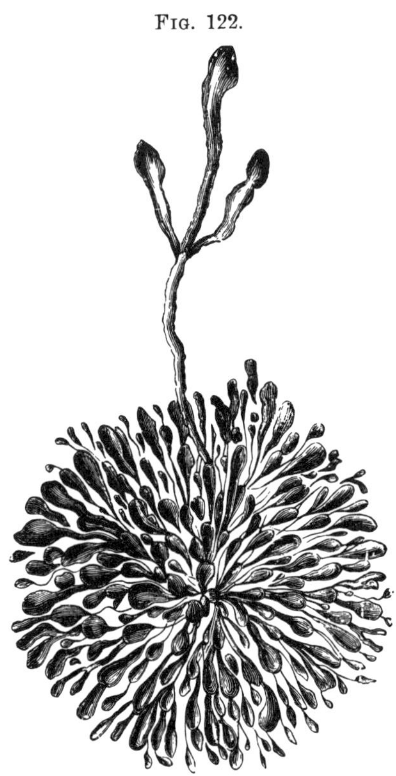

The Ray-Fungus. (Actinomyces.)
(After Ponfick.)

"The inflated bones have a pumice-stone-like appearance, caused by central osteoporosis and external hyperostosis. Most of the bulbous and conglomerated growths, which, after some length of time, often become puriform or entirely break down, and lead to the formation of ulcers, abscesses, and fistulous canals, usually attain the size of a child's head or even beyond.

"Such tumors are composed of a conglomeration of soft consistency, pale yellowish color, and juicy luster (saftigem Glanze), united by tense connective tissue. On the surface of the cut we find scattered, usually cloudy, yellowish-white, abscess-like centers, or the hard cores are of spongious structure, showing numerous hemp-seed-sized spaces and caverns in the fibrous stroma, which contain murky, yellow, thick, often cheesy pap. The mass of the tumor is infiltrated with a puriform or cheesy substance which often shows a reticular arrangement, and may be readily obtained by scraping the surface of the cut with a knife.

"The microscopical examination reveals, among other things,

numerous opaque, slightly yellow, coarsely granulated or gland-like bodies of different sizes, often resembling mulberries. These are here and there incrusted with lime, and on closer examination are found to be of fungous nature.

"This mycosis occurs not only in the jaw-bones, but also in the tongue of cattle, where it leads to the formation of erosions, ulcers, and scars, or to secondary interstitial glossitis." (Bollinger.)

Soon after Bollinger's discovery, J. Israel[225] published his observations and investigations concerning two cases of disease in human beings which showed the symptoms of chronic pyæmia. The very numerous abscesses, appearing on all parts of the body, when lanced, discharged profuse, stinking matter, strewn with yellowish millet-seed-sized grains. These corpuscles, when crushed, revealed various morphological constituents, which, as Ponfick afterward proved, were elements of the ray-fungus. Von Langenbeck made a similar observation as early as 1845.

Ponfick,[226] basing his deductions on the essential identity of the constituents of the tumors of the jaws in cattle and the neoplasms lining the cavities in human beings, but above all on the identity of the morphological elements characteristic of both, came to the conclusion that the ray-fungus is not confined to cattle, but is found in man also.

In the human mouth the ray-fungus, like many other pathogenic bacteria, seems to be able to exist without producing any signs of disease, for example in the lacunæ of the tonsils, until by some means or other (mechanical injury, etc.) a point of attack is created.

James Israel,[227] who has paid much attention to actinomycosis, and to whom we are particularly indebted for our knowledge on this subject, classified the cases of actinomycosis hominum, observed up to 1885, according to the point of entrance of the infection, into four chief groups:

1. Cases of invasion through the oral and pharyngeal cavities.
   a. Central formation of foci in the mandibula.
   b. Localization on the margin of the lower jaw in the submaxillary and sublingual region.
   c. Localization on the neck.

d. On the periosteum of the upper jaw.
e. In the region of the cheek.
2. Cases of primary actinomycosis of the respiratory tract.
3. Cases of primary actinomycosis of the intestinal tract.
4. Cases with uncertain point of entrance.

In dental literature very few cases of actinomycosis hominis have been published. I can recall only one, but unfortunately am not able to give a full description of it.

In medical literature, on the other hand, we find quite a number of cases of actinomycosis hominis. With the assistance of Baumgarten's Jahresberichte, 1885–87, I have been able to collect seventy-five cases, in addition to the thirty-eight mentioned by Israel, making a sum total of one hundred and thirteen. Of the newly-added cases, forty-eight have been described by Hochenegg,[228] Rotter,[229] Partsch,[230] Moosbrugger,[231] Roser,[232] and Braun.[233]

Of the one hundred and thirteen, about fifty-three must be placed under the first division of Israel's classification. The region of the mouth is consequently particularly prone to this infection.

Israel refers the infections of the lower jaw and neck region chiefly to the colonization of the ray-fungus in carious teeth, but minor injuries or defects of the mucous membrane may also suffice to create an entrance-point. (Ponfick, Partsch.)

We consequently have here again another dangerous source of infection in the human mouth, which the dentist and physician do well not to lose sight of.

CHAPTER XII.

SUPPLEMENTARY REMARKS ON BUD-, MOULD-, AND ANIMAL-FUNGI.

BUD-FUNGI.

BUD-FUNGI (yeast-fungi, yeast, Saccharomycetes, Blastomycetes, etc.) are microscopically small, mostly spherical, oval or cylindrical vegetable cells, with membrane and protoplasm (Fig. 123). The size of the cells varies considerably in the different kinds, from 2.5μ in thickness and 5μ in length in Saccharomyces exiguus, to 5μ in thickness and 100μ in length in Saccharomyces

FIG. 123.

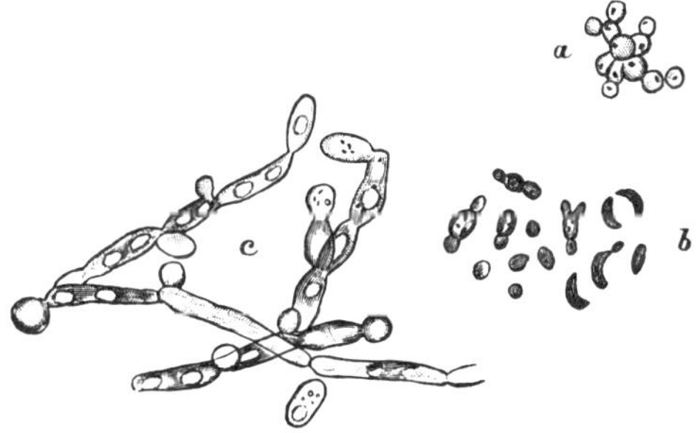

VARIOUS FORMS OF YEAST-FUNGI. *a*, colonies of round cells (Saccharomyces conglomeratus?); *b*, single cells of different forms partly forming daughter-cells; *c*, cylindrical cells of the pellicle-fungus (Saccharomyces mycoderma).

albicans (Flügge). They proliferate in the following manner: at or near one or both ends a dilatation appears; this immediately fills with the contents of the cells, gradually grows into a new cell, and finally separates itself from the old cell by means of a transverse wall. The old cell is called the mother-, the new one the daughter-cell. The latter then forms new cells in the same way. The daughter-cells either separate themselves from the mother-cell and lead an independent existence, or remain connected with it to form colonies (Fig. 123 *a*). Under certain conditions of growth, proliferation may also occur by means of spore-formation; it would lead us beyond the design of this chapter, however, to enter more in detail into the biology of the yeast-fungi. Certain species of bud-fungi, particularly Saccharomyces cerevisiæ and Saccharomyces ellipsoideus, possess the power of exciting fermentation in saccharine solution (dextrose, levulose, lactose, etc.), resulting in the production of ethyl alcohol and large quantities of carbonic acid ($C_6H_{12}O_6 = 2\,C_2H_5,HO + 2\,CO_2$). In the alcoholic fermentation many by-products are formed, and the actual decomposition is much more complicated than is represented by the simple equation given above.

Of the best-known and most important yeast-fungi I mention:

1. Saccharomyces cerevisiæ (Cryptococcus cer.), round or oval cells, 8 to 9μ long, either single or united to colonies; used in beer breweries and bread bakeries. At the higher temperature at which beer is brewed (18° to 20° C.) the fermentation progresses rapidly, and the yeast forms large branching colonies which are carried to the surface by the great quantities of carbonic acid evolved (upper yeast, Oberhefe).

At the lower temperature (4° to 10° C.) the fermentation proceeds more slowly, and the cells appear isolated or form only small complexes which fall to the bottom of the vessel (under yeast, Unterhefe).

The upper yeast is extensively used in the manufacture of bread and in the preparation of compressed yeast. Added to the dough it makes it "rise," and gives it a light, spongy character through the development of carbonic acid. Recently the chief part in this action has been assigned to bacteria, and Laurent [234] among others describes a Bacillus panificans which is said to be present during the fermentation of dough and to produce the necessary carbonic acid; others again claim that bacteria first convert the starch into sugar, which is then further decomposed by the yeast into alcohol and carbonic acid.

2. Saccharomyces ellipsoideus, wine-yeast: elliptical cells, 6μ long, single, or in small branched colonies, very widespread in nature, chief cause of the spontaneous fermentations.

3. Saccharomyces conglomeratus, on decaying grapes and at the beginning of wine-fermentation.

4. Saccharomyces mycoderma (pellicle-fungus, Kahmpilz), which forms a white, wrinkled coating on fermenting liquids, fruit-juices, etc. Cells 2 to 3μ thick and 6 to 20μ long, forming much-branched growths, which sometimes have been mistaken for moulds. It very often appears in mixtures of bread and saliva left standing for some time at 25° to 35° C., consumes the acid, and imparts an etherous smell to the mixture, especially if brought under the surface by stirring.

Bud-fungi are almost constant inmates of the oral cavity. If cultures from the acid food-particles present in dental cavities be made on slightly acid or neutral gelatine, round, rapidly-growing, opaque white colonies will usually develop, which under a low power (70 : 1) may readily be recognized as masses of yeast-cells. These organisms being widely distributed in nature, and finding their conditions of growth best fulfilled in slightly acid or fermenting media, their occurrence in the human mouth is not to be wondered at. Compared to bacteria, the bud-fungi play an insignificant part in the oral cavity. I regard them as the most harmless of all mouth-parasites.

Fig. 124.

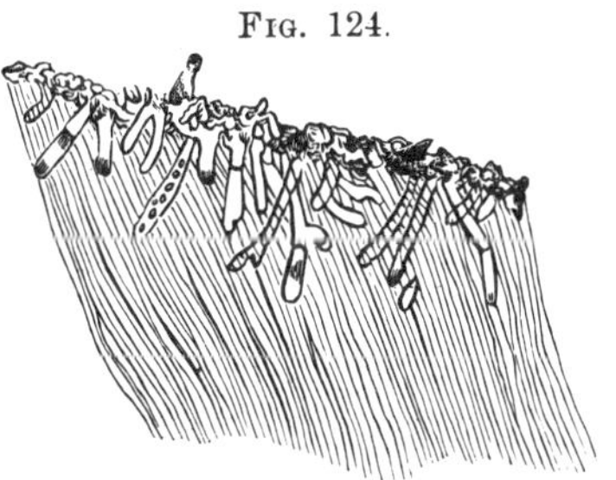

Yeast-Fungi, probably Saccharomyces mycoderma, penetrating solid dentine. 105 : 1.

On examining a piece of dentine which had been preserved in water for some time, as well as two human teeth which had been worn in the mouth as pivot-teeth, I noticed the interesting fact that the dentine had been perforated by a bud-fungus (Saccharomyces mycoderma) (Fig. 124). I described this case in 1882, at the time expressing the opinion that the fungus in question produced at its extremity an acid, "by means of which it perforates or corrodes the hardest dental tissue."

Galippe noted a similar (perhaps the same) occurrence in the teeth of an exhumed skeleton. He also thought it probable that "these microbes secrete an acid," etc.

I am not, however, convinced of the correctness of this explanation, but am now rather inclined to believe that dentine is dissolved and destroyed by this fungus, similarly as bone or dentine by the osteoclasts. It is a disputed question whether acids participate in this process or not.

The only species of bud-fungi which, according to all observations hitherto made, possesses pronounced pathogenic properties, is Saccharomyces albicans, the thrush-fungus. It was formerly classed among the mould-fungi, and called Oidium. Numerous experiments recently made by Plaut,[235] Klemperer,[236] Baginsky,[237] Grawitz,[238] Rees, etc., point, however, to the conclusion that the fungus of thrush is not a mould, but a bud-fungus, a view

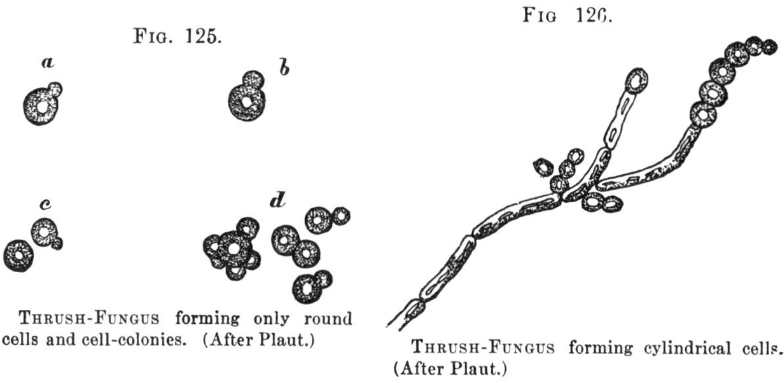

Fig. 125.

Thrush-Fungus forming only round cells and cell-colonies. (After Plaut.)

Fig. 126.

Thrush-Fungus forming cylindrical cells. (After Plaut.)

now adopted by most mycologists, while others (Baumgarten) accord the thrush-fungus a place in the class of the Torulaceæ, —*i.e.*, a middle position between the typical yeast- and mould-fungi.

The shape of the cells of the thrush-fungus depends in a high degree upon the conditions of cultivation; on acid, strongly saccharine media (plum-decoction agar), it generally appears in the form of quite spherical and oval cells (Fig. 125). In media containing but little sugar and no acid, common beef-water-peptone gelatine, the cells bud out to long threads (Fig. 126). (Compare Klemperer and Plaut.)

A question not yet definitely settled, is that concerning the identity of the thrush-fungus with other species of fungi:

Saccharomyces mycoderma, Mycoderma vini (Cienkowski), Monilia candida, etc. Plaut's numerous experiments lead him to conclude that Saccharomyces mycoderma and the thrush-fungus are not identical. "The former produces but minute fermentation, during which the cells die; it readily forms spores; its cells are somewhat spindle-shaped or ellipsoidal; it cannot produce thrush when inoculated into hens in pure culture. The thrush-fungus, on the other hand, excites pronounced fermentation, during which it grows exuberantly, forms no spores, shows somewhat spherical cells, and is able to call forth pronounced cases of thrush when transmitted to the crops of chickens." My own observations coincide with the above. Cultures of both these fungi on the same nutrient medium invariably manifested the same differences of growth, in that Saccharomyces mycoderma showed a constant tendency to form cylindrical cells, whereas the thrush-fungus in my cultures, made on exactly the same medium and in exactly the same manner, formed only round or oval cells.

Baginsky discovered that in test-tube cultures on the surface of the gelatine, *i.e.*, exposed to the air, thrush-fungi form only round or slightly oval cells, whereas those lying deeper develop into thick mycelial threads, and those still farther down into delicate ones. This is a phenomenon which characterizes the growth of the fungus occurring pathologically in the tissues.

Thrush is peculiarly a disease of children or sucklings. In adults it occurs, with very rare exceptions, only after exhausting diseases, when the mucous membrane has completely lost its power of resistance, or on the vaginal mucous membrane of pregnant women. The infection is caused by inhalation of germs from the air (the fungus of thrush being rather widely distributed), or more commonly by contact with infected objects. In children the infection is chiefly due to unclean sucking-bottles, sucking-bags, sugar-teats, etc., which, particularly when the contents are undergoing fermentation, furnish most excellent nutrient media for bud-fungi. According to Hausmann, the transmission of the disease from the vagina of the mother may also occur at the time of delivery.

The neglect to keep the mouth in a proper state of cleanliness naturally favors the proliferation of the fungus. It grows best on the juicy, porous plaster-epithelium, and its chief seat of vegetation is therefore the mucous membrane of the oral and pharyngeal cavities and of the œsophagus as far as the cardia; furthermore, that of the vulva, vagina, and anal orifice. But it also occurs in the nasal cavity, larynx, trachea, and bronchi, on the male genitals, and the nipples of the breast. The growth of this fungus is, as a rule, restricted to the mucous membrane, only exceptionally penetrating into the connective tissue or blood-vessels, so that the observation of Zenker, who found elements of the thrush-fungus in the interior of multiple abscesses of the brain of a child, still stands alone.

Klemperer, by bringing pure cultures of the thrush-fungus into the circulation of rabbits, succeeded in producing a general thrush infection, which, however, was no more accompanied by suppuration and abscess-formation, than the natural infection in the mouth, so that the observation of Zenker is probably to be accounted for by a mix-infection (Baumgarten).

The proliferation on the usually more or less inflamed mucous membrane of the mouth first appears in the form of millet-seed-sized, isolated and scattered white dots.

By the development of other centers of growth, or by the enlargement or junction of adjacent growths, a continuous thrush-membrane is produced which may line the entire oral cavity and firmly adhere to the mucous membrane. The fungal proliferation spreads itself from the oral to the pharyngeal cavity, and in rare cases also to the œsophagus; sometimes even to the mucous membrane of the stomach, to the nasal cavity, and the larynx.

The fungi may multiply to such an extent in the œsophagus that its entire lumen becomes filled, making the introduction of food impossible. If the growth extends to the larynx, hoarseness ensues, sometimes even want of breath. According to Bühl and Virchow, the aspiration of thrush-masses may lead to bronchitis and pneumonia.

The treatment of thrush must be chiefly prophylactic,—good air, good food, above all the removal of any fermentable substances from the nursery and proper cleaning of the mouth after drinking. If the fungus has already colonized, it must be combated by applying alkalies, as it, in common with other bud-fungi, does not flourish on alkaline media (repeated wiping out of the mouth with a cloth dipped into a 5 to 10 per cent. solution of bicarbonate of soda). In more serious cases hourly painting with nitrate of silver (0.1 : 20 to 50) are prescribed. Internally chlorate of potassium (1 : 100.0, every two hours a teaspoonful), and where the œsophagus threatens to become obstructed, emetics. One should guard against the inexcusable mistake of confounding thrush with leucoplakia oris.

MOULD-FUNGI.

Mould- or thread-fungi (Hyphomycetes, moulds) differ morphologically from bacteria and bud-fungi by the formation of long, branching threads (hyphæ), which, where the growth is not impeded, generally radiate from a center (the spore) and increase by peripheral growth. The hyphæ are usually divided into joints by transverse walls or partitions.

The entire development proceeding from a spore, exclusive of the fruit hyphæ, is called a *mycelium.* Sometimes it is comparatively simple, but slightly ramified, sometimes again innumerable ramifications appear, so that the mycelium forms a densely-meshed flocculent mass. Finally, when the hyphæ are very closely woven, firm, fibrous chords or bulbous, fleshy bodies of various shapes (sclerotia) are formed.

Mould-fungi reproduce chiefly by spores. Individual threads springing up from the mycelium (Fig. 127) display certain differences in form and growth in contradistinction to the others. These are the so-called fruit-hyphæ above mentioned, on which spores are produced in various ways. At this stage, the growth taken as a whole, mycelium and fruit-hyphæ, is called a *thallus.*

Mould-fungi are very common in nature. They grow on almost all kinds of organic media, and are able to send the extremities of their threads into the hardest vegetable and animal tissues, and even to perforate bones and teeth. They do not by any means excite those intense processes of decomposition in animal substances characteristic of bacteria. They have been found, on the other hand, to be the cause of a large number of devastating diseases of plants, vegetables, and cereals, as well as of various diseases of fishes and insects. Several species of Aspergillus and Mucor have proved pathogenic to mammals,

FIG. 127.

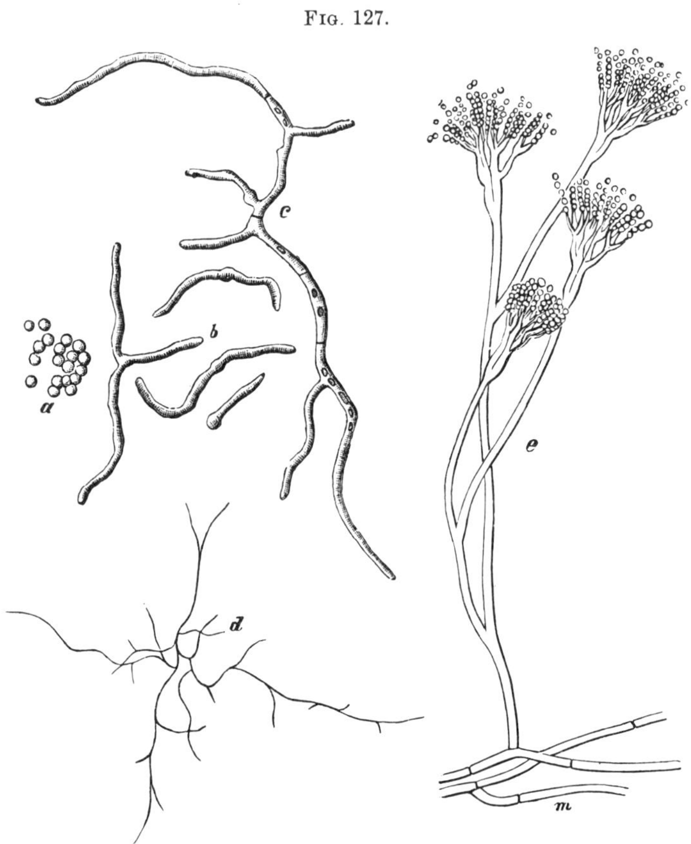

CYCLUS OF DEVELOPMENT OF THE FUNGUS PENICILLIUM GLAUCUM. *a*, spores; *b*, *c*, budding of the spores (*b* after 24, *c* after 36 hours). 500 : 1. *d*, appearance of the mycelium after 48 hours, low power (75 : 1); *m*, a small piece of the mycelium after 3–5 days, carrying a branched fruit-hypha *e*, on whose extremities the spores are being thrown off. 500 : 1.

while mould-fungi have also been shown to be the cause of a number of cutaneous diseases in man. Mould-fungi, especially Oidium lactis (milk-mould), are frequently met with in the human oral cavity. The latter fungus is almost always found in milk and butter (C. Fränkel[239]). Its frequent occurrence in the mouth is therefore easily explicable.

Cultures made from various parts of the mouth frequently develop one or more colonies of moulds. (See Fig. 15.)

The mould-fungi of the oral cavity are, however, to be considered simply as occasional intermixtures; they attain to no marked development, with the single exception, possibly, of the fungus designated by Dessois as Glossophyton, which is said to occasion a disease of the mouth called "black tongue." "Intensely black, inky stains, with rough, furry surface, which slowly spread and may disappear of their own accord, are found mostly on the back of the tongue, sometimes on the middle, sometimes in the margins, at the base, or the point. The black discoloration is said to be communicated to the epithelium by imbibition from the black fungus-spores." (Schech.) This affection seems, at best, to occur exceeding rarely, no other case to my knowledge having been observed.

MYCETOZOA, ANIMAL-FUNGI OR FUNGOUS ANIMALS.

(After Zopf[240] and de Bary.[241])

By the name Mycetozoa, de Bary has designated a group of lowest organisms, whose proper position in the natural world is still a subject of dispute, and which, consequently, have at present been assigned a place outside of, or between, the animal and vegetable kingdoms. They are, according to de Bary's conception, more nearly related to the simplest animal organisms (the Amœbæ) than to the fungi.

The Myxomycetes (Schleimpilze, slime-fungi) form the chief contingent of the Mycetozoa.

These may be frequently observed as naked, slimy, transparent, amœboidal, protoplasmic bodies, sometimes of considerable size, mostly in moist places, on dead vegetable matter (leaves, etc.), or on the trunks of trees. Their resemblance to fungi lies partly in their mode of life and nourishment, and partly in the fact that they form organs of reproduction which are structurally and biologically closely analogous to the spores of fungi. The spores of Myxomycetes, when isolated, are almost without exception of spherical shape, and present the structure of simple fungus-spores. In the process of germinating, the spores swell up in consequence of absorption of water, the spore-membrane ruptures, "and a protoplasmic body exudes or crawls slowly out of the orifice" (Fig. 128, *a*, *b*, *c*).

In this state the organism forms a naked protoplasmic body of changeable shapes, and is called a "swarmer" (Schwärmer). These "Schwärmer" (Fig. 128, *d*, *e*, *f*) are partly provided with cilia, partly without them, and manifest, according as they are with or without cilia, two kinds of movement, a hopping (hüpfende) and a crawling.

FIG. 128.

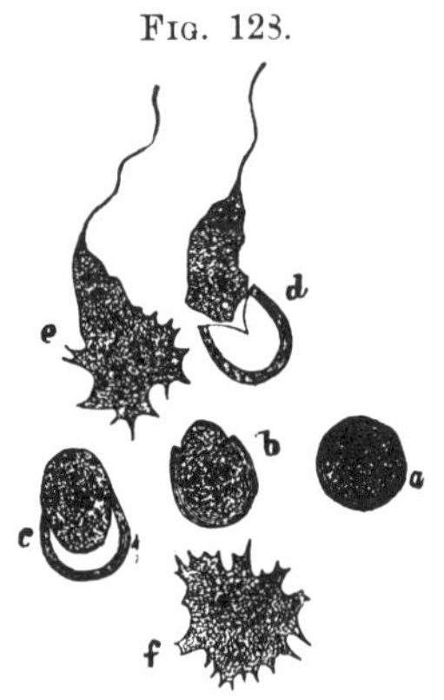

BUDDING OF A SPORE OF A MYXOMYCETES (Trichia varia). *a*, the spore at rest; *b*, *c*, *d*, rupture of the spore-membrane and escape of the "swarmer;" *e*, amœboid swarmer with, *f* without cilium. 390:1. (After de Bary.)

Zopf therefore distinguishes a "Schwärmerstadium" and an "Amœbastadium." According to him, a Schwärmer is a membraneless lump of plasm (primordial cell) in which we may distinguish plasma, nucleus, vacuoli, and cilia. The amœba also represents a primordial cell, in which plasma, nucleus, and vacuoli may be distinguished. As they further develop, the "Schwärmer" unite, forming larger motile protoplasmic bodies (Plasmodia). By the fusion of these plasmodia larger plasmodia are formed, which resemble arboreally ramified bodies or nets. The development of the plasmodium ends in spore-formation, either in the interior of sporangia or on the surface of spore-bearers, sporophores, or in the form of free reproduction-cells.

All better-known Myxomycetes are adapted to a saprophytic mode of life. They occur in moist places or dead vegetable matter, on decayed wood, on parts of trees, etc., but manifest no pathogenic properties.

I am not acquainted with any investigations concerning the occurrence of Myxomycetes in the oral cavity.

The *Acrasia*, a small group of fungous organisms belonging to the Mycetozoa, differ from the Myxomycetes in this, that they do not form true plasmodia.

Zopf and others also class among the Mycetozoa in a wider sense, the *Monadines, lower Mycetozoa*, which by many botanists are referred to the animal kingdom. They show a course of development in its principal features identical with that of the Myxomycetes. These play an important part as parasites. They attack not only all kinds of aquatic growths (algæ, fungi, etc.), but even higher plants; they have also been found in animal bodies, in the muscles of pigs, in the digestive tract of mice, etc. In the human digestive tract, especially in intestinal diseases, amœbæ (Amœba coli) have been found in enormous numbers (Lösch, Cunningham, and others); furthermore, in the urine and vaginal secretion of a girl suffering from tuberculosis of the uro-genital organs (Bälz.) Marchiafava and Colli found plasmodia in the blood of malarial patients. It has not been possible, however, to determine with certainty the pathogenic significance of these organisms in the human body, although many (Woronin,[242] Koch,[243] Eidam,[244] and others) have expressed the opinion "that the appearance and development of many pathological excrescences and swellings occurring in the animal body are brought about by small Myxamœbæ which invade the living organism, develop into plasmodia, and cause considerable irritation," etc.

Flügge[245] and Baumgarten[246] also assign a greater significance to the lower Mycetozoa as carriers of infection.

As far as I know, no investigations have been made concerning the occurrence of Monadines in the human mouth; but that they are often introduced into the oral cavity with vegetable food and water cannot be doubted.

INDEX OF AUTHORS.

(The figures in heavy-faced type refer to the table of Literature, pp. xiii-xx.)

GENERAL INDEX.

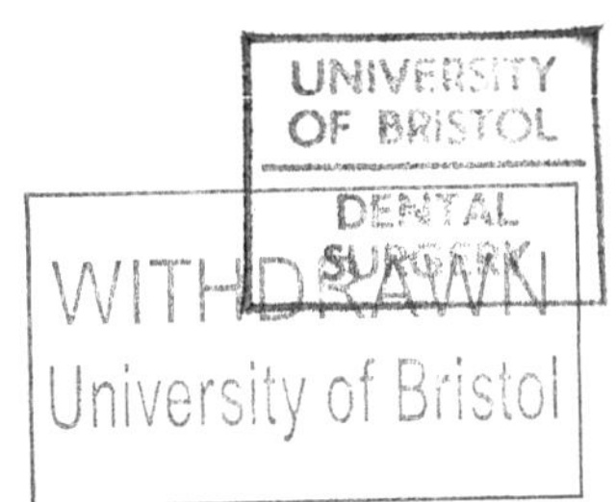

PLATE III.

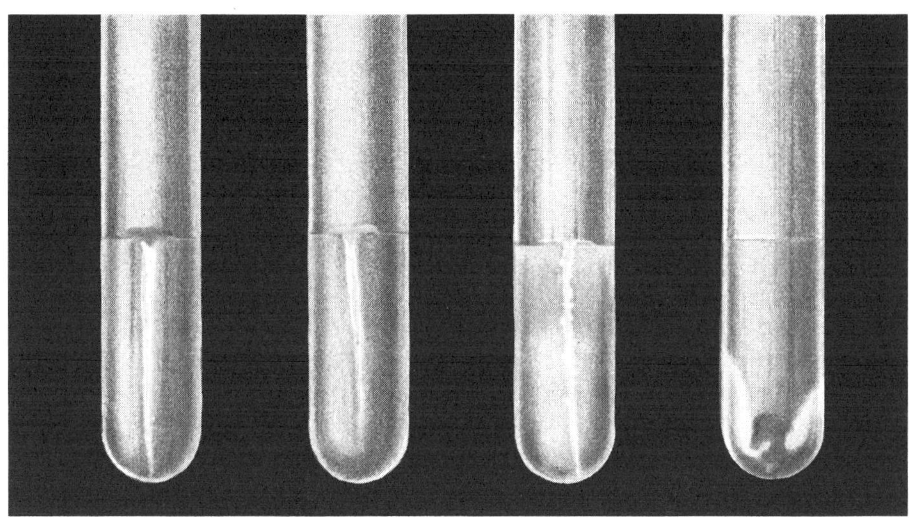

FIGS. 1-4.—Test-tube cultures of chromogenic mouth-bacteria.

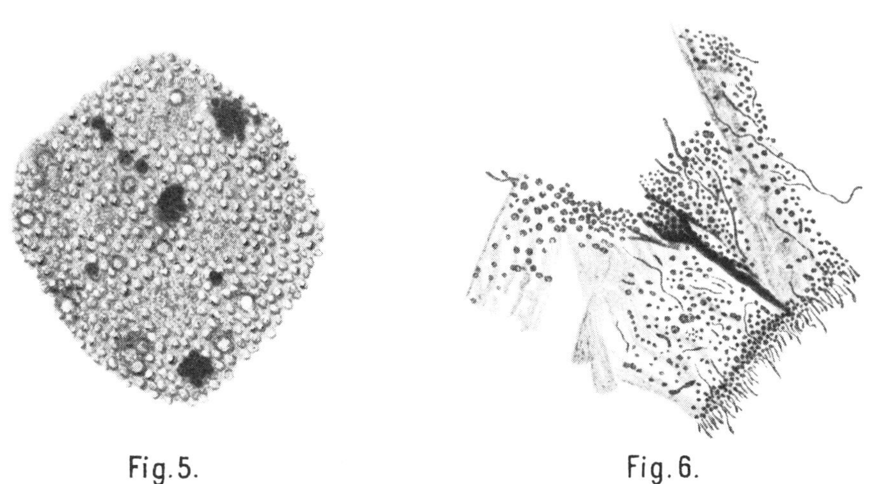

FIG. 5.—A cross-section of decayed dentine, stained with picrocarmine.

FIG. 6.—Nasmyth's membrane from a decayed tooth, stained with fuchsine 1100 : 1.